THE ENCYCLOPEDIA OF

FERTILITY AND INFERTILITY

THE ENCYCLOPEDIA OF

FERTILITY AND INFERTILITY

Carol Turkington and
Michael M. Alper, M.D.

Facts On File, Inc.

The Encyclopedia of Fertility and Infertility

Facts On File, Inc.
132 West 31st Street
New York, NY 10001

Library of Congress Cataloging-in-Publication Data
Turkington, Carol.
The encyclopedia of fertility and infertility / Carol Turkington and Michael M. Alper.
p. cm.
Includes bibliographical references and index.
ISBN 0-8160-4154-7 (alk. paper)
1. Reproductive health—Encyclopedias. 2. Fertility, Human—Encyclopedias.
3. Infertility—Encyclopedias. 4. Human reproductive technology—Encyclopedias.
I. Alper, Michael M. II. Title.

RG133.5.T87 2001
616.6′92′003—dc21   00-067749

Facts On File books are available at special discounts when purchased in bulk quantities for businesses, associations, institutions or sales promotions. Please call our Special Sales Department in New York at (212) 967-8800 or (800) 322-8755.

You can find Facts On File on the World Wide Web at http://www.factsonfile.com

Text design and cover design by Cathy Rincon

Printed in the United States of America

VB FOF 10 9 8 7 6 5 4 3 2 1

This book is printed on acid-free paper.

CONTENTS

FOREWORD

If you are having trouble conceiving or know of someone who is, then you are not alone. In fact, one out of six couples of reproductive age who is trying to have a baby is unable to do so. Since the birth of the world's first "test tube baby" in 1978, there has been an explosion of information about human reproduction. Hundreds of thousands of couples around the world have benefited from medical advances that have resulted from this new information.

Yet it's often confusing for couples struggling with infertility to understand the medical terminology associated with reproductive medicine. This book will help couples faced with infertility as well as individuals who work in the field of reproductive medicine to understand the field better.

It's not unusual for those who are first confronted with infertility to be overwhelmed with the array of new terminology, treatments, and biological facts associated with the condition. Our parents were often not expert in their explanation of human reproduction to us! Sometimes the most basic information that we have about the reproductive process is incorrect. This book will hopefully serve as a resource to navigate through a potentially complicated field of knowledge.

Having been involved in the care of the infertile couple for 20 years, I remain amazed at the complexity and the miraculousness of the process. How two tiny cells transform themselves into a human being is mind boggling. As medical director of the largest fertility center in the United States (Boston IVF), I feel privileged to have watched many couples' dreams come true. And the longer I practice within this field of medicine, the more in awe I become.

Yet as amazing as the past 20 years have been, the future will bring advances that will literally transform the field of medicine. For example, human embryos (stem cell research) will allow us to understand how cells differentiate and will allow us to develop tissues to be able to treat many afflictions facing humans.

Fortunately, the vast majority of patients who seek treatment are successful. But we should not forget that many patients who suffer from infertility do not ever receive care. It has been estimated that less than 10% of couples with infertility actually get treatment. This is due to lack of awareness of the treatments available, failure of health care providers to recognize that the condition exists, as well as other factors such as the cost of treatments.

Both the medical community and society as a whole need to understand that there are effective treatments available for infertile individuals. Education is sorely missing. For those who have been blessed to have children and can understand the importance of family, we should never take this for granted and never forget the disappointment of those who are having difficulty.

Several countries around the world and states within the United States have laws requiring insurers to cover infertility. This book is dedicated to those couples who need fertility care but do not seek it for lack of awareness or lack of resources. And to the thousands of couples who are undergoing fertility treatments, we hope this book brings you a better understanding of the treatments you are undergoing. We wish you good luck!

—Michael M. Alper, M.D.

INTRODUCTION

Five million Americans who desperately want children can't conceive—or if they conceive, can't carry a baby to term. Because the drive to become parents is so strong, many couples are prepared to go to extraordinary lengths to have a baby. To meet this demand, a veritable industry of fertility services has developed in the last 20 years, a multibillion dollar effort to sell hope to these couples. More than 15% of all American women have taken advantage of these advances and received some type of infertility service.

Fortunately, almost every month brings still more advances in the field of fertility and infertility—and the more knowledge a couple has, the better off they'll be. For the fact remains that when a woman is trying to have a baby, every day counts as she approaches a time when her biological time clock has run out. Yet for many people, understanding today's cutting-edge technology can be a daunting task as it becomes more difficult to find accurate information and guidance. Moreover, the topic of infertility is filled with old maids' tales and half-truths. Many people don't understand even the basics of fertility, how to plan a family, the best ways to control contraception, newer methods, or updates on health risks.

The Encyclopedia of Fertility and Infertility presents the newest information on fertility and infertility with the most up-to-date treatment for infertility, the most recent reproductive technologies, and the latest information on birth control and understanding fertility.

The Encyclopedia of Fertility and Infertility takes the reader on a guided tour through the human reproductive system, looking at structure, function, and causes and treatments of infertility. An extensive glossary explains medical terms related to fertility, and a detailed index helps locate important entries. Appendixes include extensive listings of self-help organizations related to fertility and infertility, hotlines, helpful books to learn more about specific problems, tips on how to select a fertility specialist, and questions to ask providers.

Although information presented in this book comes from the most recent sources available, readers should keep in mind that changes can occur very rapidly in medicine and technology—and fertility treatments are very high tech indeed. The very latest technical information on fertility and infertility should come from a couple's own specialist. No medical information in this book should be substituted for prompt medical attention.

—Carol A. Turkington

ACKNOWLEDGMENTS

Thanks to everyone who gave their time and advice about fertility and infertility, including staffers at the National Adoption Information Clearinghouse; Planned Parenthood; DES Action USA; the Endocrine Society; the National Adrenal Diseases Foundation; Boston IVF; the Endometriosis Association; the American Urological Association; the Impotence Information Center; the American College of Obstetricians and Gynecologists Resource Center; the American Fertility Society (AFS); the International Council on Infertility Information Dissemination; RESOLVE, Inc.; Compassionate Friends; the Center for Study of Multiple Birth; Mothers of SuperTwins; the Polycystic Ovary Syndrome Association; the Association of Reproductive Health Professionals; the American Society for Reproductive Medicine; the Society for Assisted Reproductive Technology; the Society for Reproductive Endocrinologists; the American Association of Tissue Banks; the American Surrogacy Center; the Organization of Parents Through Surrogacy; the American Urological Association; and the National Women's Health Network.

Finally, my thanks to my agents Bert Holtje and Gene Brissie at James Peter Associates, to Dr. Michael Alper, to the very patient Jim Chambers at Facts On File, and to Michael and Kara.

—Carol Turkington
Cumru, Pennsylvania

ENTRIES A–Z

abdominal ultrasound aspiration A procedure in which the egg is removed from the ovary with the help of external ultrasound as a guide. This was the first procedure that was developed to replace laparoscopic collection of eggs for IN VIT-RO FERTILIZATION. During the aspiration, a needle is inserted through the abdominal wall into the ovarian follicle to collect the egg. This procedure has been replaced with VAGINAL ULTRASOUND EGG RETRIEVAL.

abortion, habitual A term that refers to repetitive (three or more) MISCARRIAGES.

abortion, incomplete An abortion after which some tissue remains inside the uterus. A dilation and curettage (D&C) must be performed to remove the tissue and prevent complications.

abortion, missed The term for a situation in which the pregnancy fails to progress, but there is no bleeding or cramping. A missed abortion usually occurs in the first trimester, and a D&C (dilation and curettage) will be needed to remove the fetal remains and prevent complications.

abortion, surgical A medical procedure that ends a pregnancy. Abortion services are offered in hospitals and clinics, and usually are performed before 12 weeks of gestation. Abortions performed after 11 to 12 weeks carry higher complication rates.

The most common technique is to use suction to remove the uterine contents; if the pregnancy has progressed beyond 15 weeks, the process is more complicated because of the size of the fetus.

After a surgical abortion, the woman will experience cramps and light to medium bleeding over 5 to 7 days. Most doctors recommend not having sex until the cervix has closed (usually when the bleeding stops). After an abortion, a woman should call her doctor immediately if she notices heavy bleeding or any signs of infection, such as fever and chills.

abortion, therapeutic A procedure used to terminate a pregnancy. See also ABORTION, SURGICAL.

abortion, threatened Spotting or bleeding that occurs early in the pregnancy. This type of bleeding may stop and restart in a normal pregnancy, or it may progress to a spontaneous abortion (MISCARRIAGE).

abortion, spontaneous A pregnancy loss during the first 20 weeks of gestation (MISCARRIAGE).

abortion pill See RU-486.

absolute infertility See STERILITY.

acrosome A membrane covering a sperm's head. This membrane contains enzymes that, when released, allow the sperm to pierce the coating around an egg and penetrate and fertilize the egg. See also ACROSOME REACTION; ACROSOME REACTION TEST.

acrosome reaction   A chemical change that enables a sperm to penetrate an egg. The coating of the egg bursts in response to the enzyme covering a sperm's head (ACROSOME), enabling the sperm to push through the egg's "shell" (called the ZONA PELLUCIDA).

acrosome reaction test   A sperm function test that determines if the covering of a sperm head (the ACROSOME) can undergo the chemical changes necessary to dissolve and penetrate an egg's tough outer "shell" (ZONA PELLUCIDA).

During fertilization, just before the sperm penetrates the egg it goes through the ACROSOME REACTION, in which the membranes of the front portion of the sperm ruptures, releasing various enzymes. This exposes surface antigens that were previously hidden inside the cell.

A positive acrosome reaction test result may indicate the need for INTRACYTOPLASMIC SPERM INJECTION (ICSI) or use of a donor sperm.

activated partial thromboplastin time (APTT)   A coagulation test performed by adding an activating substance such as silica or calcium to blood and measuring the time it takes to clot (a "normal" reading is from 25 to 35 seconds). This test is often used to measure the ability of the blood to coagulate, such as when patients are on medications that thin blood.

acupuncture   For many years practitioners of Chinese medicine have used acupuncture and Chinese herbs to treat infertility, believing that it boosts sperm count and improves the sperm's ability to move. Several Chinese studies have found that acupuncture can be effective.

Some patients prefer to use acupuncture treatments as an adjunct to more traditional infertility treatment. Typically, patients will visit a certified acupuncture specialist twice a week for treatments lasting between 20 minutes and an hour. The average cost of acupuncture for this type of problem is between $50 and $100 per treatment.

ACTH   See ADRENOCORTICOTROPIC HORMONE.

adenohypophysis   The part of the pituitary gland that produces the following hormones: FOLLICLE-STIMULATING HORMONE (FSH); LUTEINIZING HORMONE (LH); PROLACTIN, growth hormone; THYROID-STIMULATING HORMONE (TSH); and ADRENOCORTICOTROPIC HORMONE (ACTH).

adenomyosis   An abnormal uterine condition (similar to fibroids) in which the cells from the uterine lining grow into the muscle of the uterine wall. This may occur after a woman has had several pregnancies; instead of sloughing off during the menstrual period, some uterine tissue invades the wall and thickens in response to hormonal changes. The condition may begin with small areas of uterine scarring or it may involve large areas of the uterus.

Symptoms
Many symptoms of adenomyosis are similar to ENDOMETRIOSIS. They include swelling of the uterus, pain during periods, and heavier flow. If this swelling is limited to one area, it is called an adenomyoma and can be very similar to a fibroid.

In severe cases, the uterine tissue extends through the entire uterine wall and interferes with the implantation of an embryo. It may also affect an embryo's ability to grow, so that the pregnancy ends in MISCARRIAGE.

Treatment
Unlike a fibroid, an adenomyoma is not easy to remove during surgery because it's not easy to separate from surrounding tissue. If symptoms are severe, a HYSTERECTOMY may be recommended. See also FIBROIDS AND INFERTILITY.

adhesion, pelvic   Scar tissue that may be located in the abdominal cavity, FALLOPIAN TUBES, or inside the uterus. Adhesions can interfere with the transport of the egg and implantation of the embryo in the uterus, and are thus a cause of infertility.

Cause

The surface of the organs in the pelvis is covered with a slippery surface called the peritoneum, which keeps the organs from sticking together. When there is a break in this covering, a bit of scar tissue can form as healing occurs. This resulting adhesion (scar) can cause two adjoining organs to stick together.

Most adhesions in the pelvic area are caused by either PELVIC INFLAMMATORY DISEASE or injury during surgery. As inflammation causes the peritoneal tissue to break down it forms scars (adhesions). Even if the inflammation is not located in a reproductive organ but in a neighboring area (such as the appendix), the inflammation can cause an injury that nonetheless causes either an ovary or fallopian tube to stick together.

In addition, any surgical injury to any of the organs in the pelvic area can damage the peritoneal surface, such as a simple procedure to treat an inflamed appendix or cystic ovary. This risk to future fertility during surgery is why a woman should try to choose LAPAROSCOPY instead of LAPAROTOMY and find the most qualified surgeon to perform the techniques. Laparoscopic surgery is less traumatic than a laparotomy, which reduces the risk of scars. If a woman must have a laparotomy, microsurgery instead of standard surgery carries less risk of subsequent adhesions. Using microsurgery means that the surgeon uses magnification so that no tiny blood vessels or adhesions are missed; microinstruments are designed to cause the smallest possible cuts and trauma to normal tissue.

Treatment

Once an adhesion forms, it can be very difficult to separate the organs linked by the scar tissue. They must be removed surgically, ideally with laparoscopy to avoid further trauma to the pelvic area. Only in extreme cases of pelvic adhesions should laparotomy be used.

adoption Although medical treatment for infertility is an excellent choice for many infertile couples, not everyone who seeks treatment will become pregnant and deliver a child, even with advanced reproductive technologies. As a result, some couples choose adoption instead. Adoption ends childlessness and can be a satisfying means of building a family. Nearly 70,000 children are adopted in the United States each year, including 8,000 international children and 10,000 children with special emotional or physical needs.

The option of adoption should be considered as part of the infertility evaluation. Adoptions may be arranged independently or through an adoption agency. An independent adoption usually requires an adoption attorney or counselor, physician, or minister. When deciding to adopt, couples should allow themselves time to accept their fertility-related losses before adopting.

Adoption laws vary significantly from state to state. Adopting between states or from a foreign country also is possible, but it's more complex. Many prospective parents want to adopt healthy babies who come from a similar background, but in the United States there are very few healthy Caucasian infants available. Most Caucasian infants are placed through agencies and independent adoptions.

African-American, Hispanic, and mixed-race infants are available both through public and private adoption agencies. However, the adoption of Native American children of all ages by non-Indians is strictly limited by the Federal Indian Child Welfare Act (P.L. 95-608).

Many children with "special needs" are available for adoption. These children may be older; they may have physical, emotional, or mental disabilities; or they may have brothers and sisters who should be adopted together. Usually children like these are being cared for by the state and are placed in foster care. Both public agencies and some private agencies place children with special needs.

However, families can get help in adopting a child with special needs from national, regional, and state adoption exchanges. Adoption exchanges and agencies usually have photo listings and descriptions of available children, and many now provide information about waiting children on the Internet. In many cases, adoption subsidies are available to help parents pay for the legal, medical, and other costs that can occur when caring for a child with special needs.

International Adoption

Some parents may prefer to give a home to a child from another country. Most foreign-born children adopted in the United States come from Russia, China, Korea, India, and countries in Eastern Europe, Central America, and South America. More than 700 private U.S. agencies place children from foreign countries; a few countries allow families to work with attorneys rather than agencies.

However, it's not necessarily easier to look outside the borders of the United States for a child. There are strict immigration requirements for international adoptions, as well as substantial agency fees, and transportation, legal, and medical costs.

Prospective parents should consider the emotional and social implications of adopting a child of a different nationality. Agencies seek families who will help a child learn about and appreciate the native culture.

Types of Agencies

An "agency adoption" is allowed in many states and includes adoption through a local public agency or a licensed private agency. Many states also allow a couple to use an attorney or other intermediary; some states allow the use of adoption facilitators. Because adoption laws vary from one state to the next, an adoption across state lines must comply with the laws in both states. The Interstate Compact for the Placement of Children governs how children can be placed across state lines.

Agency adoptions offer the most assurance of monitoring and oversight, since agencies are licensed and are required to follow certain procedures. A couple who chooses an independent adoption by an attorney at least is assured that the attorney must follow the standards of the Bar Association; some attorneys who specialize in adoption are members of the American Academy of Adoption Attorneys, a professional membership organization with standards of ethical practice. Adoptions by facilitators are the riskiest, since they involve the least amount of supervision.

Open Adoption

Not so long ago, almost all U.S. adoptions were anonymous, but today many couples prefer open adoption. In an open adoption, there is an exchange of information and contact between the birth and adoptive parents. This is becoming more popular in the United States, since experts stress that keeping adoption a secret from an adopted child is generally not a good idea.

Costs

Fees and waiting times for infants vary tremendously, depending on the type of adoption involved. Public agency adoptions are often less expensive than private agency or independent adoptions, although private adoptions may take less time. Costs of adopting a healthy infant in the United States through a private agency range from $15,000 to $30,000. Foreign adoptions can be expensive as well; families pay between $10,000 and $20,000 in fees, and that may not include travel and living expenses while in the foreign country.

It is not expensive to adopt a child with special needs; often the agency has a sliding fee scale, and there may be little or no cost. After the adoption, the child may receive subsidies to cover medical and other expenses, although the family is still likely to incur costs for ongoing care. Couples should obtain a written disclosure of all adoption fees and costs before going ahead with the adoption.

Who Can Adopt

Agencies recognize that many different kinds of people can be loving, effective parents. People considering adoption should be stable, sensitive, and be able to give a child love, understanding, and patience. An adoptive parent may be married or single, childless or already a parent. It's possible to adopt even if a person is divorced, has had marital problems, received counseling, or has a disability—if the person can still care for a child. Agencies usually ask for proof of marriage, divorce, or death of a spouse, and applicants are generally asked to have a physical examination to document that their health permits them to care for a child.

The adoptive parent does not have to own a home or have a high income to provide permanence, stability, a lifetime commitment, and a chance to be part of a family. Children need one or more caring and committed individuals willing to meet their needs and raise them in a nurturing family environment.

More and more agencies and some foreign countries place children with single applicants, who can be as mature, independent, and supportive as couples. In fact, single adoptive parents are often the placement of choice for children who have trouble dealing with two parents due to a history of abuse or neglect.

For many infant adoptions in the United States, however, agency criteria for applicants are more restrictive. Often agencies will consider only couples married for at least 1 to 3 years, who are between ages 25 and 40, and who have good, stable jobs, although some agencies accept applicants who are older than 40.

Some agencies are more restrictive, requiring that the couple

- have no other children
- be infertile
- have one at-home parent for at least 6 months after the adoption

In some states a minor is allowed to adopt. A few states have special requirements for prospective adoptive parents: There must be a certain age differential between the child and the adoptive parents; the adopting parent must live in the state for a certain period of time before being able to adopt; or the prospective adoptive parents and adoptee must live together for a period of time prior to the adoption. In most states,

adoption by "preferred" relatives or stepparents is simpler; waiting periods, home studies, and even the adoption hearing may be waived.

The Adoption and Safe Families Act of 1997 requires state agencies to speed up a child's move from foster care to adoption by establishing time frames for permanency planning and guidelines for when a child must be legally freed for adoption. The bill also removes geographic barriers to adoption by requiring that states not delay or deny a placement if an approved family is available outside the state. The 1995 Multi-Ethnic Placement Act bars any agency that receives federal funding and is involved in adoption from discriminating because of race when considering adoption opportunities for children.

Gay men and lesbians are adopting children both at home and abroad, as well as adopting younger children through private and international adoptions. The Family Pride Coalition and the Adoption Resource Exchange for Single Parents (see Appendix I) can provide more information about single parent and nontraditional adoption.

The Process

When an adoption is being considered, a social worker will visit the home to assess the potential adoptive parents physically, emotionally, and financially. This homestudy usually involves a series of meetings to provide more in-depth information about adoption and help prepare an applicant for parenting an adopted child. Social workers want to be sure that a person or couple can provide a safe and nurturing environment for a new child in their home.

The home study process varies from agency to agency. Some conduct individual and joint interviews with a husband and wife; others conduct group home studies with several families at one time. Most ask applicants to provide written information about themselves and their life experiences.

There is a waiting period for all adoptions. The time frame, like the cost, varies with the type of child being adopted. The wait is typically between 2 and 7 years for a healthy infant. Children with special needs can often be adopted quickly, within a few months, if the prospective family has a completed home study.

Once an adoptive child is placed in the home, a legal application must be filed for an adoption with the court. After the child has been living in the home for some time, a social worker will visit the home again for a followup visit. After the adoption petition has been filed, a court hearing is held to review the case and grant the final adoption decree.

Birth parents must relinquish legal custody for a child to be adopted. With most agency adoptions, a child is already legally free for adoption before a placement occurs. While cases where a parent changes his or her mind (usually before an adoption is finalized) are highly publicized, they occur very rarely. See also ADOPTION RESOURCE EXCHANGE FOR SINGLE PARENTS, INC.

Adoption Resource Exchange for Single Parents, Inc., The A nonprofit organization founded in 1994 to help single people adopt special-needs children. ARESP provides direct services to the Washington, D.C., area but also serves single adults nationwide. The group is a member of the North American Council on Adoptable Children, Adoption Exchange Association, Adoptive Families of America, and Families Adopting Children Everywhere.

The group advocates and promotes the adoption of older and special-needs children in the foster care system while supporting the rights of single adoptive and foster parents. The organization provides information on the process of adoption, the home study process, and the search for waiting children; maintains listings and profiles of waiting children; and gathers resources to be made available to prospective parents.

ARESP operates an Adoption Help Line (703-866-5577), publishes a quarterly newsletter, offers seminars for prospective adoptive parents and workshops at major adoption conferences, and helps prospective parents in the search for children. The organization believes that every child has a right to a loving and caring home and that any person willing to give a child love and support should be considered a prospective adoptive parent regardless of age, sex, race or ethnicity, creed, marital status, or sexual orientation. Contact: ARESP at 8605 Cameron Street, Suite 220, Silver Spring, MD 20910; phone (301) 585-5836; website: http://www.aresp.org.

adrenal gland A gland lying over each kidney that is important in the production of male hormones (androgens) in women. The adrenal gland is also responsible for producing the stress hormone cortisol.

adrenal hyperplasia, congenital (CAH) This condition present at birth is characterized by high levels of male hormones (androgens). Female children may be born with ambiguous genitalia from the excess production of male hormone. This common disease occurs in two forms: severe ("classical") or mild ("nonclassical").

Symptoms

Girls with classical CAH are born with masculine-appearing external genitals but with female internal sex organs. Boys with classical CAH look normal at birth, so a diagnosis of CAH is sometimes missed. People with classical CAH are likely to have trouble retaining salt, a condition that can cause life-threatening adrenal crises.

In addition, girls with either classical or nonclassical forms of the disease also have unusually high levels of the male sex hormone testosterone in their blood, which can lead to early and excessive growth of hair, acne, and infertility.

CAH carriers may have mild forms of the disease, with less severe symptoms similar to those with classical disease that appear at any time.

Cause

Congenital adrenal hyperplasia is an autosomal recessive genetic disease, which means that a child with CAH must have two parents who carry the defective gene. Occurring in 1 in every 1,000 people, the nonclassical mild form of CAH is the most common of all autosomal recessive diseases. Its incidence is higher in certain ethnic groups, affecting 1 in every 27 Ashkenazic Jewish people, 1 of every 53 Hispanics, 1 of every 63 Yugoslavs, and 1 of every 333 Italians. The classical severe form occurs in 1 in every 12,000 people.

Treatment

Beginning at birth, people with classical CAH must be treated with steroids to restore normal hormone levels and prevent dangerous and potentially fatal adrenal crises. However, careful monitoring of treatment is critical, especially during childhood, when growth can be affected by excessive steroids.

The symptoms experienced by people with a milder form of CAH also respond well to steroid treatment, although other treatment options are also available.

Prenatal Treatment

After a woman gives birth to a child born with classical CAH, doctors will perform a prenatal screen for the condition in any subsequent pregnancies. CAH can be diagnosed with amniocenteses or chorionic villi sampling early in pregnancy. Early treatment—before birth—may help minimize some of the manifestations of the disease and possibly spare affected girls from the corrective surgery they would otherwise need after birth.

Newborn Diagnosis

Some states now require newborn blood-screening programs to identify CAH in infants during the first few days of life.

In the Future

New research on CAH focuses on locating the precise amino acid defects in the genes, treating infants before birth, and discovering improved methods of diagnosis and treatment.

adrenocorticotropic hormone (ACTH)   A hormone produced by the pituitary gland that stim-

ulates the adrenal glands to produce ANDROGENS (male sex hormones) and cortisol.

age and assisted reproductive technology
Age plays a very important part in the success of any assisted reproductive technology (ART) procedure, because a woman's ovarian function is directly related to age. A woman over age 40 has less of a chance of producing many good-quality eggs and embryos per cycle.

The ART specialist can predict how well a woman may respond to hormonal stimulation by testing ovarian function. Because multiple eggs are required for ART procedures, a woman's ability to produce these eggs is important. A blood test on the second or third day of a woman's cycle will show that if the FSH level is less than 15 mIU/ml and the ESTRADIOL level is less than 75 pg/ml, there is a good chance the woman will respond to controlled ovarian hyperstimulation. However, a normal test doesn't guarantee that the eggs will be healthy. This is why doctors recommend that women 43 or older consider egg donation as an alternative.

IN VITRO FERTILIZATION for women over age 40 results in a live birthrate per transfer of embryo of between 10% and 12%.

age and infertility   Age directly affects the ability to conceive. While age is not an absolute barrier to getting pregnant, it is true that a woman's ability to become pregnant lessens with time. This is probably directly due to the age-related decline in the number of eggs remaining in a woman's ovaries as she gets older.

A woman is born with all the eggs she will ever have, and they begin to be depleted at birth. Ovulation further depletes the store; most eggs are simply absorbed by the body over time. By her 50s or 60s, most women have lost all their eggs (OVARIAN FAILURE). If this process begins early so that all a woman's eggs are depleted before age 40, it is called premature ovarian failure.

There are many factors that influence the decline of the ability to get pregnant. Over the past 20 years, there has been a tendency to postpone having children until later in life. For many couples this means a relatively shorter time in which to conceive, since both men and women experience reduced fertility with age. A decrease in sexual activity with age also may lead to declining fertility. In addition, as a woman gets older her hormone levels begin to fluctuate, which can lead to irregular cycles and infrequent ovulation.

Sometimes as a woman ages her ovaries release an egg but don't produce enough progesterone afterward. Progesterone is responsible for preparing the lining of the uterus to receive the fertilized egg; if the progesterone levels drop, the egg won't be able to implant in the uterus. This is called LUTEAL PHASE deficiency.

Even if eggs are produced, they may not be of such good quality in older women. The eggs may not fertilize as well, and they're less likely to survive if they do get fertilized. Because eggs are some of the longest-living cells in the body (since they are present at birth), there is a greater risk that the eggs may become defective with each subsequent year of life.

Finally, there is a greater chance of spontaneous MISCARRIAGE in later life. Up to age 30 the risk is about 10%, but this rises to 18% as women approach the end of their 30s, further rising to 34% for women in their 40s.

However, age isn't just a woman's problem; advancing years also affect a man's fertility. Age can interfere with testicular function and decrease hormonal levels as well as sperm production. Men may find that their ejaculate quality drops as they have sex less often. Some men experience a drop in testosterone levels and a subsequent loss of interest in sex. Sperm movement and appearance also can deteriorate with age. While 75% of men under 25 can impregnate their female partners within 6 months, only about 33% of all men over 40 can do this within the same amount of time.

Still, men continually produce such a large number of sperm that their decline in fertility is not as pronounced as it is in women; a man produces millions of sperm each day, and millions more are found in each ejaculation.

If a known infertility-related problem exists, or if a woman is older than age 35, an infertile couple should be encouraged to seek infertility treatment after 6 months of trying to conceive.

alcohol and infertility   Even moderate drinking can interfere with fertility in both men and women. In one recent Danish study, women who drank less than five alcoholic beverages a week were twice as likely to conceive within 6 months as women who drank more than 10 drinks a week. Even women who drank only five drinks a week had less chance of conceiving than did women who had less than five drinks.

While the association is not clear, experts suggest that a woman who drinks a few glasses of wine a week will experience an increase in the hormone prolactin. Excessively high prolactin levels interfere with the ovulation cycle, leading to problems in getting pregnant. Occasionally, a level of prolactin may rise so high it can lead to hyperprolactinemia ("too much prolactin"), making a woman become essentially infertile until the level drops.

Men who drink alcohol also can experience fertility problems, because the alcohol lowers the quality of sperm and interferes with libido and potency. Long-term male alcoholics whose drinking has damaged their liver may experience higher estrogen levels in the blood, which can interfere with testosterone, necessary to maintain libido and sperm quality.

Severe alcoholism can lead to testicular shrinkage, failure of the testosterone-producing cells of the testes (LEYDIG CELLS), and lower production of testosterone. Affected men also may experience a loss of facial and pubic hair, shrinkage of the prostate, and overdevelopment of the male breasts.

Very limited drinking, such as one beer or alcoholic drink a day, will probably not cause higher estrogen levels.

amenorrhea The lack of a menstrual period for 6 months or more. "Primary amenorrhea" refers to a woman who has never menstruated; "secondary amenorrhea" refers to a woman who has menstruated at one time but who has not had a period for 6 months or more.

American Association of Tissue Banks A scientific, nonprofit organization founded in 1976 that sets guidelines for sperm banking systems and ensures the safety and availability of high-quality transplantable human tissue. The reproductive tissues most commonly provided by members of the AATB are human sperm and embryos.

Organizations such as sperm or embryo banks attain AATB membership by undergoing a process of inspection and accreditation by adhering to the published standards of the group. The AATB further promotes the quality and safety of tissues and cells for transplantation through its program of voluntary inspection and accreditation of tissue banks. Attaining AATB accreditation is a high achievement for any tissue bank. Contact: American Association of Tissue Banks, 1350 Beverly Road, Suite 220-A, McLean, VA 22101; phone 703-827-9582; website: http://www.aatb.org. See also SPERM BANK.

American College of Obstetricians and Gynecologists The nation's leading group of professionals who provide health care for women. Founded in Chicago in 1951, ACOG today has more than 40,000 physician members. This nonprofit membership organization aims to serve as an advocate for quality health care for women, supports continuing education for members, and promotes patient education and understanding. For more information, contact The American College of Obstetricians and Gynecologists, 409 12th Street, S.W., PO Box 96920, Washington, DC 20090-6920. Internet address: http://www.acog.org.

American Fertility Society The former name for the AMERICAN SOCIETY FOR REPRODUCTIVE MEDICINE.

American Foundation for Urological Disease, The A nonprofit organization dedicated to the research, prevention, and cure of urological diseases. The foundation provides a variety of programs to keep medical professionals, patients, and the public informed about urologic disorders, the latest treatment options, and up-to-date research findings. The Sexual Function Health Council of the AFUD educates patients, the public, and health care providers on sexual health issues, including IMPOTENCE. Contact: 1128 North Charles Street, Baltimore, MD 21201; phone: (410) 468-1800; website: http://www.afud.org.

American Infertility Association Headquartered in New York City, this national organization is dedicated to helping women and men facing decisions related to family building and reproductive health—from prevention and treatment to social and psychological concerns. The mission of the AIA is to serve as a lifetime resource for men and women needing reproductive information and support and to promote the causes of adoption and reproductive health through advocacy, education, awareness building, and research funding. The group offers support groups, educational seminars, infertility libraries and resources, medical advisory board, the largest annual infertility symposium in the country, online chats, educational meetings, a newsletter, physician referrals, a 24-hour phone helpline, and an Internet message board. Contact: American Infertility Association, 666 Fifth Avenue, Suite 278, New York, NY 10103; e-mail address: info@americaninfertility.org; phone: (718) 621-5083; website: http://www.americaninfertility.org.

American Society for Reproductive Immunology   A society founded in 1980 to foster the development of reproductive immunology research, increase intellectual exchange between clinical and basic branches of reproductive immunology, and assist new scientists interested in reproductive immunology. The society itself includes clinical and basic scientists in molecular biology, microbiology, mucosal immunology, genetics, pediatrics, infectious diseases, endocrinology, obstetrics, gynecology, pathology, veterinary medicine, and animal science.

The society sponsors the *American Journal of Reproductive Immunology,* one of two journals devoted to publishing reproductive immunology research. Prior to the founding of the journal, there were no publishing outlets that were specifically oriented toward reproductive immunology. Contact: website http://theasri. org.

American Surrogacy Center, Inc.   A website established in March 1996 for the primary purpose of disseminating information on the third-party reproductive options of surrogacy and egg donation via the Internet and World Wide Web. The website's mission is to offer information, professional resources, hope, and the opportunity to connect with others who are pursuing these family-building options. In February 1997, the group launched several online support and e-mail discussion groups that include password-protected 24-hour "Live Chat" bulletin boards for members only and virtual seminars hosted by professionals in various fields related to the topic. Contact: http://www. surrogacy.com.

American Urological Association   A scientific and educational organization for urologists founded in 1902 that supports research in urology and offers UROLOGIST referrals. Today, as the world's preeminent urological association, the AUA conducts a wide range of activities to ensure that more than 13,000 members stay current on the latest research and best practices in the field of urology. An educational nonprofit organization, the AUA pursues its mission of fostering the highest standards of urologic care by providing a wide range of services, including publications, an annual scientific forum, continuing medical education, and health policy advocacy, and works with other medical associations to improve medical education and patient care. On its website, the AUA provides a referral service called Find A Urologist to help patients look for a urologist near their home. Contact: AUA, 1120 North Charles Street, Baltimore, MD 21201; phone: (410) 727-1100; website: http://auanet.org.

anabolic steroids and infertility   Use of anabolic steroids (synthetic derivatives of TESTOSTERONE) is one cause of MALE FACTOR INFERTILITY, because using these drugs can cause a profound drop in sperm production that may be irreversible. Anabolic steroids, which have often been used by athletes trying to enhance their physical performance, have been linked to testicular shrinkage and depressed gonadotropin secretion. While these effects may be temporary, they also may lead to permanent infertility.

androgens   Male sex hormones produced by the testes and ovaries, which in high concentrations may cause fertility problems in both men and women. Androgens include TESTOSTERONE, which is the primary androgen in both men and women, and ANDROSTENEDIONE, a weaker androgen produced in women by the adrenal glands and the ovaries. Much higher levels of androstenedione are produced in the testis.

High levels of androgens in women may lead to the formation of male secondary sex characteristics, and may be found in women with POLYCYSTIC OVARIES, or (rarely) with a tumor in the pituitary gland, adrenal gland, or ovary. A high androstenedione level points to a malfunctioning adrenal gland. Adrenal gland overproduction of hormones can be controlled by treatment with such steroids as prednisone or dexamethasone. These drugs lower the secretion of ACTH from the pituitary, which lowers the adrenal production of hormones.

If the ovaries are producing too many androgens, the drug spironolactone can bind to the androgens and lower the amount of androgens that can affect specific tissues, such as skin.

andrologist   A physician (often a UROLOGIST) who performs evaluations of male fertility. An andrologist is usually affiliated with a fertility treatment center working on IN VITRO FERTILIZATION. Often, andrologists direct procedures for handling sperm in larger clinics, where they work closely with the embryologist to prepare sperm up to the point of fertilization.

Urologists with a subspecialty in andrology are the most highly qualified physicians to deal with all aspects of MALE FACTOR INFERTILITY. These doctors have often completed a fellowship training in andrology.

androstenedione   A weak male sex hormone that is produced by women in the ovary and the adrenal glands; in men it is produced in much higher levels in the male testis.

anejaculation   The absence of EJACULATION. This condition, which is characterized by the inability to ejaculate, can be caused by a psychological or physical problem.

Types of Anejaculation
"Psychological anejaculation" is not usually accompanied by orgasm. Men with "situational anejaculation," however, can ejaculate in some situations but not in others. For instance, a man may be able to ejaculate and attain orgasm with one partner but not with another. This usually occurs when there is a psychological conflict or a relationship difficulty with one partner. Situational anejaculation also can occur in stressful situations, such as when a man is asked to collect a sample of semen in the laboratory for infertility treatment.

In cases of total anejaculation, the man is never able to ejaculate when awake. Deep-rooted psychological conflicts are usually the cause. Such men, however, usually have normal night sleep emissions.

"Physical anejaculation," which includes retrograde ejaculation, can occur due to obstructions. Diabetes is an important cause of physical anejaculation.

Treatment
Treatment depends on the cause of the ejaculation problem, and may include psychosexual counseling, drugs such as ephedrine and imipramine, vibrator therapy, or ELECTROEJACULATION (a procedure in which an electrical current is applied to the ejaculatory organs to trigger ejaculation). Physical obstructions will require surgery.

anovulation   The failure to ovulate. This is the most common cause of female infertility. It can be caused by several factors, including hormonal imbalances, premature ovarian failure, or POLYCYSTIC OVARY SYNDROME. The failure to have any ovulation is anovulation; an irregular ovulatory cycle is called oligo-ovulation.

There are many different causes for the failure to ovulate, including problems with the central nervous system or pituitary gland, and abnormalities within the follicles or ovaries.

Pituitary Problems
Some women fail to ovulate because of a malfunctioning pituitary gland, sometimes related to anorexia or too much exercise or stress. These women don't produce enough LH and FSH to stimulate any follicles in the ovaries to maturity. This problem can be treated by administering CLOMIPHENE to stimulate the pituitary or to simply replace the missing LH and FSH directly.

Premature Ovarian Failure
Other women don't ovulate because they have few or no eggs left in their ovaries. If this happens before age 40, it is referred to as premature

ovarian failure (premature menopause). This could happen as a result of earlier chemotheraphy or radiation treatment, removal of the ovaries, or genetic problems. Usually, however, there is no clear reason why a woman has no eggs left. Ovulation-inducing medications aren't effective when there are few or no eggs remaining in the ovaries. See OVARIAN FAILURE, PREMATURE.

Polycystic Ovarian Disease

Most women who don't regularly ovulate have a normal pituitary gland and plenty of eggs. For these women, the problem appears to be the relationship between the effects of LH and FSH released from the pituitary and the response from the follicles.

Many of these women have many immature eggs, giving the ovaries a cystic appearance (hence the term polycystic ovary syndrome). Often, these women don't have enough FSH stimulation to keep their follicles developing to maturity. In these cases, treatment usually focuses on boosting FSH levels so that follicles can grow and develop, ultimately releasing a healthy, mature egg.

anovulatory cycles   Menstrual bleeding not associated with ovulation.

anovulatory dysfunctional uterine bleeding Unusually heavy bleeding during irregular periods triggered by fluctuating levels of ESTROGEN, but without ovulation. An anovulatory menstrual period may be painless and vary in length and amount from one period to the next.

A normal menstrual period in which ovulation occurs, on the other hand, is triggered by a drop in PROGESTERONE and is more predictable. Such a period usually is accompanied by some degree of period pain on the first day and is usually about the same length of time and amount from one period to the next.

Antagon   Trade name for GANIRELIX ACETATE.

antibodies   Chemicals made by the body to target and attack specific proteins called "antigens" identified by the immune system as invasive and threatening. See ANTICARDIOLIPIN ANTIBODY; ANTINUCLEAR ANTIBODY; ANTIPHOSPHOLIPID ANTIBODIES; ANTISPERM ANTIBODIES.

anticardiolipin antibody   A substance produced by a woman's immune system that attacks the components in a cell's membrane. This is a possible cause of recurrent MISCARRIAGE.

anti-Mullerian hormone (AMH)   A hormone produced by an embryo's SERTOLI CELLS in the testes that suppresses the development of the fetal structures that form the uterus (MULLERIAN DUCTS).

antinuclear antibody   A substance produced by a person's immune system that attacks components in the nucleus of the person's own cells, sometimes triggering an autoimmune disease. Presence of antinuclear antibodies is a possible cause of recurrent MISCARRIAGE and for the autoimmune disease systemic lupus erythematosus.

antiphospholipid antibodies   A class of proteins that in some cases appears to attack an early developing pregnancy, causing either a MISCARRIAGE, intrauterine growth retardation, or even fetal death.

Under normal circumstances, antibodies are proteins made by a person's immune system to fight substances recognized as foreign by the body (such as bacteria and viruses.) For unclear reasons, sometimes the body's own cells are interpreted as "foreign," and induce antibody formation.

In some cases, the body recognizes phospholipids (part of a cell's membrane) as foreign and produces antibodies against them. Antibodies to phospholipids are called "antiphospholipid antibodies"; these can be found in the blood of some people with lupus, but they are also seen in people without any known illness. Lupus anticoagulant and anticardiolipin antibody are the two known antiphospholipid antibodies that are associated with recurrent pregnancy loss.

Among women with recurrent pregnancy losses, antiphospholipid antibodies have reported to be present in between 11% and 22% of cases. Lupus anticoagulant and/or anticardiolipin antibodies have been associated with first, second, and third trimester pregnancy losses. The association is even higher when several recurrent antiphospholipid antibody tests are positive.

Although experts don't know exactly how antiphospholipid antibodies affect pregnancy, one theory is that they may cause microscopic blood clots that may occur in the blood vessels of the placenta. Because the placenta provides nourishment to the baby, any interruption in this process can threaten the pregnancy.

Antiphospholipids may raise the risk of miscarriage, poor fetal growth, high blood pressure during pregnancy, and stillbirth. It has yet to be proved, but many researchers think the antiphospholipid antibodies may go into remission or exacerbation similar to other diseases such as lupus, rheumatoid arthritis, and multiple sclerosis.

Women should be tested for antiphospholipid antibodies in addition to other routine tests if they have

- a history of recurrent pregnancy losses.
- a history of unexplained poor fetal growth.
- early onset of severe high blood pressure in pregnancy.
- unexplained placental abruption.
- a history of clots in the blood vessels, stroke, heart attack, or low platelet count.
- presence of other autoimmune disorders such as lupus.

Testing for these antibodies is a basic part of the workup for recurrent pregnancy loss. However, while they seem to be linked to miscar-

riage, it's not clear if these antibodies play any role in the ability to *conceive*. Some physicians believe that the presence of antiphospholipid antibodies may decrease the chance for pregnancy through IN VITRO FERTILIZATION.

This remains a controversial subject. One of the largest studies that looked for these antibodies in women undergoing in vitro fertilization found that they were no more likely to be detected in those who did not become pregnant as in women who did conceive.

Treatment
The drug of choice is heparin, an injection to prevent blood from clotting together with low-dose aspirin. In certain cases, prednisone and low-dose aspirin are used to treat the antiphospholipid antibodies. These pregnancies should be monitored closely by ultrasound every month to check on fetal growth, beginning at 32 weeks gestation. Although there are successful pregnancies without treatment, the majority of researchers have reported a 70% to 75% success rate with treatment.

antisperm antibodies Antibodies that can attach to sperm and possibly inhibit their ability to fertilize an egg. Normally, antibodies prevent infection, but when they attack the sperm or fetus, they may cause infertility.

Men produce antisperm antibodies only when their sperm come in contact with their blood, such as after surgery or an injury to the testicles. Under normal circumstances, sperm are kept separated from the immune system by a natural mechanism called the blood-testes barrier, which maintains close connections between the cells lining the male reproductive tract so that immune cells can't reach the sperm within. Normally, sperm develop in the testicles and aren't exposed to blood. If contact is accidentally made, such as during an injury that breaks down this barrier, the immune system has access to sperm. When this happens, the body misinterprets the sperm as intruders and develops antibodies against them.

Antisperm antibodies can be produced by the immune system of either a man or a woman. Once formed, the antibodies may interfere with the sperm's movement and ability to penetrate a woman's cervical mucus, or they can directly affect the sperm's ability to penetrate and fertilize an egg, depending on where on the sperm the antibodies attach themselves. Antibodies may also cause the sperm to clump together.

Antisperm antibodies have been found in about 10% of infertile men, compared to less than 1% of fertile men. The likelihood of antibodies rises dramatically in men who have had surgery on their reproductive tract; nearly 70% of men who have had a VASECTOMY reversal will have antibodies on their sperm.

Women have a much lower chance of developing antibodies to sperm; less than 5% of infertile women have antisperm antibodies. It isn't clear which women are at risk for antibodies.

Risks

Anything that interferes with the normal barrier between blood and testes can lead to the formation of antisperm antibodies, including the following conditions:

- CRYPTORCHIDISM (undescended testicles)
- infection (ORCHITIS, prostatitis)
- inguinal hernia repair before puberty
- TESTICULAR BIOPSY
- TESTICULAR CANCER
- TESTICULAR TORSION (twisting of the testicle)
- VARICOCELE (dilation of the veins around the spermatic cord)
- VAS DEFERENS, CONGENITAL ABSENCE OF
- vasectomy reversal

Despite these many risk factors, most men with antisperm antibodies have not had any of the conditions listed above. INTRAUTERINE INSEMINATION (placing washed sperm into the uterus) has not been shown to trigger the formation of antisperm antibodies.

Diagnosis

Over the years many tests have been developed to detect antisperm antibodies. In women, blood tests for antisperm antibodies may be more practical than trying to measure antibodies in the cervical mucus, which is the primary place where the immune system interacts with sperm. The POSTCOITAL TEST, a standard part of the infertility evaluation, may suggest the presence of antisperm antibodies. By examining the cervical mucus after intercourse near the time of ovulation, antisperm antibodies may be observed to cause either a lack of sperm or sperm that do not swim but simply shake in place.

In men, a direct examination of their sperm for attached antibodies is more reliable than testing blood. Two commonly used tests are the IMMUNOBEAD TESTS and the mixed agglutination reaction (MAR). Both tests use antibodies bound to a small marker, such as plastic beads or red blood cells, which will attach to sperm that have antibodies on the surface. The results are read as a percentage of sperm bound by antibodies.

Treatment

The exact role of antisperm antibodies is unclear. It is not certain whether the antibodies contribute to the infertility. Most treatments are unproven. Suppressing the immune system with corticosteroids may decrease the production of antibodies, but this can also cause serious side effects. Current approaches to the treatment of antisperm antibodies include methods of sperm processing to remove surface antibodies, such as rapid washing, freeze-thawing, and enzyme cleavage. However, all of these methods have only modest (if any) success rates.

INTRAUTERINE INSEMINATION (IUI) (with or without FERTILITY DRUGS) has been used to establish a pregnancy despite antisperm antibodies. IN VITRO FERTILIZATION (IVF), with or without sperm processing, may provide a better alternative for couples with antisperm antibodies. It appears to be the best way for a couple to become pregnant if there are antisperm antibodies, especially when there are very high levels of antibodies (near 100% of sperm are bound by antibodies). There is no clear guidance on whether INTRACY-TOPLASMIC SPERM INJECTION (ICSI) (injecting one sperm into an egg) is necessary in the presence of antisperm antibodies, unless there had been a complete absence of fertilization on a prior attempt at in vitro fertilization.

antisperm antibody test The antisperm antibody test can detect the presence of antisperm antibodies that attach themselves to the surface of the sperm. Once attached, the antibodies may interfere with the sperm's ability to move, to make their way through the woman's cervical mucus, or to fertilize an egg, depending on where they attach.

Normally, the immune system produces antibodies to help fight off foreign substances and diseases, but sometimes the body's own immune system mistakenly begins to attack its own tissues. This is what occurs when certain antibodies attack sperm.

Over the years many tests have been developed to detect antisperm antibodies, which can be measured in semen or blood. However, the value of these tests in the infertility evaluation is controversial.

The two most common tests directly examine a man's sperm for attached antibodies, which is more reliable than testing blood. The IMMUNO-BEAD and the mixed agglutination reaction (MAR) both use antibodies bound to a small marker, such as plastic beads or red blood cells, which will attach to sperm that have antibodies on the surface. The results are read as a percentage of sperm bound by antibodies.

In women, blood tests for antisperm antibodies may be more practical than trying to measure antibodies in the cervical mucus, which is the primary place where the immune system interacts with sperm. The POSTCOITAL TEST, a standard part of the infertility evaluation, may suggest the presence of antisperm antibodies. By examining the cervical mucus after intercourse near the time of ovulation, antisperm antibodies may

cause either a lack of sperm or sperm that don't swim but simply shake in place.

artificial insemination Placing sperm into the vagina, uterus, or fallopian tubes through artificial means instead of by intercourse. The technique is used to treat fertile women whose husbands are infertile due to low sperm count, poor sperm movement, and so on. The technique is also often used to overcome sexual performance problems, infertility due to cervical mucus problems, or for using donor sperm.

INTRAUTERINE INSEMINATION (the most common insemination technique) is a simple and painless procedure that can be performed in a doctor's office without anesthetic. Sperm is first washed and then injected through a catheter or cannula into the uterus. This procedure is used for both donor and husband's sperm.

Asherman's syndrome A gynecological condition causing scars inside the uterus that interfere with normal uterine lining development by creating fibrous bands between the walls of the uterine cavity. Intrauterine scarring can happen spontaneously or, more commonly, as a result of trauma to the uterus after surgery (usually dilation and curettage—D&C. In the United States, D&Cs are most commonly done for therapeutic ABORTIONS, after a MISCARRIAGE, or to treat bleeding related to hormonal problems. Asherman's also may occur after a cesarian section.

The scars begin to form as raw or infected surfaces heal. Scarring in the lower part of the uterus may block the cervical opening so that menstrual flow lessens or stops completely.

Symptoms

A doctor will suspect Asherman's syndrome if a woman's periods become very light or stop after a D&C or other uterine surgery. The condition can range from very mild to severe, causing irreversible damage to the uterine cavity, including abdominal pain and infertility.

Diagnosis

The most common way to diagnose the condition is by placing a small viewing device into the uterus to see the inside of the organ (a technique called HYSTEROSCOPY). The condition also can be diagnosed by an X ray of the uterus called a HYSTEROSALPINGOGRAM (HSG), as long as this X ray is performed using a small tube placed just inside the cervix. Some experts prefer to use a procedure called saline hysterosonography, which combines ultrasound with the insertion of a tiny catheter into the cervix; after injecting saline (saltwater) into the uterus, the ultrasound is repeated.

Treatment

The best treatment is really prevention—avoiding infection. In severe cases, a D&C can remove the scar tissue. For those women with only slight scarring, surgery to remove the bands often can be completed in the same setting as the diagnosis. For more severe cases in which the margins of the uterus can't be easily determined, ultrasound or LAPAROSCOPY (in which the viewing device is inserted through a small cut in the abdomen) may be used to accurately locate the limits of the uterine cavity.

Treatment success rates are above 85% with small adhesions. However, if scar tissue has replaced most of the uterine cavity, there is little hope of restoring normal uterine function.

aspermia   An absence of semen during male orgasm.

aspirin and infertility   Low-dose aspirin (80 to 100 mg) may be used to treat infertility in women who produce antibodies that trigger blood clots in vessels that lead to the developing baby.

Typically, women with antibodies are prescribed a very low dose of aspirin (between 70 and 81 mg daily) together with injections of heparin, an anticoagulant prescribed to prevent blood clots. However, these treatments have not been well studied or proved.

assisted conception   See CONCEPTION, ASSISTED.

assisted hatching (AH or AZH)   A new MICROMANIPULATION procedure in which an opening is made into the hard outer surface of the egg with the use of chemicals, mechanical techniques, or lasers to improve implantation after the embryo is transferred into the uterus.

Getting the embryo to implant is one of the greatest challenges in IN VITRO FERTILIZATION (IVF). When embryos are replaced into the woman's uterus, they are covered by a tough outer coating, which must dissolve in order for the embryo to be able to "hatch." This hatching is a necessary step if implantation is to take place.

Unfortunately, implantation is less likely to occur naturally in women who are over age 38 and who have high FSH levels, or who have failed to get pregnant in an earlier IVF cycle.

Procedure

To perform assisted hatching, a microscopic glass tube is used to place a tiny amount of a dissolving fluid on the outer coating of the embryo on the third day after egg retrieval. Some experts believe that women may benefit from treatment with steroids to suppress the immune system and antibiotics to kill germs in the uterus. Steroids and antibiotics are given for 4 days only, beginning the day of egg retrieval. This helps a normal growing embryo to emerge from the egg covering and implant in the uterus.

Many scientists believe that there is a higher implantation rate with assisted hatching, especially for older women. However, well-controlled studies are lacking to support its use.

Side Effects

Rare side effects from the steroids can include high blood pressure, salt or water retention, a higher susceptibility to infection, mood swings, insomnia, osteoporosis, nausea, and allergic reactions. However, many of these side effects occur only with long-term steroid use. The antibiotic (usually tetracycline) may increase skin sensitivity to sunlight and may predispose a woman to vaginal yeast infections.

Risk Factors

Assisted hatching has been used extensively, but there is a small potential risk of damaging an embryo and preventing its replacement in the uterus.

assisted insemination   This term refers to insemination techniques such as INTRACYTOPLAS-MIC SPERM INJECTION (ICSI) that help sperm penetration into the egg.

assisted reproductive technology (ART)   A group of "high tech" treatment methods used to improve fertility, which involves collecting the eggs and putting them in direct contact with sperm. Together they form an alphabet soup of techniques including

- IVF (IN VITRO FERTILIZATION)
- GIFT (GAMETE INTRAFALLOPIAN TRANSFER)
- ZIFT (ZYGOTE INTRAFALLOPIAN TRANSFER)
- ICSI (INTRACYTOPLASMIC SPERM INJECTION)
- ASSISTED HATCHING

This new field was established in 1978 with the development of IVF, a process that allows fertilization to occur in the lab, followed by the transfer of the embryo (or embryos) into the uterus, bypassing the fallopian tubes. Louise Brown, born in 1978, was the first child born as the result of IVF, known at the time as the world's first "test tube baby." (See BROWN, LOUISE.)

Since that time, other ART procedures have been developed that further refined IVF; all of these procedures are no longer considered experimental but are established medical treatments for infertility. These new techniques include

- transfer of cryopreserved embryo, a procedure in which embryos frozen from an earlier IVF cycle are thawed and transferred into the uterus.
- gamete intrafallopian transfer (GIFT), a procedure in which the sperm and eggs are surgically transferred into the fallopian tubes, where fertilization is then allowed to occur. GIFT may be appropriate only when the woman has at least one normal fallopian tube.
- zygote intrafallopian transfer (ZIFT), also called TUBAL EMBRYO TRANSFER (TET). This is a hybrid of IVF and GIFT. The eggs retrieved from the woman's ovaries are fertilized in the lab, and the embryos are replaced in the fallopian tubes rather than in the uterus.
- intracytoplasmic sperm injection (ICSI). In this microinsemination procedure, a single sperm is injected directly into an egg.
- assisted hatching. In this microsurgical procedure, a small area of the shell surrounding the embryo (ZONA PELLUCIDA) is chemically dissolved to help the embryo hatch and implant.
- Egg donation, for women who may have impaired ovaries or carry a genetic disease that can be transferred to the offspring. Eggs are donated by another healthy woman and fertilized in the lab with the male partner's sperm before being transferred to the partner's uterus.

A number of factors are taken into account to determine if a couple should be a candidate for an ART procedure and which procedure is best, including the couple's age, the condition of ovaries, fallopian tubes, uterus, and condition of sperm. Other important factors for couples to consider are the time commitment and cost of ART, insurance, religious beliefs, emotional stress, and risk of multiple births. Unfortunately, even with modern medicine and the sophisticated ART techniques, there is no guarantee of success.

There are more than 70,000 babies born in the United States as a result of all these types of assisted reproductive technologies, including 45,000 as a result of IVF alone. About two-thirds of births from ART procedures are single births. Of the rest, almost all are twins, with about 6% resulting in the birth of triplets or more.

Most ART procedures involve in vitro fertilization, in which an egg is removed from a woman's ovary, fertilized in the lab, and transferred back into the uterus. To boost the chances of a successful conception, doctors generally prescribe hormonal therapy to stimulate the ovaries to produce multiple eggs.

These medications include

- CLOMIPHENE CITRATE (Serophene or Clomid). This drug prompts the brain to trigger release of pituitary hormones that stimulate the ovaries. It should not be used for more than six months, according to the American Society for Reproductive Medicine.

- HUMAN MENOPAUSAL GONADOTROPINS (hMG) (Humegon), the injected form of two hormones, FSH (FOLLICLE-STIMULATING HORMONE) and LH (LUTEINIZING HORMONE), which stimulate the ovaries to produce more follicles, thereby increasing the number of eggs produced.

- FSH (Metrodin or Fertinex). This hormone is used to stimulate the ovaries to produce more follicles, which may increase the number of eggs.

- HUMAN CHORIONIC GONADOTROPIN or hCG (Pregnyl, Profasi). This hormone matures the egg in the follicle and also triggers its release. It also may boost sperm production in men.

- PROGESTERONE, a hormone that stimulates the lining of the uterus to thicken in preparation for implantation of an embryo.

- LEUPROLIDE ACETATE (Lupron). This drug suppresses hormone LH and FSH production from the pituitary, needed to develop follicles and release eggs. It can suppress the body's own hormones to allow better control over the stimulation of the ovaries when other hormone medications are given.

How It Works

Over time, in vitro fertilization has become the most popular type of ART due to its simplicity and effectiveness. A typical cycle begins as the ovaries are temporarily shut down, using a GNRH AGONIST such as Lupron (leuprolide). After about 2 weeks of this medication, the ovaries temporarily shut down. Then the ovaries are stimulated with a potent drug such as Pergonal, given for about 10 days. When the eggs are ready to harvest, hCG is given to induce final egg maturation.

The eggs are then harvested from the vagina; under heavy sedation, a thin needle guided by ultrasound is inserted into the ovaries, and between 5 and 15 eggs are suctioned from the follicles. The eggs are then fertilized by adding approximately 100,000 sperm to each egg. If the sperm won't fertilize the eggs naturally, intracytoplasmic sperm injection (ICSI) may be used. In this procedure, the egg is punctured under a microscope and one sperm is injected into the egg.

The next day after retrieval, fertilization is documented. The embryos are observed for 3 to 6 days, and then 3 or 4 embryos are placed in a catheter and transferred through the cervix into the uterus. It is also possible to perform blastocyst embryo transfers. Because these embryos are more mature, fewer of them need to be transferred.

Two weeks later, a pregnancy test can document a successful pregnancy, and 2 weeks after that an ultrasound can detect the fetal heartbeat.

If more embryos are obtained than can be replaced, freezing (CRYOPRESERVATION) can save these additional embryos for later use. It's cheaper to store frozen embryos for future replacement than conduct another IVF cycle.

Although in vitro fertilization is probably the most effective technique to treat infertility when compared with others on a monthly basis, it's not without controversy. IVF is expensive (one cycle can cost $6,000 to $7,000), and there's no guarantee it will work. The technique also carries a risk of multiple pregnancies, although the risk varies with age. Younger patients need to have fewer embryos replaced and older patients need more.

The Program

Of course, ART programs differ from one clinic to the next, but the basic services are quite similar. Many clinics offer a team approach, which usually includes a REPRODUCTIVE ENDOCRINOLOGIST responsible for OVULATION stimulating, EGG RECOVERY and embryo transfer, and for monitoring the LUTEAL PHASE once the embryos have been returned to the uterus. The laboratory director is responsible for preparing the eggs and sperm, for the embryo culture, and for any required CRYOPRESERVATION, thawing and ICSI. The nurse coordinator interacts with the patients and the other team members. Many clinics also include mental health counseling in addition to ultrasound experts and endocrine lab staff.

Large clinics usually offer a wide range of services, although smaller programs with smaller patient loads may achieve good results as well. The AMERICAN SOCIETY FOR REPRODUCTIVE IMMUNOLOGY is affiliated with the Society For Assisted Reproductive Technology (SART), which registers almost all the clinics in the United States and Canada. Data for each of these clinics are available at www.cdc.gov/nccdphp/drh/art.htm. Each year in North America, information about the success rates of various ART procedures is collected by SART. This group has established a voluntary registry for all ART clinics to report their data; the results are then summarized and published. Couples can obtain this information either from their doctor, the American Society for Reproductive Medicine, or SART. However, it is important that SART statistics not be used to compare IVF programs, since there are many variables among each different IVF center.

Most patients are referred to an ART program by their doctor. Once the couple decides on a procedure (usually in consultation with a doctor or nurse at the program), an orientation to learn about IVF is available. Some additional tests may be required.

Ovarian Screening

While menopause usually occurs at about age 51, menopause in the early 40s is not unusual. About 6 years before the end of menstruation, women tend to be more infertile, and their miscarriage rate is quite high. Since the average age of patients in ART programs is 35, many programs screen all women over age 35 for ovarian function. The standard test measures FSH on day 3 of the menstrual cycle.

Results

While most couples are very interested in the results of any one program, ART results are not standard. Pregnancy may be reported per cycle initiated, per retrieval, or per transfer. In addition, if a couple doesn't conceive on their first try, statistics show that their chances of conceiving in a second or subsequent cycle remain the same.

asthenozoospermia　A term used to describe sperm that can't move forward very well (weak sperm motility).

Atlee brothers　Two brothers who grew up in Pennsylvania played an active role in gynecological medicine in the 19th century. John Atlee (1799–1885) was a founder and president of the Lancaster County Medical Society, the Pennsylvania Medical Society, and the American Medical Association. His younger brother, Washington, was instrumental in the formation of the American Gynecological Society.

Together, the brothers revived the procedure involving surgical removal of an ovary. Washington performed the first successful surgical removal of a fibroid tumor of the uterus (myomectomy) in 1844. He also followed his brother's footsteps as president of the Pennsylvania Medical Society and the AMA.

autoimmunity and infertility   See IMMUNE SYS-
TEM AND INFERTILITY.

azoospermia   Semen that contain no sperm,
either because the testicles can't make sperm or
because the man's reproductive tract is blocked.
Obstructive azoospermia is caused by a block in
either the epididymis, vas deferens, seminal
vesicles, or ejaculatory ducts. Sperm production
may be normal (which may be verified through
testicular biopsy), but the obstruction prevents
the sperm from being ejaculated. Some causes of
obstructive azoospermia are VASECTOMY, the absence of vas deferens from birth, scarring from
past infections, or past hernia operations.

Nonobstructive azoospermia refers to
severely impaired or nonexistent sperm production in the testis. This problem can be overcome
by extracting sperm directly from the testicles
(TESTICULAR SPERM EXTRACTION), followed by IN
VITRO FERTILIZATION using INTRACYTOPLASMIC
SPERM INJECTION.

balanced translocation (BT) The crossover of genetic material from one chromosome to another (translocation). The person with a balanced translocation is normal, but the abnormal translocation can be passed on to a child.

Chromosomes occur in pairs in all cells except sperm and eggs. If part of one chromosome is in a completely different chromosome, it's "translocated" but since the person still has the same amount of genetic material, the translocation is "balanced" and there is no negative result. However, when that person makes eggs or sperm, some of these will have too much or too little genetic material, as will the resulting embryo. In this case, the embryo will have a chromosomal translocation that is unbalanced and the embryo will be miscarried.

The problem can be inherited from one parent and then balanced out by the other, but if both parents have similar translocation problems, recurrent MISCARRIAGE may occur.

barrier methods A type of birth control that prevents pregnancy by providing a physical barrier that can stop sperm from getting into the uterus. When used with SPERMICIDE, barrier methods are among the safest and cheapest ways to prevent pregnancy, and they can also help reduce the risk of being infected with certain sexually transmitted diseases, PELVIC INFLAMMATORY DISEASE, and perhaps even cervical cancer. However, if they aren't used consistently and correctly, barrier methods have a relatively high failure rate.

Barrier methods include CONDOMS, DIAPHRAGM, CERVICAL CAP, SPONGE, and the VAGINAL CONTRACEPTIVE FILM. See also BIRTH CONTROL METHODS.

basal body temperature (BBT) The body temperature when taken at its lowest point, usually in the morning before getting out of bed. Charting a woman's BBT is used to document ovulation. If the BBT pattern rises about a half degree during the latter half of the menstrual cycle, it suggests that ovulation has taken place. If a woman's body temperature remains relatively constant throughout the cycle, this suggests that ovulation is not taking place.

During the first half of her cycle (The FOLLICULAR PHASE) a normal BBT pattern will show only slight variations in temperature (under 98 degrees). In response to progesterone produced at midcycle by the corpus luteum, the BBT will rise about a half degree (to about 98.4) and should remain high until the next period starts.

Therefore, the 2 or 3 days before the temperature rise is a woman's most fertile time. Once her temperature rises, the odds of getting pregnant are slight. By checking these data for 2 to 3 months, a woman can usually predict her most fertile days.

However, BBTs are not quite as accurate if a woman is taking fertility medications. For example, Clomid often causes elevated BBTs around the time when the medication is taken. Other types of ovulation monitoring are more reliable when a woman is on medication. See also BASAL BODY TEMPERATURE CHART; BASAL BODY TEMPERATURE THERMOMETER.

basal body temperature chart A daily record of the body's temperature at rest (known medically as the BASAL BODY TEMPERATURE) over several months to pinpoint when OVULATION has taken place. While not without error, the chart is popular because it is cheap and simple. During ovulation, the body's temperature will rise about 0.6°F to 0.8°F and stay elevated for about 14 days until the period starts.

A woman should measure her basal (resting) body temperature in the morning, even before getting out of bed. She should start taking her temperature on the morning her menstrual period ends. When taking a resting temperature, a woman should not smoke, eat, drink, or get up for any reason before taking a temperature reading.

A woman also can record on the chart the days she menstruates, the days she has sex, when she feels MITTELSCHMERZ (the twinge of pain associated with ovulation), and days when she is ill. When carefully tracked, this record can provide valuable information for planning a couple's fertility treatment.

If a woman's temperature remains relatively constant throughout a cycle, ovulation may not have occurred. On the other hand, a sustained rise in temperature beyond the date for the next period indicates a probable pregnancy. See also BASAL BODY TEMPERATURE THERMOMETER.

basal body temperature thermometer A special thermometer designed to take a basal body temperature. This type of device is more reliable and more accurate than regular glass mercury thermometers designed to measure a fever, which are only accurate to .2°F.

A basal body thermometer needs to be accurate to .1°. The BBT digital is more accurate for some people, and it takes only 30 to 60 seconds, which can matter if a woman is waiting to go to the bathroom first thing in the morning. The digital BBTs are harder to break and can retain the temperature reading.

BBT See BASAL BODY TEMPERATURE.

beta hCG test A blood test used to detect very early pregnancies and to evaluate the development of the embryo. A beta hCG test measures HUMAN CHORIONIC GONADOTROPIN (hCG), which is secreted by the placenta after implantation. It can be measured in the urine as a positive or negative, or the amount of hCG can be measured in the blood.

bicornuate uterus A malformation of the uterus during fetal development resulting in two separate cavities, each with a separate connecting fallopian tube. It occurs when the unborn baby's MULLERIAN DUCTS don't join correctly, resulting in a doubling of the upper portion. Each of the two sides is smaller than a normal uterus.

If the uterus is divided into two parts by a thin sheet of tissue, it is called a SEPTATE UTERUS, which may look heart-shaped or like an upside-down triangle.

Women with a bicornuate uterus can still get pregnant and carry a baby to term. However, because the uterus is half the normal size, the baby may be born prematurely.

biking and infertility The off-road sport of mountain biking may cause lower sperm counts and infertility as a result of scrotum problems such as benign tumors, swelling, and pain. In recent studies, Austrian researchers found that 96% of the serious bikers they studied had scrotal abnormalities, compared with just 16% of the nonbikers. The problems among the bikers included painful benign tumors, sperm-containing cysts capable of causing infections, fluid-filled cysts, and calcification of the sperm-storing epididymis that can cause infection and swelling. Some of these changes could lead to potential fertility problems.

Previous studies have found that long-distance bike riding can cause decreased sperm counts.

Bike seats constructed with holes or shaped like a "Y" to alleviate pressure may help somewhat, as might wearing a support. But full-suspension bikes with shock absorbers are probably more helpful because the bike, rather than the body, absorbs the shock.

birth control methods Today couples have a wide variety of birth control methods from which to choose that are very effective in preventing pregnancy. Of the 58 million women in the United States between age 15 and 44, about 39 million are sexually active and can become pregnant unless they use some form of birth control.

Among the 35 million women who use contraception, 39% rely on sterilization, 31% on pills, 20% on barrier methods, and 2% on intrauterine devices (IUDs).

Each year, 10% of teenage girls and women between ages 15 and 44 become pregnant. More than half of these pregnancies are unplanned and result because contraception was not used or because it failed.

Birth control methods include

- *barrier methods.* CONDOMS, DIAPHRAGMS, CERVICAL CAPS, and SPONGES work by physically preventing sperm from getting into the reproductive system and fertilizing an egg.

- *intrauterine devices.* IUDs are physical devices that are inserted into a woman's uterus to prevent pregnancy, but exactly how they work is controversial and little-understood.

- *hormonal methods.* Hormone implants and injections work by interfering with ovulation, conception, or implantation.

Natural Methods

For many reasons (mostly religious or health), some women rely on natural family planning as their main method of contraception. The rhythm method is the most popular form of natural birth planning. Basically, this means not having sex on the days when a woman is most fertile.

Because sperm may live in a woman's reproductive tract for up to 7 days, and the egg remains fertile for about 24 hours, it's possible to get pregnant from 7 days before ovulation to 3 days after. A woman needs to figure out her fertile time by using a method based on her menstrual cycle, changes in cervical mucus, or changes in body temperature.

Withdrawal is another type of natural family planning, in which a man pulls his penis out of the vagina before he ejaculates. In theory, this works because pregnancy can't occur if sperm is kept out of the vagina. Of every 100 women whose partners use withdrawal, 19 will become pregnant during the first year of typical use. Of every 100 women whose partners use withdrawal, 4 will become pregnant during the first year of perfect use.

Withdrawal fails because fluids that leak from the penis before ejaculation can contain enough sperm to cause pregnancy. Pregnancy is also possible if semen or pre-ejaculate is spilled on the vulva.

Withdrawal offers no protection against sexually transmitted infections. In addition, some men can't tell when they are going to ejaculate, and some ejaculate very quickly.

Barrier Methods

Barrier methods of birth control physically stop sperm from getting into the uterus (and the spermicide used with many methods also kills sperm). When used with spermicide, barrier methods are among the safest and cheapest ways to prevent pregnancy—and they can also help reduce the risk of being infected with certain sexually transmitted diseases, pelvic inflammatory disease, and perhaps even cervical cancer. However, if they aren't used consistently and correctly, barrier methods have a relatively high failure rate.

Condom: His and Hers

Both male and female versions of the condom are designed as a latex or polyurethane barrier to sperm; the male version fits over the erect penis, the female variety is inserted into the vagina, covering the cervix inside and the lips of the vagina outside. Condoms (both his and hers) can be used only once. Some have spermicide added (usually nonoxynol-9 in the United States) to kill sperm, although spermicide doesn't seem to provide more contraceptive protection beyond the condom alone. Because condoms act as a mechanical barrier, they prevent direct vaginal contact with semen, infectious genital secretions, and genital lesions and discharges.

Other than not having sex at all, latex condoms are the most effective way to lower the risk of infection from HIV, the virus that causes AIDS, and other STDs. Most condoms are made from latex rubber (hence their nickname "rubber"). Polyurethane condoms, marketed in the United States since 1994, are an alternative method of STD protection for those who are allergic to latex.

A small percentage of condoms are made from lamb intestines ("lambskin" condoms). Unlike latex or polyurethane condoms, lambskin condoms don't always prevent STDs because they're porous and may permit passage of viruses like HIV, hepatitis B, and herpes.

Some condoms are prelubricated, but these lubricants don't provide more birth control or STD protection. Non-oil-based lubricants (such as water or K-Y jelly), can be used with latex or lambskin condoms, but oil-based lubricants such as petroleum jelly (Vaseline), lotions, or massage or baby oil should not be used because they can weaken the condom material.

Used alone, the male condom has an expected failure rate of 2% and a typical failure rate of 12% (mostly because it can slip or break during withdrawal). Used with spermicide, the failure rate can be reduced almost to zero.

Female condoms, approved by the FDA in 1993, are sold under the brand names Femidom and Reality. Less likely to slip or burst than the male version, the female condom is a lubricated polyurethane sheath with a closed flexible ring at one end and a larger open ring at the other. The closed ring is inserted into the vagina, fitting over the cervix, leaving the open end hanging outside the vagina where it partially covers the labia. It must carefully be removed after sex; a fresh condom must be inserted for each subsequent act of sexual intercourse. If these rules are followed, the female condom seems to be as effective as the diaphragm or cervical cap. A female condom should not be used together with a male condom because they may not both stay in place.

Diaphragm

Available by prescription only and sized by a health professional to achieve a proper fit, the diaphragm uses a dual mechanism to prevent pregnancy. A dome-shaped rubber disk with a flexible rim covers the cervix so that sperm can't reach the uterus, while the spermicide applied to the diaphragm before insertion kills sperm.

The diaphragm protects for 6 hours; after that time (or for repeated intercourse within this period), fresh spermicide must be inserted into the vagina with the diaphragm still in place. It must remain in place for at least 6 hours after the last intercourse, but no more than 24 hours because of the risk of toxic shock syndrome (TSS), a rare but potentially fatal infection. Used consistently and correctly, the diaphragm carries a failure rate of about 6%, but the typical failure rate is more like 18%.

Diaphragm fit should be checked at an annual gynecological exam

- whenever a woman gains or loses 10 pounds or more
- after an abortion
- after a miscarriage
- after a full-term pregnancy

Cervical Cap

The cap is a soft rubber cup about the size of a thimble with a round rim, sized by a health professional to fit snugly around the cervix. It's available by prescription only and, like the diaphragm, is used with a small amount of spermicide. The spermicide may be enough to help prevent the spread of certain STDs, but it doesn't guarantee safety.

The cap protects for 48 hours and for multiple acts of intercourse within this time. Wearing it for more than 48 hours is not recommended because of the low risk of toxic shock syndrome. With prolonged use of 2 or more days, the cap may cause an unpleasant vaginal odor or discharge in some women.

The cap is basically a smaller diaphragm that fits over the cervix and is held in place by suction. Because it can be difficult to insert and doesn't fit all women, it's a less popular method than the diaphragm. On the other hand, it can be left in place longer than the diaphragm and can be used to collect menstrual blood.

The Sponge

The Today sponge is a donut-shaped polyurethane device containing the spermicide nonoxynol-9 that is inserted into the vagina to cover the cervix, much like a diaphragm. A woven polyester loop is attached for easy removal. The sponge is a low-cost, nonprescription product that protects for multiple acts of sex for 24 hours. It must be left in place for at least 6 hours after sex for contraceptive protection, but no more than 30 hours after insertion because of the slight risk of toxic shock syndrome.

Once so popular a form of birth control that it became a joke on the *Seinfeld* TV comedy ("Are you spongeworthy?"), the Today sponge was taken off the market in 1995 for financial—not health—reasons. The sole manufacturer (Whitehall Laboratories of Madison, N.J.) had decided it would cost too much to correct manufacturing problems the FDA had discovered at the old factory where the sponge was made. (The FDA stressed that there never was any problem with Today's safety, just with the factory.)

Some 116,000 American women had been using Today in 1995 when its manufacturer stopped production, which had made it the most popular choice among methods that didn't require a doctor's visit. The only other woman-controlled nonprescription choices were spermicide and the female condom; unlike those options, the sponge could be inserted up to 24 hours before sex and didn't require new applications for repeated intercourse. With its low risk of side effects, the sponge was attractive to women who didn't want to have to be fitted by a doctor, who had problems with prescribed hormonal contraceptives, or who enjoyed its ease of insertion.

Competing sponges were sold in France, Canada, and a few other countries, but once Today was off the U.S. market, no plans were made to bring back the contraceptive sponge in this country until 1999, when Allendale Pharmaceuticals of New Jersey decided to reintroduce it in the United States. Because the FDA never revoked the Today's approval, getting it back on the market was a quick process.

Allendale's sponge is available in Canada under the name of Today; a competing sponge (Protectaid) is also available in Canada and some European countries. At press time, the FDA was preparing to conduct final inspections of the plant, which must be completed before the sponge can be sold again in this country.

Spermicide

Vaginal spermicides are inserted into the vagina where they kill sperm on contact. They're most effective when combined with a barrier method of birth control such as a diaphragm or condom. Vaginal spermicides are available as a foam, cream, jelly, film, suppository, or tablet.

While all products contain a sperm-killing chemical, it's important to follow package instructions because some products require a 10-minute wait or more after inserting the spermicide before having sex. Once it's been inserted, one dose of spermicide is usually effective for 1 hour; for repeated intercourse, more spermicide needs to be applied. After sex, the spermicide must remain in place for at least 6 to 8 hours to ensure that all sperm are killed (this means the woman should not douche or rinse the vagina during this time).

According to a 1996 FDA advisory committee panel, some vaginal spermicide containing NONOXYNOL-9 may reduce the risk of GONORRHEA and CHLAMYDIA transmission. However, nonoxynol-9 may cause tissue irritation, boosting the risk of some STDs, including HIV.

The only birth control methods that definitely protect against sexually transmitted diseases are latex or polyurethane male and female condoms together with spermicide. BIRTH CONTROL PILLS, NORPLANT (birth control implants), DEPO-PROVERA (birth control injections), IUDs, and lambskin condoms don't protect against STD infection.

Intrauterine Device (IUD)

An IUD is a T-shaped device inserted into the uterus by a health care professional. Today there are only two types of IUDs legally available in the United States: the Paragard Copper T 380A and the Progestasert Progesterone T. The Paragard IUD can remain in place for 10 years; the Progestasert IUD must be replaced every year.

During the 1970s, an IUD known as the Dalkon Shield was taken off the market because it was associated with a high incidence of pelvic infections and infertility, and some deaths. Today, serious complications from IUDs are rare, although IUD users may be at increased risk of developing PELVIC INFLAMMATORY DISEASE. Other side effects can include perforation of the uterus, abnormal bleeding, and cramps. Complications occur most often during and immediately after insertion.

It's not entirely clear how IUDs prevent pregnancy. They seem to prevent sperm and eggs from meeting by either immobilizing the sperm on their way to the fallopian tubes, or altering the uterine lining in some way so that the fertilized egg cannot implant in it.

IUDs have one of the lowest failure rates of any contraceptive method. In the population for which the IUD is appropriate (those in mutually monogamous, stable relationships who aren't at a high risk of infection), the IUD is a very safe and very effective method of contraception. It has an expected failure rate of between 1% and 2% depending on the type, and a typical failure rate of about 3%. Still, menstrual cramps and excessive bleeding led a sizable minority of women to have their IUDs removed during their first year. Because women who haven't yet had children experience a higher risk of developing pelvic inflammatory disease with the IUD, most clinicians won't use one with a woman who is still interested in having children.

Hormonal Contraception

Given in the form of injections, pills, or implants, hormones can interfere with normal ovulation, conception, and implantation very effectively. Unfortunately, they also can cause a range of side effects:

- headaches
- acne
- weight changes
- excess hair or hair loss
- nausea and vomiting
- depression
- menstrual irregularities

Despite these problems, for many women the benefits of hormonal methods—they are the most easy to use and among the most effective—make them a popular choice. Implants and injections in particular can be a good choice since they are estrogen-free and they are easy to use.

The Pill

Oral contraceptives have been on the market for more than 35 years and are the most popular form of reversible birth control in the United States. The pill works by suppressing ovulation (the monthly release of an egg from the ovaries) as a result of the combined actions of the hormones estrogen and progestin. If taken daily as directed, there is an extremely small chance of becoming pregnant. But the pill's effectiveness may be reduced if a woman takes certain other medications (such as some antibiotics) at the same time. If a woman forgets a pill, she should use a backup method of birth control for the next 2 days to be sure she's protected against pregnancy.

Birth control pills also can affect other medications or lab test results. The estrogen and progestin in birth control pills can affect liver function. If taken together with other drugs that are metabolized by the liver, there may be higher blood levels of the birth control pill, causing more toxic side effects. These effects might be strongest in pills with large amounts of progestin.

In the past, strong versions of the pill containing high doses of estrogen made this type of contraception dangerous for women over age 35; newer, safer forms are now highly effective and reasonably safe for most nonsmoking women up to age 45. Still, the long-term effect of taking these pills is not clear, because not enough women have taken them for that long.

Besides preventing pregnancy, the pill offers additional benefits. The pill can

- make menstrual periods more regular
- protect against pelvic inflammatory disease
- protect against ovarian and endometrial cancers

While birth control pills are safe for most women (safer even than delivering a baby), they do carry some risks for some women. The pill may contribute to high blood pressure, blood clots, and blockage of the arteries. One of the biggest questions has been whether the pill increases the risk of breast cancer in past and current pill users. An international study published in the September 1996 journal *Contraception* concluded that women's risk of breast cancer 10 years after going off birth control pills was no higher than that of women who had never used the pill.

During pill use and for the first 10 years after stopping the pill, women's risk of breast cancer was only slightly higher in pill users than nonpill users.

Most health experts advise that some women not take the pill, including the following:

- women who smoke—especially those over age 35
- women with a history of blood clots
- women with a personal history of breast or endometrial cancer
- women with heart disease
- women over age 45

Some women object to the pill not because of health concerns but because of side effects, which include nausea, headache, breast tenderness, weight gain, irregular bleeding, and depression. While the problems may subside after a few months, some women experience continued problems.

Another type of oral contraceptive called the "minipill" is taken daily, but it contains only the hormone progestin, with no estrogen. These pills work by reducing and thickening cervical mucus to prevent sperm from reaching the egg. They also keep the uterine lining from thickening, which prevents a fertilized egg from implanting in the uterus.

Because they lack estrogen, these pills are slightly less effective than combined oral contraceptives. Women who take the minipill late (even by as little as 3 hours) have a higher chance of pregnancy.

Minipills can decrease menstrual bleeding and cramps, as well as the risk of endometrial and ovarian cancer and pelvic inflammatory disease. Because they contain no estrogen, minipills don't present the risk of blood clots associated with estrogen in combined pills. They are a good option for women who can't take estrogen because they are breast feeding or because estrogen-containing products cause them to have severe headaches or high blood pressure. Side effects of minipills include menstrual cycle changes, weight gain, and breast tenderness.

Contraceptive Implants

One of the newest types of birth control options is contraceptive implants (NORPLANT)—small, matchstick-sized tubes containing a progestin or levonorgestrel—inserted just under the skin of a woman's arm. Once in place, the implants release a small amount of hormone each day for 5 years, blocking ovulation and thickening cervical mucus. Other than vasectomies, the implants are probably the most effective method of contraception available. Once the implants are removed, a woman can become pregnant again.

The implants can be inserted during an office visit. First, the doctor numbs the skin with local anesthetic, then imbeds the tubes under the skin of the upper arm. They must be surgically removed (which may be difficult).

Some women may experience inflammation or infection at the site of the implant. Other side effects include menstrual cycle changes, weight gain, breast tenderness, or loss of bone mass.

While implants are very effective, they can cause all of the side effects typically related to hormonal types of birth control. Some serious symptoms include

- arm pain
- pus or bleeding at the insertion site (it could be an infection)
- expulsion of the implant
- delayed menstrual periods after a long time of regular periods

Women should not use implants if they

- are (or might be) pregnant
- have unexplained unusual vaginal bleeding
- take antiseizure drugs
- take the antibiotic rifampin
- have blood clots
- have had blood clots in the lungs

Birth Control Injections

Some women don't like the idea of having tubes inserted into their arms; they prefer hormone injections. These injections, which are considered to be safe and effective, involve a long-acting type of progesterone that is injected every 3 months. The method (DEPO-PROVERA) uses a progestin that is normally injected into the buttocks.

The injections work by preventing ovulation; when taken as scheduled, it's more than 99% effective and completely reversible once the hormone is eliminated from the body. A shot should be scheduled within 5 days of the start of a menstrual period to get full protection from pregnancy right from the beginning.

Women should not have the injections if they are (or might be) pregnant, or if they have unexplained unusual vaginal bleeding any time in the preceding 3 months.

After taking the injections for several cycles, a woman actually has a bit more protection (a few weeks longer than 3 months); this provides a "safety period" until the next shot. However, once a woman has gotten the injection, there is no way to become fertile again until it wears off about 3 months later.

Because the injections aren't metabolized in the liver, some of the side effects from pills are avoided. However, the injections may cause

- abdominal discomfort
- nervousness
- decreased sex drive
- depression
- acne
- dizziness
- weight gain
- menstrual cycle disruption
- bleeding and spotting

Serious symptoms include

- heavy bleeding
- severe headaches

- depression
- frequent urination
- severe lower abdominal pain (rare)

Sterilization

Surgical sterilization is a contraceptive option intended for people who don't want children. It's considered permanent because reversal requires major surgery that is often unsuccessful. In general, VASECTOMY is less expensive and less risky than female sterilization.

If one of a couple has been sterilized and now is considering reversal, the other partner should be examined for infertility before the reversal operation is attempted.

Female Sterilization

In female sterilization, the doctor blocks the fallopian tubes with various surgical techniques so that the egg can't travel to the uterus. Sterilization is usually done under general anesthesia, with laparoscopy to cauterize both fallopian tubes so that the egg released each month by an ovary can't come in contact with sperm.

The doctor will introduce gas into the abdomen to push the intestines away from the uterus and fallopian tubes, and then insert a lighted tube (laparoscope) through the same incision. Next, instruments are inserted through the laparoscope (or a smaller second incision at the pubic hairline). The doctor then seals the fallopian tubes using one of these methods:

- electrocoagulation: burning the walls of the fallopian tubes with electrical energy so that the two parts of the tubes are blocked

- mechanical blocks: clips or bands that block and crush the fallopian tubes

Complications are rare, but they may include infection or damage to the bowel or blood vessels, or problems related to general anesthesia. Some studies suggest that sterilization may cause changes in a woman's menstrual cycles or lead to abdominal pain later.

Male Sterilization

In male sterilization (vasectomy), a doctor seals, ties, or cuts the vas deferens (the tube that carries the sperm from the testicle to the penis). Vasectomy is a quick operation (usually under 30 minutes), with only minor postsurgical complications such as bleeding or infection.

A man can have sex a few days after surgery, but there may still be some mature sperm in the reproductive tract, so pregnancy could still result. Typically, a man should ejaculate 15 times after a vasectomy before he's infertile. It's best to use some sort of backup birth control method until a doctor can verify that the sperm count is zero.

Some studies have suggested that a man who's had a vasectomy is more likely to get prostate cancer than one who hasn't, but more research is needed.

Emergency Contraception

An EMERGENCY CONTRACEPTIVE PILL refers to a method that can prevent pregnancy after unprotected sex, after birth control fails, or after a rape. The ECP method involves a higher doses of combined oral contraceptives for use as "morning after" pills to be taken within 72 hours of unprotected intercourse to prevent the possibly fertilized egg from reaching the uterus. While there's no guarantee, ECP probably cuts the chances of getting pregnant by 90% to 95%.

The "morning after" pill has been officially recognized as safe and effective by the Food and Drug Administration as of February 1997. Scientists aren't sure exactly how it works, but they suspect that the large doses of hormones prevent the lining of the uterus from getting thick enough to allow an egg to implant or that they interfere with ovulation in some way, slowing the way the egg travels through the fallopian tube.

On the other hand, the larger dose of hormones may cause side effects similar to (but stronger than) the side effects after a regular dose of birth control pills. If nausea is severe and a woman gets so sick she vomits, she may lose the pills before they can work. The doctor may suggest taking another dose in this event. A woman's next period may be late because of the pills, but if a period doesn't begin within three weeks of treatment a woman should contact her doctor to make sure she's not pregnant.

When Birth Control Fails . . .

Very few birth control devices are 100% foolproof—and too many times, people don't use the methods correctly or consistently. In the event of an unwanted pregnancy, a woman has the choice of ending the pregnancy or carrying the baby to term. The sooner a decision is made, the better for the woman (if she decides to terminate) and the better for both mother and child if she decides to continue the pregnancy.

If a woman decides to terminate, she should seek help from an experienced abortion provider, since the earlier a pregnancy is aborted the less dangerous. Although abortion is currently legal in the United States, some states do have mandatory waiting periods, some require parental involvement for minors, and some require that a doctor show graphic material designed to discourage abortion.

RU 486 (Mifepristone)

Abortions using the "French abortion pill" (MIFEPRISTONE, or RU 486) were approved by the FDA in September 2000. Unlike surgical abortion, which is often not done before the seventh or eight week of gestation, medical abortion can be used earlier—as soon as pregnancy is determined.

The drugs contain antiprogestins that block the action of natural progesterone; without progesterone's effects, the uterine lining softens and breaks down, leading to menstruation. This is most effective when used in the first weeks after fertilization and implantation, when progesterone is being produced mostly by the ovaries. As pregnancy proceeds, the placenta takes over progesterone's role, and the antiprogestins are less effective.

The process is this:

1. Between 49 and 63 days after the first day of a woman's last menstrual period, she swallows the drug and stays in the clinic for an hour.
2. Two days later she returns to the clinic for an oral dose of prostaglandin, which boosts uterine contractions.
3. After staying at the clinic for 4 hours wearing a sanitary pad, most women experience a shedding of the uterine lining, passing the fertilized egg or embryo. (The process continues for a day.)
4. She then returns to the clinic 2 weeks later for a follow-up visit.

About 4% of women don't abort; they require a surgical abortion.

Surgical Abortion

This is another type of FDA-approved abortion available in the United States, but in some states it's very hard to obtain. Abortion services are offered in hospitals and clinics, and usually are performed before 12 weeks of gestation. Abortions performed after 11 to 12 weeks carry higher complication rates. If the pregnancy is beyond 15 weeks, the process is more complicated because of the size of the fetus. After a surgical abortion, women will experience cramps and light to medium bleeding over 5 to 7 days. Most doctors recommend not having sex until the cervix has closed (usually when the bleeding stops). After an abortion, a woman should call her doctor immediately if she notices heavy bleeding or any signs of infection, such as fever and chills.

Methods That Don't Work

There are also a number of methods that don't work very well in preventing pregnancy. These include

- sex during a woman's menstrual period (there's still a slim chance a woman can get pregnant this way).

- douching after sex: It's not possible to destroy all the sperm by douching; in fact, douching may force the sperm higher into the uterus.

- urinating after sex: Urine and sperm travel in two separate parts of a woman's body, so urinating won't have any affect on sperm traveling up the vagina.

- washing after sex: No matter how fast a woman washes after ejaculation, sperm are already swimming quickly through the cervix, where they won't be destroyed by washing.

- early withdrawal: Even if the penis is removed before ejaculation, there is usually some sperm in the pre-ejaculatory liquid. The penis doesn't even need to be inside the vagina for some sperm to make it through the cervix and fertilize an egg.

birth control pill Oral contraceptives, also known simply as "The Pill," a birth control device that revolutionized contraception in the 1960s. The birth control pill, in various forms, has been on the market for more than 35 years and is the most popular form of reversible birth control in the United States.

The pill works by suppressing ovulation (the monthly release of an egg from the ovaries) as a result of the combined actions of the hormones ESTROGEN and progestin. If taken daily as directed, it protects a woman almost completely from getting pregnant. But the pill's effectiveness may be reduced if a woman takes some other medications (such as certain antibiotics) at the same time. If a woman for-gets a pill, she should use a backup method of birth control for the next 2 days to be sure she's protected against pregnancy.

Birth control pills also can affect other medications or lab test results. The estrogen and progestin in birth control pills can affect liver function, for example. If taken together with other drugs that are metabolized by the liver, there may be higher blood levels of the birth control pill, causing more toxic side effects.

These effects might be strongest in pills with large amounts of progestin.

Safety

In the past, strong versions of the pill containing high doses of estrogen made this type of contraception dangerous for women over age 35; newer, safer forms are now highly effective and reasonably safe for most nonsmoking women up to age 45. Still, the long-term effect of taking these pills is not clear, because not enough women have taken them for that long.

Besides preventing pregnancy, the pill offers additional benefits. The pill can

- make menstrual periods more regular

- protect against pelvic inflammatory disease

- protect against ovarian and endometrial cancers

Risks

While birth control pills are safe for most women (safer even than delivering a baby), they do carry some risks for some. The pill may contribute to high blood pressure, blood clots, and blockage of the arteries.

One of the biggest questions has been whether the pill increases the risk of breast cancer in past and current pill users. An international study published in the September 1996 journal *Contraception* concluded that women's risk of breast cancer 10 years after going off birth control pills was no higher than that of women who had never used the pill. During pill use and for the first 10 years after stopping the pill, women's risk of breast cancer was only slightly higher in pill users than nonpill users.

Most health experts advise that some women not take the pill, including the following:

- women who smoke—especially those over age 35

- women with a history of blood clots

- women with a personal history of breast or endometrial cancer

- women with heart disease
- women over age 45

Side Effects

Some women object to the pill, not because of health concerns but because of side effects, which include nausea, headache, breast tenderness, weight gain, irregular bleeding, and depression. While the problems may subside after a few months, some women experience continued problems.

Minipill

Another type of oral contraceptive called the "minipill" is taken daily, but it contains only the hormone progestin, with no estrogen. These pills work by reducing and thickening cervical mucus to prevent sperm from reaching the egg. They also keep the uterine lining from thickening, which prevents a fertilized egg from implanting in the uterus.

Because they lack estrogen, these pills are slightly less effective than combined oral contraceptives. Women who take the minipill late (even by as little as 3 hours) have a higher chance of pregnancy.

Minipills can decrease menstrual bleeding and cramps, as well as the risk of endometrial and ovarian cancer and pelvic inflammatory disease. Because they contain no estrogen, minipills don't present the risk of blood clots associated with estrogen in combined pills. They are a good option for women who can't take estrogen because they are breast feeding or because estrogen-containing products cause them to have severe headaches or high blood pressure. Side effects of minipills include menstrual cycle changes, weight gain, and breast tenderness.

blastocyst   A stage of embryonic development that occurs about 5 days after fertilization, when the embryo consists of two different cell types (those that will form the placenta and those that will form the fetus) and a central cavity. The sur- face cells become the placenta, and the inner cell mass becomes the fetus.

A healthy blastocyst should hatch by the end of the sixth day. Within about 24 hours after hatching, it loses its protective coating and begins to implant into the lining of the uterus.

blastocyst transfer   Following IN VITRO FERTILIZATION, the embryos are allowed to reach BLASTOCYST stage (usually at 5 days) before being transferred into the uterus, instead of being transferred after the second or third day.

Traditionally, embryos are transferred to the uterus after initial embryonic cell division on the second or third day of development. This was done to minimize the exposure of the embryos to culture media, which in the past could only sustain growth for 2 to 3 days. Today, however, researchers have developed new culture solutions rich in nutrients that help the embryos develop longer in vitro.

The benefit of allowing the embryos to grow into blastocysts is that this gives the cells of the embryo time to divide and differentiate. The inherent "health" of any embryo will dictate its ability to continue to grow and divide. Although several eggs may have initially been fertilized, only a few will progress to the four-cell stage, fewer still to the eight-cell stage, and even fewer will develop into blastocysts—a type of survival of the fittest.

In the past, if a woman has 15 eggs retrieved, only about 10 will fertilize by the first day. It's impossible to determine at this point which of these 10 are most likely to develop into a baby. On the traditional day of embryo transfer (day 3) only 5 of the 10 embryos may be developing into vibrant, growing embryos. The others may have slowed or stopped their development altogether.

Of the 5, however, it's impossible to know which ones are the best choice to transfer. Two additional days in the blastocyst culture medium allows the natural elimination process to continue, so that after 5 days of growth in the lab, only 2 or 3 of the original 10 embryos may be viable. It's then clearer which are the best embryos to transfer.

Embryos transferred at the blastocyst stage have survived key growth processes and usually offer a better chance of implanting. Transferring only one or two blastocysts to the mother instead of the typical three or four early embryos also cuts down on the risk of high-order multiple pregnancy, which carries many potential risks. In addition, if there are more than two available blastocysts at the time of transfer, those remaining may be preserved for future use.

On the other hand, there is no advantage to blastocyst transfer for women who have had fewer eggs retrieved, fewer fertilized embryos, or fewer dividing embryos by day 3. In general, freezing blastocyst embryos is not as successful as freezing earlier stage embryos, which may limit its usefulness. Further research is needed to determine the precise role of blastocyst culture in IVF.

blastomeres   Cells that make up the BLASTOCYST.

blighted ovum   An old-fashioned term for an embryo that has not developed normally after fertilization. The amniotic sac may only contain fluid and no fetal tissue when the MISCARRIAGE occurs.

blood group antibody screen   A test done to measure red blood cell A, B, or other antigens and to see if antibodies to the antigens exist.

blood pressure medication and infertility Medications used to treat high blood pressure may interfere with potency and the ability to ejaculate, and they may be associated with retrograde ejaculation. Reducing the dose or changing the medication will usually reverse the effects, but doing so may take many weeks to show an improvement. See also EJACULATION DISORDERS.

blood tests for infertility   Blood tests are valuable in assessing infertility and in monitoring most kinds of assisted reproduction, helping to pinpoint fluctuating hormone levels, and screening for infections.

Hormone levels must be tracked through a series of tests throughout an IVF cycle. Blood tests include ESTRADIOL (E2), LUTEINIZING HORMONE (LH), FOLLICLE-STIMULATING HORMONE (FSH), or PROGESTERONE.

Estradiol (E2)

Estradiol is one of many forms of estrogen released by the developing follicle. In general, as follicles develop, estradiol levels increase; therefore, low levels of estradiol may indicate that the follicle does not contain a healthy egg.

The use of ovulation induction drugs such as FSH necessitates several estradiol measurements. These measurements provide the physician with information needed to make dosage adjustments. Low levels of estradiol may indicate a need to increase dosage, and high levels may signal an increased risk of OVARIAN HYPERSTIMULATION SYNDROME.

LH Kits

The LH kit measures the level of luteinizing hormone (LH) in the urine. A sudden large release of LH from the pituitary gland culminates in the release of a mature egg from the follicle (OVULATION) about 36 hours after the surge begins.

FSH Assay

FSH is a hormone produced by the pituitary gland responsible for the development of the egg in the female and sperm in the male; it's also the active ingredient in the injectable drugs used to stimulate ovulation. FSH is measured in women on day 3 of the menstrual cycle. A high FSH level may indicate that there are fewer healthy eggs within the ovary.

Progesterone

Progesterone is secreted after ovulation by the corpus luteum (the follicle becomes a corpus luteum after the egg is released). One of progesterone's major functions is to influence the uterine lining. This female hormone can be measured to determine if ovulation has occurred. Progesterone is produced in small amounts in developing follicles, so low levels can be detected at most times during the stimulation phase of treatment.

Blood is drawn 4 to 9 days after predicted ovulation. At that time, progesterone levels should be elevated consistent with ovulation. Also, progesterone is usually administered to supplement ovarian production for 2 weeks after an ART cycle to help support the growth of the developing embryo.

If the levels of progesterone rise during FSH administration within an IVF cycle, it may indicate that follicle development is not proceeding smoothly, and the eggs may be of poor quality.

Blood Tests in Men

If a semen analysis is abnormal, blood tests can measure levels of reproductive hormones. However, less than 3% of cases of male infertility are caused by primary hormone defects.

Blood tests known as radioimmunoassays (RIAs) are used to measure levels of the reproductive hormones testosterone, LH, FSH, and prolactin, which interact with each other in an intricate balance. Testosterone, which is produced by the LEYDIG cells of the testes, is directly regulated by LH, a secretion of the pituitary gland. LH, in turn, is controlled by GONADO-TROPIN-RELEASING HORMONE (Gn-RH), which is produced by the hypothalamus. Prolactin, another pituitary hormone, affects Gn-RH release from the hypothalamus.

Although blood levels of estradiol (a form of estrogen) are not routinely monitored, they may be measured in men with gynecomastia (enlarged breasts). Prolactin levels may be measured in infertile men who experience sexual dysfunction and show signs of pituitary disease.

body mass index   An estimate of a person's amount of fat. It is calculated by dividing the weight in kilograms by the square of the height (in meters). It should normally be between 20 and 25 (although the upper limit increases with age). Extremes of BMI can cause menstrual irregularity.

Boston IVF   The largest fertility treatment facility in the United States. Established in 1986, Boston IVF is considered to be one of the most successful advanced fertility treatment facilities in the country. Boston IVF is affiliated with the Beth Israel Deaconess Medical Center, a major teaching hospital of Harvard Medical School; and has pioneered innovative protocols and research projects in the field of reproductive medicine.

breakthrough bleeding   Light bleeding or spotting while taking the BIRTH CONTROL PILL or while taking a PROGESTOGEN. In the first few months of pill use, this type of light spotting is common, but if it occurs after many months of pill use that could mean that the pill is not working well. Breakthrough bleeding occurs either because of an illness (such as diarrhea), antibiotic use, other medications that boost the pill's action, or a problem with the uterus or cervix.

bromocriptine (Parlodel)   A medication used to lower PROLACTIN levels. Prolactin is a hormone normally elevated only during breast feeding, but when high at other times it may interfere with normal ovulation. When prolactin levels return to normal, ovulation usually returns, and chances of pregnancy also return to normal. The drug, which has a direct effect on prolactin-producing cells in the pituitary gland, also can reduce the size of a pituitary tumor (which can lead to high prolactin levels). This medication is usually administered by mouth, but it also is effective when the tablet is placed into the vagina.

Side Effects

Bromocriptine is usually started at bedtime to reduce side effects, which can include dizziness, upset stomach, and vomiting. Treatment usually begins with a small dose, which is gradually increased as needed. Other side effects include nasal stuffiness and constipation. Although elevations in blood pressure, hallucinations, gastric bleeding, and the worsening of Raynaud's syndrome have been reported, these side effects occur very rarely.

Brown, Louise   The first child born from a successful IN VITRO FERTILIZATION, Louise Brown was born in Great Britain in 1978. Her mother's fallopian tubes were irreparably blocked, and this type of tubal damage became the first—and for a while, the only—indication for IVF. In Brown's case, her mother's egg and her father's sperm were combined in a lab to produce an embryo that was later implanted in her mother's uterus.

When Louise was born 9 months later, she became known around the world as a technological miracle, the world's first "test tube baby." Today, Brown lives in England and works at a daycare center.

Today IVF is the most common of the high-tech infertility treatments, accounting for more than 70% of all ASSISTED REPRODUCTIVE TECHNOLOGY (ART) procedures.

brucellosis   A rare disease in which inflammation of the testicles (ORCHITIS) develops in between 2% and 20% of men with the disease. Orchitis can lead to infertility.

Cause

It is caused by contact with farm animals carrying the Brucella bacteria, which infects cattle, goats, dogs, and pigs. Transmission of the disease to humans occurs by contact with infected meat, the placenta of infected animals, or drinking unpasteurized milk. The illness may be chronic and persist for years. Brucellosis is rare in the United States, except in the western states and in visitors or immigrants from countries where it is common, such as Spain, Mexico, and South America. Between 100 to 200 cases occur in the United States each year. People working in occupations requiring frequent contact with animals or meat—such as slaughterhouse workers, farmers, and veterinarians—are at high risk.

Symptoms

Acute brucellosis may begin with mild flu-like symptoms or with fever, chills, sweating, muscle aches (myalgia), joint aches (arthralgia), and malaise. Characteristically, fever spikes every afternoon to levels around 104°F. Its nickname ("undulant fever") originates from this undulating (fluctuating) fever.

Diagnosis

Brucellosis is diagnosed by examining cultures of blood, urine, bone marrow, and spinal fluid, in addition to testing for the brucellosis antigen.

Treatment

A combination of antibiotics, such as doxycycline and rifampin or an aminoglycoside, is recommended to treat the disease and prevent relapse. Longer treatment may be required for complications. However, relapse may occur and symptoms may persist for years.

caffeine and infertility Many studies have been conducted to determine the effects of caffeine intake on fertility in women, but results are inconclusive. Most studies found that moderate caffeine intake does not affect fertility or increase the chance of having a miscarriage or a baby with birth defects. However, some studies did find a relationship between caffeine intake and fertility or miscarriages—especially in women who drank large amounts of coffee (5 or more cups daily).

Moderate caffeine intake (1 or 2 cups a day) does not appear to boost a woman's chances of having a miscarriage, according to a study published in the *New England Journal of Medicine*. One small study in 1988 suggested that caffeine, equivalent to the amount consumed in 1 or 2 cups of coffee daily, might decrease female fertility. However, the researchers acknowledged that delayed conception could be due to other factors they did not consider, such as exercise, stress, or other dietary habits. Since then, larger, well-designed studies have failed to support these findings.

Higher amounts may cause more problems, however. In one study, pregnant women who drank the equivalent of 5 or more cups of coffee a day were twice as likely to miscarry.

In 1990, researchers at the Centers for Disease Control and Prevention and Harvard University examined the association between the length of time to conceive and consumption of caffeinated beverages. The study involved more than 2,800 women who had recently given birth and 1,800 women with the medical diagnosis of primary infertility. Each group was interviewed concerning caffeine consumption, medical history, and lifestyle habits. The researchers found that caffeine consumption had little or no effect on the reported time to conceive in those women who had given birth. Caffeine consumption also was not a risk factor for infertility.

Supporting those findings, a 1991 study of 11,000 Danish women examined the relationship among number of months to conceive, cigarette smoking, and coffee and tea consumption. Although smokers who consumed 8 or more cups of coffee per day experienced delayed conception, nonsmokers did not, regardless of caffeine consumption.

California Cryobank The best-known U.S. SPERM BANK that was founded in 1977 to provide physicians and their patients an accessible and comprehensive resource for semen storage and specialized reproductive services. Now one of the largest laboratories of its kind, the bank is accredited by the AMERICAN ASSOCIATION OF TISSUE BANKS.

California Cryobank offers a choice of standard donor specimens for intracervical inseminations or prewashed processed donor specimens for INTRAUTERINE INSEMINATIONS. The company produces a new donor catalog with more than 200 choices each month and offers an extensive medical history on each donor. Quality control measures include color coding donor specimens by race and an electronic identification system to obtain positive donor identification prior to each deposit.

All shipments are sent in liquid nitrogen dry-shipper tanks, where specimens can survive for 7 days. See also CRYOS; CRYOPRESERVATION.

capacitation An invisible process that helps sperm become able to fertilize an egg. After ejaculation, the sperm go through capacitation as they travel through the woman's reproductive tract, which helps them move quicker and penetrate the egg. Capacitation is brought about naturally as sperm swim through the uterus and fallopian tubes, or it can be triggered in the lab by spinning and washing the sperm through a series of solutions.

carbon dioxide test An old-fashioned test used to tell whether the fallopian tubes are blocked. Although it's an old test, it's still used by some doctors today. To perform the test, the doctor guides a catheter into the cervix and then passes carbon dioxide into the uterus and fallopian tubes. If the tubes are open, the carbon dioxide will flow through and out of them, settling under the diaphragm. When this occurs, the patient will feel shoulder pain. If the shoulder pain occurs on both sides, both fallopian tubes are believed to be open; pain in only one side is believed to indicate that only one tube is open.

The drawback to this test is that it is extremely painful, and because pain is not an exact science, it's possible that a woman could feel pain on both sides even though only one tube is blocked. Since the test doesn't allow the doctor to actually see the fallopian tubes, findings aren't as accurate as those obtained from a HYSTEROSALPINGOGRAM (HSG). The only accurate way to assess the uterus and fallopian tubes is by looking at them with an HSG. See also FALLOPIAN TUBES.

Center for the Evaluation of Risks to Human Reproduction This government center brings together experts to evaluate data indicating that a chemical or mixtures of chemicals could impair human reproduction and development. The center does not conduct research or provide counseling or medical treatment. Instead, it convenes panels of 10 to 15 scientists with expertise in reproduction, toxicology, and related areas to review information on the effects of a chemical on reproduction and development. Panel meetings are open to the public.

The center reviews two or three chemicals or mixtures a year that are nominated by the public, scientists, industry, workers, and government agencies. Expert panels prepare consensus reports on the strength of scientific evidence that an exposure poses a hazard to reproduction and the health of children. Reports are written in terms that can be understood by those who are not scientifically trained and are published in the journal of the National Institute of Environmental Health Science (NIEHS) and on the Internet linked to the NTP and NIEHS websites (http://cerhr.niehs.nih.gov).

Nominations of chemicals and of panel members can be sent to the attention of John Moore, DVM, 1800 Diagonal Road, Suite 500, Alexandria, VA 22314-2808; (703) 838-9440.

See also ENVIRONMENTAL FACTORS AND INFERTILITY.

cerclage A surgical stitch to keep the cervix tightly closed that is used to prevent premature birth in women with an incompetent cervix. See also CERVICAL INCOMPETENCE.

cervical canal atresia A condition in which a baby is born without a cervical canal. In cases of cervical canal atresia, a uterus and cervix is usually normal, but no connecting canal forms. As a result, there is no way for sperm to get from the vagina into the uterus. This extremely rare problem causes problems early in a girl's life, when menstrual blood has no way to escape. In this case, doctors must stop bleeding by suppressing the hormones.

It is possible to surgically create a cervical canal and create a pregnancy with INTRAUTERINE INSEMINATION.

cervical cap A type of birth control for women, consisting of a soft latex dome-shaped device about the size of a thimble with a round rim, sized by a health professional to fit snugly around the cervix. Like the DIAPHRAGM, the cap is a barrier that blocks passage of sperm from the vagina through the cervix into the uterus and tubes where they can fertilize the ripened egg. The cap is basically a smaller diaphragm that fits over the cervix and is held in place by suction. How well a cap fits is critical to contraceptive effectiveness, so it is important to have a proper fit initially and then insert it correctly with every use. It's available by prescription only and, like a diaphragm, is used with a small amount of SPERMICIDE. The spermicide may be enough to help prevent the spread of certain STDs, but it doesn't guarantee safety.

The cap protects against pregnancy for 48 hours and for multiple acts of intercourse within this time. Wearing it for more than 48 hours is not recommended because of the low risk of toxic shock syndrome. With prolonged use of 2 or more days, the cap may cause an unpleasant vaginal odor or discharge in some women.

Recent studies have confirmed that the cap's effectiveness is about the same as a diaphragm's. Pregnancies are due primarily to incorrect placement or inconsistent use. Women who have not been pregnant who use the cap correctly each time can expect 91% effectiveness, but the typical effectiveness rate of the cap is about 82%. The cap is less effective for women who have had one or more vaginal deliveries.

Because it can be difficult to insert and doesn't fit all women, it's a less popular method than the diaphragm. On the other hand, it can be left in place longer than the diaphragm and can be used to collect menstrual blood.

Some women shouldn't use the cap, including those women who have

- an unusually long or short cervix
- a history of cervical lacerations or scarring
- current cervicitis
- an unusually shaped cervix
- current pelvic, tubal, vaginal, or ovarian infection

- an abnormal Pap smear
- history of toxic shock syndrome

A woman should use a backup method of birth control during the first month of cap use. If it dislodges more than once, it should be reported to the practitioner who fitted the cap. See also BIRTH CONTROL METHODS.

cervical incompetence A weakness of the cervix, which begins to dilate and thin before the pregnancy has reached full term. Occurring in the second or third trimester, cervical incompetence is a cause of late miscarriage and premature birth.

When a cervix is called "incompetent," it means that the muscle of the cervix is weak and the pressure of the growing baby causes the cervix to open early. There are no contractions. If the doctor knows that a woman has a weak cervix (usually because of a problem in an earlier pregnancy), measures can be taken to reduce the risk of miscarriage or premature birth in subsequent pregnancies. Cervical incompetence occurs in only 1% to 2% of all pregnancies, but it is the cause of up to a quarter of all miscarriages in the second trimester.

There are several risk factors, including

- previous surgical procedure involving the cervix (such as a D&C)
- malformed cervix
- maternal exposure to DES
- damage to the cervix during a prior difficult delivery
- multiple fetuses

Symptoms
Often there are no symptoms until the waters break, when it is too late to treat. If they do occur, symptoms include vaginal bleeding or spotting and pressure or heaviness in the lower abdomen.

Diagnosis

There is no way to diagnose an incompetent cervix before a pregnancy occurs; once it has been diagnosed, it will be a factor for all future pregnancies.

Treatment

If a woman's cervix begins to dilate and the problem is caught early, the doctor may try to delay birth, but it's hard to prevent delivery for very long once the cervix begins to dilate. If a woman has been diagnosed with cervical incompetence in the past, the doctor may stitch the cervix to keep the opening closed during subsequent pregnancies. A stitch placed around the cervix can strengthen and support it enough so that the pregnancy can continue to term. Called a CERCLAGE, stitches are placed above the opening of the cervix to narrow the canal and reinforce the cervical muscle. The sutures may stay in place or be removed as the pregnancy approaches term, depending on the type of cerclage that was used. Cerclage is usually done before 20 weeks of pregnancy, but even with this procedure a woman with an incompetent cervix has a 25% risk for preterm birth. Usually a woman requires bed rest and treatment for preterm labor during the pregnancy.

cervical mucus   A sticky, thick mucus produced by glands in the cervical canal that plugs the opening of the cervix. Most of the time this thick mucus plug prevents sperm and bacteria from entering the womb unless ovulation is about to take place. At this time, under the influence of estrogen, the mucus becomes thin, watery, and stretchy so that sperm can pass into the womb.

Mucus varies from dry, to sticky, to creamy, to egg white before ovulation in most women. "Creamy" mucus may look white and feel somewhat like lotion; this mucus can be fertile but isn't always. "Egg-white cervical mucus" is given this name because it resembles raw egg whites. It's either clear or streaked and stretches an inch or more.

After ovulation it is normal to have some dry, sticky, or creamy mucus, and some women have watery mucus or a little egg white again, right before their menses begin.

cervical mucus test   There are several tests of the cervical mucus that can help determine whether sperm can move through the woman's reproductive tract. The first, the SPINNBARKEIT TEST, a woman can do by herself simply by examining mucus characteristics. Because cervical mucus changes in consistency throughout the menstrual cycle, it's possible to tell if ovulation is about to occur by taking a small sample of mucus from the vagina. If it's watery and stretchable, it's a good chance that ovulation is approaching.

The second cervical mucus test is also known as the POSTCOITAL TEST (or the Sims-Huhner or sperm-mucus interaction test). This test is planned to take place close to OVULATION, when a woman's cervical mucus is thin and watery so that the sperm are better able to swim through the cervix and fertilize the awaiting egg. The test must be performed just prior to ovulation so that the mucus will be thin and stretchy.

After the couple has sex the night before, the woman is examined in the doctor's office the next morning, and a small sample of mucus is removed from the cervix. This mucus is evaluated under a microscope; at least six to 10 moving sperm indicate a good sperm/mucus interaction. The physician will inspect the female's cervical mucus to see whether enough semen was delivered to the cervix, whether sperm are healthy, and whether they are swimming energetically through the cervical mucus.

If no sperm are found in the cervical mucus, but they are present in the vagina, hostile vaginal factor or sperm factor may be suspected, especially if the man's semen analysis is normal. In such cases, the woman may be inseminated with washed sperm to overcome such factors and to help the sperm pass into the cervix.

If many shaking, motionless, clumped, or dead sperm are found in the cervical mucus, the sperm and mucus may be incompatible, or something in the mucus may be attacking the sperm. Reactions can be caused by external factors, such as the use of vaginal lubricants, or by internal factors, such as an allergic response to the sperm by the woman or the production of ANTISPERM ANTIBODIES by the man.

The most common explanation for a poor test is improper timing; the test should be done 24 to 36 hours before ovulation, as determined by urinary LH testing.

The practical value of mucus tests such as the postcoital test is unclear. Studies to date have not reliably shown it to be helpful in treating infertility.

cervical problems and infertility Normally, the cervix (the lower part of the uterus that opens into the vagina) allows sperm to move from the vaginal canal into the uterine cavity. During ovulation, the sperm move through the opening and into the uterus via clear, watery mucus produced by special cells in the cervix walls. The mucus in the cervix should be thick and impenetrable to sperm until the follicular phase of the menstrual cycle, when the egg and follicle are maturing in the ovary. Right before ovulation, rising levels of estrogen trigger these cells to produce the mucus. The timing of this mucus production is crucial to pregnancy.

If there are problems with a woman's cervix (called "cervical factor infertility") a couple may be timing sex correctly but healthy sperm aren't able to move into the uterus. About 15% of couples have some type of problem with the cervix.

Some such problems are caused by a malformed cervix, which can either be present from birth or caused sometime alter, as a result of medical treatment. Sometimes the cervix is not positioned correctly (although this is very rare). There may not be enough mucus-producing cells in the cervix walls, or the cells may not produce enough mucus. Hormonal problems may mean that the cervix doesn't get enough estrogen to trigger the mucus production. Infections also may produce poor quality mucus. Finally, it's also possible that the cervix could be damaged after procedures such as CONIZATION, CONE BIOPSY, cauterization, or CRYOSURGERY. (Most of these procedures are usually performed after an abnormal Pap smear.) Some cervical problems are never explained. Although a woman may have cervical problems, it does not necessarily mean that the couple won't be able to have a baby together.

Congenital Problems

Problems with the cervix which are present at birth are usually caused by a drug that the mother took during pregnancy. It's also possible that the baby's cervix simply doesn't develop properly during the pregnancy for unknown reasons.

If the mother took DIETHYLSTILBESTROL (DES) during the pregnancy, the drug could have caused cervical abnormalities in the unborn child. DES was often prescribed for women in the 1940s who had MISCARRIAGE problems, and by the 1960s doctors recognized the problems that DES caused. By 1971 the FDA had recommended that the drug not be used during pregnancy.

DES exposure causes malformations of the baby's cervix, which in turn can affect cervical mucus production. Abnormalities of the baby's uterus also can occur (the so-called T-shape uterus).

Although these abnormalities can lead to miscarriage and infertility in adulthood, the vast majority of women exposed to DES during fetal development have no reproductive problems.

Medical Problems

The most common cervical factor conditions are caused by medical procedures that damage a woman's cervix so that it no longer functions. For example, if a woman has had many therapeutic abortions, she might have a damaged cervix which can lead to an incompetent cervix (a weakened cervix that won't stay closed and allows a pregnancy to proceed to term). See CERVICAL INCOMPETENCE.

Hormonal Problems

It's possible that cervical factor infertility could be related to hormones—perhaps the woman isn't producing enough estrogen to stimulate the mucus-producing cells.

Unexplained

About 15% of women have problems with the cervix that can't be identified. It's possible to treat this condition by improving the sperm transport by giving hormones or bypassing the cervix entirely.

Diagnosis

A POSTCOITAL TEST performed about 8 hours after sexual intercourse can determine whether sperm can survive in the cervical mucus. The test is scheduled for the midpoint of the menstrual cycle, when the estradiol level is highest and the woman is ovulating. Normally, the mucus is clear and can be stretched to 3 to 4 inches without breaking.

Under a microscope, the mucus has a fernlike appearance, and at the highest magnification at least five active sperm should be visible at one time. Abnormal results include overly thick mucus, no sperm, and sperm clumping together because the mucus contains antibodies to the sperm. However, abnormal results don't always indicate a problem with the mucus. Sperm may be absent only because they were not deposited into the vagina during intercourse, and the mucus may be overly thick only because the test wasn't performed at the proper time in the menstrual cycle. Although this test is widely used, it's not highly accurate.

Treatment

There are several ways to deal with cervical mucus problems. Intrauterine insemination involves placing semen directly in the uterus to bypass the mucus and giving drugs to thin the mucus, such as guaifenesin—a common ingredient of cough syrups. However, there is no proof that these measures increase the likelihood of pregnancy.

cervical polyp   A fragile growth hanging from a stalk that projects outward into the canal of the cervix and that can cause bleeding after sex. Cervical polyps are relatively common, especially in women over age 20 who have had children. Typically, polyps are benign and easily removed.

Doctors don't completely understand what causes these polyps, but they are often the result of an infection. They may be associated with chronic inflammation, an abnormal response to higher levels of estrogen, or congestion of cervical blood vessels in the cervix. Most of the time polyps occur alone, but occasionally two or three are found together. They are rare before the onset of menstrual periods.

Symptoms

Signs of a cervical polyp include abnormal vaginal bleeding after sex or douching, between periods, or after menopause. A polyp also may cause an abnormally heavy period or white or yellow mucous discharge.

Diagnosis

A pelvic exam and a pathological examination of the polyp confirm the diagnosis.

Treatment

A doctor can remove the polyp during a simple outpatient procedure; often, gentle twisting of a cervical polyp is enough to remove it. Although most cervical polyps are benign, the tissue should be sent to a pathologist for confirmation; some cervical cancers may first appear as a polyp.

cervical smear   A sample of the cervical mucus examined under a microscope to assess the presence of estrogen and white blood cells, which would indicate an infection.

cervical stenosis   A narrowing or blockage of the cervical canal caused by a birth defect or from complications of surgical procedures.

cervicitis An inflammation of the cervix usually caused by an infection. In this situation, sperm may have trouble getting through the cervical mucus.

cervix The opening into the uterus and the vagina. The cervical mucus plugs the cervical canal and normally prevents foreign materials from entering the reproductive tract. The cervix remains closed during pregnancy and dilates during labor and delivery to allow the baby to be born.

cervix, incompetent See CERVICAL INCOMPETENCE.

chemical pregnancy A pregnancy verified by lab tests but which fails before a gestational sac is seen on an ultrasound. This is a very early MISCARRIAGE, and often occurs before the woman misses a period.

chemicals and infertility Many chemicals have toxic effects on reproduction, and have been implicated in lowering a man's sperm count. Some experts believe that a decline in fertility may be due to the exposure of male fetuses during pregnancy to environmental chemicals with estrogenlike effects. Such chemicals include pesticides such as DDT, aldrin, dieldrin, PCPs, dioxins, and furans. Although tests of single chemicals containing estrogen have reported little danger, other studies indicate that combinations of estrogen-containing chemicals may be very harmful. Overexposure to estrogen reduces the number of SERTOLI CELLS (the cells necessary for the initial development of sperm). In addition to the effect on fertility, some researchers believe such overexposure may also contribute to testicular cancers.

Aside from the estrogenlike chemicals, other environmental pollutants can interfere with sperm quality and count, although the effects of most have not been proved. One British study did find that phthalates, a plasticlike chemical added to powdered baby milk in England, can impair male fertility.

Women
Environmental chemicals such as certain pesticides, aldrin, dieldrin, PCPs, dioxins, and furans can be especially harmful to female fertility because of their estrogenlike effects. Although tests of single chemicals containing estrogen have produced mixed results, effects of combinations of these drugs can be very harmful. For example, studies have suggested an increased risk for infertility in women who work on farms, probably due to exposure to pesticides, and among health care workers who handle chemotherapy drugs.

Once a woman gets pregnant she is at even higher risk since exposure to certain chemicals may damage her developing baby. For example, chemicals such as carbon dioxide, ethylene oxide, and vinyl chloride are capable of being transported across the placenta from the bloodstream of the mother to her baby, causing miscarriage or birth defects.

Chemicals that may cause sterility include

- arsenic
- benzene
- cadmium
- carbon disulfide
- carbon monoxide
- epichlorohydrin
- ethylene dibromide
- lead
- manganese
- mercury
- phosphorus
- trichloroethylene
- radiation

Chemicals that may cause impotence include

- carbon disulfide
- carbon monoxide

- lead
- manganese
- mercury
- trichloroethylene

Chemicals that may lead to miscarriage include

- antimony
- arsenic
- cadmium
- carbon disulfide
- ethylene dichloride
- lead
- mercury
- polychlorinated biphenyls
- trichloroethylene
- vinyl chloride
- radiation

Chemicals that cause birth defects, mutations and fetal damage include

- antimony
- cadmium
- carbon disulfide
- cellosolve chlorinated hydrocarbons
- ethylene dibromide
- ethylene dichloride
- lead
- mercury
- nitrous oxides
- polychlorinated biphenyls
- trichloroethylene
- vinyl chloride
- radiation

See ENVIRONMENTAL FACTORS AND INFERTILITY.

chlamydia   A type of organism (especially *Chlamydia trachomatis*) that is sexually transmit-

ted and can cause infertility. Chlamydia functions like a virus in some ways and like a bacterium in others. This infection can damage the fallopian tubes and cause infertility. In men, the infection can cause nonspecific urethritis.

Symptoms
In men, the urethritis can cause a feeling of burning during urination or a yellow-colored discharge from the penis. In women there can be a vaginal discharge or mild to moderate abdominal pain. Chlamyidal infection is suspected whenever there is yellow-colored mucus in the cervix during a Pap smear. It's also possible that the infection will cause no symptoms in either sex.

Diagnosis
Tests of cell scrapings from the cervix or the urethra will reveal the infection.

Treatment
When this infection is diagnosed, both sex partners should be treated with antibiotics such as tetracyclines or erythromycin.

chocolate cyst   A cyst in the ovary that is filled with blood. It is known medically as an "endometrioma," because it resembles melted chocolate. A chocolate cyst forms when ENDO-METRIOSIS implants invade the ovary and bleed.

Symptoms
Often, women with these large cysts don't have any symptoms.

Treatment
If the cyst ruptures or the ovary containing the cyst twists, emergency surgery may be necessary. Usually treatment can be carried out using a LAPAROSCOPE.

cigarette smoking and infertility   See SMOKING AND INFERTILITY.

cilia   Tiny hairlike projections lining the inside surface of different organs, including the FALLOP-

IAN TUBES. In the fallopian tubes, the waving action of these "hairs" sweeps the egg toward the uterus.

Clomid A brand name of CLOMIPHENE CITRATE.

clomiphene citrate (Clomid, Serophene) One of the simplest, most useful synthetic hormones used to treat FEMALE FACTOR INFERTILITY (and which also can be used to boost sperm production in men). Clomiphene citrate acts on both the hypothalamus and the pituitary to induce ovulation. It has revolutionized the field of infertility since its introduction in the late 1950s. If patients are well screened, about 65% to 90% of women with irregular and absent periods or polycystic ovary syndrome will ovulate when given this drug, and 40% of those will become pregnant. As with any treatment, the ovulation rates may be lower depending on the woman's age, the presence of other factors, and the precise reason she is being treated.

Clomiphene is classified as an antiestrogen. That is, it blocks the action of estrogen and tricks the pituitary into believing that the ovary's follicles aren't producing enough ESTRADIOL. As a result, the pituitary secretes more FOLLICLE-STIMULATING HORMONE (FSH) and LUTEINIZING HORMONE (LH). The rising FSH levels boost the follicle development, which then starts to secrete more estrogen. When therapy is stopped, the hypothalamus signals the pituitary to begin the LH production and egg release.

This drug is used to stimulate ovulation in women who don't have many periods or who have long cycles or LUTEAL PHASE DEFECT. It's also one of the oldest and least expensive of all the FERTILITY DRUGS.

Usually a woman takes this drug every day for 5 days in a row, beginning several days after the start of a menstrual period, depending on a woman's particular hormone profile. If successful, a woman should ovulate about a week after the last tablet is taken. If ovulation is not achieved, then the amount of clomiphene can be increased until ovulation occurs or the patient is considered to be nonresponsive to this medication.

Most pregnancies in women who aren't ovulating occur in the first three cycles of clomiphene citrate. After the first six cycles of the medication, the success rate falls dramatically. About 90% of women who will conceive while taking clomiphene will do so within the first six cycles of treatment.

Side Effects
The higher the dose, the more likely (and more severe) the possible side effects. Some women experience hot flashes or mood swings; later in the cycle, side effects may include mood changes, breast tenderness, and nausea. Vision problems or severe headaches should be immediately reported to the doctor. If eye symptoms persist, therapy should be stopped and a complete eye examination carried out.

Most common side effects are ovarian cysts and ovarian enlargement. Some women experience "throbbing" in the ovaries near ovulation, and occasional insomnia and irritability have been reported.

To minimize adverse reactions, the smallest dose should be given first and may be increased after several cycles if ovulation does not occur. LH levels in the urine should be measured daily beginning day 11 or 12 of the cycle; the doctor should be contacted when an LH surge occurs, since ovulation usually occurs the next day.

Sometimes transvaginal ultrasound is used to verify pending ovulation and to determine if the ovaries are overly enlarged or cystic.

Risks
There is no more increased chance of multiple births with this drug than with other fertility drugs. The chance of a twin is about 5% to 10%, falling to 1% for the chance of more than two.

Who Responds Best
If a woman is menstruating (even irregularly), clomiphene is usually effective, particularly if her follicles aren't reaching normal size. Just

before a mature follicle ruptures and releases its egg, it should be about the size of a small grape. If it's not, clomiphene may help small, immature follicles grow to maturity.

A woman who ovulates infrequently (at 6-week intervals or less) is also a good candidate for clomiphene therapy, since this drug will induce ovulation more often. The more a woman ovulates, the more opportunities her mature eggs have to be exposed to her husband's sperm and, therefore, the greater her chance to become pregnant. Clomiphene is also often effective for a woman with luteal phase defect (LPD).

Contradictions

Clomiphene should not be given to women with liver disease. In cases of abnormal or irregular uterine bleeding, abnormalities of the endometrium or cervix should first be ruled out. It should not be given to women with ovarian cysts, since further enlargement may occur. It should not be given to any woman who may already be pregnant, although harmful effects on the fetus haven't been proved.

clomiphene citrate challenge test (CCCT, CCT)

A test to determine a woman's fertility in which 100 mg of CLOMIPHENE CITRATE is given on menstrual cycle days 5 through 9. Blood levels of FSH are measured on cycle day 3 and again on cycle day 10. High blood levels of FSH on cycle day 3 or cycle day 10 are associated with diminished fertility potential.

cloning   A method of replicating the genetic material of one person to produce an exact copy of that person. Unlike normal reproduction, cloning perpetuates the genetic material of only one individual, not two.

The first mammal cloned from an adult body cell was a sheep named Dolly, born at the Roslin Institute in Scotland in 1996. In this type of cloning, the animal's genetic material (the full DNA complement in the nucleus of one cell) is placed into a female's egg that has been stripped of all its DNA. The experiment that produced Dolly showed that the donor nucleus is "reprogrammed" so that it can generate an entirely new individual. But instead of having the same genetic age as the animal from which it was copied, the nucleus almost miraculously was made young again. As a result, it became fully active in all its genes and capable of developing into an entire individual.

After the success with cloning Dolly from an adult ewe, scientists moved on to clone calves, mice, and pigs. Monkeys, dogs, or cats have not yet been cloned from adult cells. However, scientists note that many cloned animals have many defects and don't survive.

The next step—cloning humans—is something that has been deeply feared and emphatically denounced by almost all scientists around the globe—on both medical and ethical grounds. Medically, the concerns center around the fact that the risks of failure and serious birth defects are quite high. Animal clones have been born with oversized organs and malfunctions, and some experts believe clones may prematurely age.

Ethicists argue about the merits and morality of human cloning. So far, an almost universal disapproval of cloning has kept scientists from getting involved. Soon after Dolly's birth, President Bill Clinton issued an executive order banning federal funding of human cloning. A proposed federal law, however, failed to pass mainly because scientists were concerned it would hamper legitimate research. Since then, four states (Rhode Island, Michigan, California, and Louisiana) have passed cloning bans.

There are still some critics who favor clones. One is a religious cult that believes in UFOs and aliens, whose leaders say they will soon try to clone cells from a recently deceased young child. Another is a maverick physicist who shocked the world when he announced in 1998 his plans to buy property in Japan to establish a cloning laboratory.

While no one has taken the dreaded yet often-predicted further step (as far as anyone knows) of cloning a star athlete or dictator, many ethicists worry that scientists may begin to tiptoe past social and legal boundaries. A British government advisory committee recently recommended that scientists be allowed to create human embryos through a cloning process to obtain embryonic stem cells that could develop into any tissue of the body. The panel firmly stated that these cloned embryos could be kept for no more than 14 days, and that they would be discarded after the stem cells were removed. Critics worry that some unethical scientist might instead place such an embryo into a woman's uterus, where it could develop into a fetus to be born.

cocaine and infertility Cocaine use may contribute to MALE FACTOR INFERTILITY, since chronic users of cocaine may have impaired levels of TESTOSTERONE and sperm production, as well as lower libido. Males exposed to cocaine before conceiving were linked to abnormal development in offspring. The suspected cause is that cocaine binds onto the sperm and finds its way into the egg at fertilization. See also MARIJUANA AND INFERTILITY.

coffee and infertility See CAFFEINE AND INFERTILITY.

coitus interruptus See WITHDRAWAL; BIRTH CONTROL METHODS.

computer-assisted semen analysis (CASA) The computerized measurement of sperm number, shape, and movement. A computer can accurately determine sperm counts and movement. Generally, sperm are scanned by a computer and microscope. The computer has been programmed to understand how normal sperm look and move. When the computer analyzes sperm under the microscope, it is able to draw a digitized picture of each individual sperm, including the speed and path this sperm takes while moving under the microscope.

However, the method is not foolproof; small changes in the computer program can significantly change the sperm calculations. Abnormal sperm must be verified by manual counting.

conception The fertilization of an egg by sperm that leads to the creation of a baby. It is diagnosed by a positive pregnancy test that detects HUMAN CHORIONIC GONADOTROPIN.

conception, assisted A group of treatments for infertility ranging from INSEMINATION to IN VITRO FERTILIZATION.

condoms A type of birth control made of latex, polyurethane, or animal tissue that physically prevents the sperm from contacting an egg. Condoms can be used only once; the male version fits over the erect penis, while the female variety (which is less commonly used) is inserted into the vagina, covering the cervix inside and the lips of the vagina outside.

Condom use is on the rise by both men and women due to concerns about loss of fertility or death from sexually transmitted diseases (STDs), such as HIV infection. When used with SPERMICIDE, condoms are among the safest and cheapest ways to prevent pregnancy; they can also help reduce the risk of being infected with certain STDs, PELVIC INFLAMMATORY DISEASE, and perhaps even cervical cancer. However, if they aren't used consistently and correctly, barrier methods have a relatively high failure rate.

Male Condoms

Because condoms act as a mechanical barrier, they prevent direct vaginal contact with semen, infectious genital secretions, and genital lesions and discharges. Other than not having sex at all, latex condoms are the most effective way to lower the risk of infection from HIV, the virus that causes AIDS and other STDs.

Most condoms are made from latex rubber (hence their nickname "rubber"), but polyurethane condoms, marketed in the United States since 1994, are an alternative method of STD protection for those who are allergic to latex. A small percentage of condoms are made from lamb intestines ("lambskin" condoms). Unlike latex or polyurethane condoms, lambskin condoms don't always prevent STDs because they're porous and may permit passage of viruses like HIV, hepatitis B, and herpes.

Some have spermicide added (usually NONOXYNOL-9 in the United States) to kill sperm. Some are prelubricated, but these lubricants don't provide more birth control or STD protection. Non-oil-based lubricants (such as water or K-Y jelly) can be used with latex or lambskin condoms, but oil-based lubricants such as petroleum jelly (Vaseline), lotions, or massage or baby oil should not be used because they can weaken the condom material.

Latex condoms come in different thicknesses; the newest, thinnest products are just as strong as thicker ones, but they can be harder to put on than thicker ones. All condoms are packed with an expiration date. Latex and urethane deteriorate over time, and a condom that has passed its expiration date should not be used.

Condoms with reservoir ends are a good choice because the reservoir is an extension of the condom that is narrower than the penis and will collect semen after ejaculation, rather than forcing the ejaculate back along the length of the penis, where it could leak.

To put a condom on properly, it should first be unwrapped but not unrolled. Holding the reservoir end with the thumb and forefinger, the man places the rolled-up condom on the head of the erect penis. The man then unrolls it over the head of the penis, making sure that there is no air in the condom. (If there is, it should be squeezed out.) It is then unrolled down the shaft of the penis. If for any reason it is removed before ejaculation (such as having to urinate or being unable to put it on properly), it should be thrown away and a new condom unrolled.

Condoms break either because air gets trapped inside or because lubricants are used improperly. If the vagina isn't lubricated well enough during sex, friction can cause the condom to break. This is why it's important for the vagina to be lubricated properly.

The penis should be removed from the vagina immediately after ejaculation, before the penis softens and sperm has a chance to spill.

If a condom breaks, the woman should wash thoroughly and use a spermicidal jelly or foam, and then urinate. There is morning-after emergency birth control available. Although washing the genitals has not proved an effective method for preventing STDs, if a condom breaks, both the man and woman should wash thoroughly and then urinate.

Used alone, the male condom has an expected failure rate of 2% and a typical failure rate of 12% (mostly because it can slip or break during withdrawal). Used with spermicide, the failure rate can be reduced almost to zero.

Female Condoms

Female condoms, approved by the FDA in 1993, are sold under the brand names Femidom and Reality. Less likely to slip or burst than the male version, the female condom is a lubricated polyurethane cylinder with a closed flexible ring at one end and a larger open ring at the other. The closed ring is inserted into the vagina, fitting over the cervix, leaving the open end hanging outside the vagina about an inch, where it partially covers the labia. It must carefully be removed after sex; a fresh condom must be inserted for each subsequent act of sexual intercourse. If these rules are followed, the female condom seems to be as effective as the diaphragm or cervical cap. A female condom should not be used together with a male condom because they may not both stay in place.

Sex should be stopped if the penis slips between the pouch and the wall of the vagina or if the outer ring is pushed inside the vagina. Some movement of the pouch is normal. Extra lubricant can be used, and then the pouch reinserted. All instructions explaining proper use of the female condom should be read carefully.

condom therapy A type of treatment designed to reduce the number of a woman's sperm antibodies by using a condom during sex for 6 months or more. At the same time, the woman must refrain from all skin contact with her partner's sperm. With this behavior, the woman's antibody level may fall to levels that will not harm the sperm. However, this treatment remains unproved and is rarely recommended.

cone biopsy A surgical procedure used to remove abnormal cells from the cervix for further testing. This procedure obtains a larger sample that can be obtained by a cervical punch biopsy. The test is performed after results of a cervical biopsy indicate precancerous cells or cervical cancer. A cone biopsy may also be done if a cervical biopsy did not reveal the cause of an abnormal Pap smear.

This diagnostic surgical procedure is usually performed in an outpatient or hospital surgical facility under anesthesia. During surgery, a small cone-shaped sample of tissue is removed from the cervix and examined under a microscope for any signs of cancer. This biopsy may serve as the treatment as well if all of the diseased tissue is removed.

Risks

There is a slight risk of bleeding and infection after surgery. Cervical scarring may result from the procedure, occasionally causing painful menstrual periods or making it more difficult to evaluate an abnormal Pap smear. The procedure may cause problems with a later pregnancy, or the procedure may make it more difficult for a woman to become pregnant if it damages the cervix and disrupts normal mucus production. It could also cause an incompetent cervix, which may open prematurely during pregnancy.

congenital abnormalities and infertility There are a number of abnormalities present since birth in either a man or woman that can lead to infertility. In a man, these include the congenital absence or obstruction of the vas deferens or epididymis, or undescended testicles. A woman may experience infertility if she is born with a malformed uterus, such as a divided (septate) uterus, or an abnormal cervical canal. See SEPTATE UTERUS; CRYPTORCHIDISM.

conization Another name for a CONE BIOPSY.

contraception See BIRTH CONTROL METHODS.

contraceptive injections See HORMONAL BIRTH CONTROL; BIRTH CONTROL METHODS.

Copper T-380A One of the most effective, long-acting reversible INTRAUTERINE DEVICES (IUD) available. It has more copper surface (380 sq mm) than any other marketed IUD and is one of the most advanced of the family of T-shaped copper birth control devices. The Copper T-380A IUD is inserted high in the uterus, providing enhanced contraceptive protection for up to 10 years.

Copper-bearing IUDs may show discoloration inside their sterile packaging, but this is harmless. The copper tarnishes because air passes through the sterile package, causing a film to form on the surface. IUD packaging has to be permeable to gases used to sterilize the devices. If the package is not damaged, and the package date hasn't expired, the IUD will be sterile even if the copper on the device is tarnished. Laboratory studies show the tarnishing does not affect the safety or effectiveness of the IUD.

More than 50 million Copper T-380A IUDs have been distributed in more than 70 countries. The U.S. Food and Drug Administration approved marketing of the Copper T-380A in the United States in 1984; the IUD was introduced into the United States in 1988, where it is marketed by Ortho-McNeill Pharmaceutical, Inc., under the name Paragard T-380A Intrauterine Copper Contraceptive. Manufacturers of the Copper T-380A are based in Finland, India, and the United States; producers for local use are located in China, Indonesia, and Mexico.

corpus luteum   A yellow-colored cyst that forms from the ovarian follicle after it releases an egg. Once formed, the cyst produces ESTROGEN and PROGESTERONE to prepare and support the uterine lining for implantation. It is progesterone that causes the half-degree basal temperature elevation noted at midcycle.

If the corpus luteum functions poorly, the uterine lining may be thin due to lack of progesterone and may not support a pregnancy. If the egg is fertilized, a corpus luteum of pregnancy forms to maintain the endometrial bed and support the implanted embryo.

A deficiency in the amount of progesterone produced (or the length of time it is produced) by the corpus luteum can mean that the endometrium is unable to sustain a pregnancy. This is called a LUTEAL PHASE DEFECT (LPD).

Crinone progesterone vaginal gel   This new form of natural progesterone taken vaginally is now available for patients to use as a supplement during ART cycles and into early pregnancy. This allows women to avoid a potentially painful intramuscular injection of progesterone, which has previously been the standard in IVF cycles.

While progesterone suppositories or capsules have been used for some time, Crinone is less messy and is absorbed better in the vagina. Women taking Crinone in an IVF cycle apply the gel once daily at bedtime; for egg donation recipients it is used twice daily.

cryopreservation   Freezing tissues or cells and then storing them in liquid nitrogen at very low temperatures. This process is used to store sperm, embryos, and, more recently, unfertilized eggs. They are stored in small vials or straws that can last for decades.

Sperm have long been frozen and used for preservation of future fertility, in part because the use of sperm presented less of a technical challenge. Sperm are much smaller than eggs and survive the freezing and thawing process unharmed.

Also, many ART centers have the ability to preserve for future use embryos that haven't been used in a particular ART cycle. Once they are frozen and stored, they can be viable for a long time. About half of frozen embryos will survive thawing and can be transferred into a woman's uterus. About 18% of frozen embryos result in pregnancy. Freezing some embryos means that it's possible to use some in the ART cycle while storing others for future use in a natural cycle without needing to resort to hormonal stimulation.

Cryopreservation of embryos also lowers the cost of subsequent ART procedures, since the first stages of ovarian stimulation and egg retrieval don't have to be repeated.

The use of frozen eggs is also being developed. Freezing and thawing an egg can damage the outer shell of the egg to which the sperm must normally bind before penetrating. IN VITRO FERTILIZATION with frozen eggs is still considered experimental, however, and is reserved for women undergoing medical treatments that directly affect their fertility. These include patients with cancer, lupus, scleroderma, or other diseases that require chemotherapy or radiation, which are toxic to the ovary. In addition, women who have their ovaries removed because of ENDOMETRIOSIS or other conditions can choose to have their eggs frozen before surgery, although this is still in the experimental stage.

Because freezing eggs is a new process, it's not known how long they can be stored and yet still produce a viable pregnancy. In contrast, some pregnancies have resulted from embryos that have been frozen for up to 10 years.

Women also have the option of having a portion of their ovary removed and frozen for future use. While no pregnancies have ever been reported from this process, in the fall of 1999 the removal, freezing, thawing, and replacement of ovarian tissue in a woman's body was reported.

The ovary did show some signs of function, and the woman ovulated and had a menstrual period.

Cryos The largest sperm bank in the world, founded in the Danish city of Aarhus in 1987. The bank has more than 200 donors and revenues nearing $1 million. Founded by Danish entrepreneur Ole Schou, the controversial sperm repository signed a special agreement with British authorities that will allow it to send bulk shipments to a Scottish clinic that can't find donors because of rigorous British standards.

In Europe, the mishmash of conflicting rules and regulations—or lack of regulation at all— has allowed Cryos to flourish. For example, Britain requires that a single donor can father only 10 children because of the genetic risks. But Denmark, whose population is much smaller than Britain's, sets that limit at 25.

Sperm bank laws in Sweden and Austria allow children to seek the identity of their fathers when they reach 18, which has led to a severe donor shortage; in contrast, Cryos does not keep donor names; instead it relies on a coded identification number. Nor does the bank keep exhaustive profiles of donor characteristics as do banks in the United States. While arguing against a sort of "designer approach" to selecting sperm donors, Cryos only tests for diseases, not hobbies or IQ scores.

cryptomenorrhea The apparent lack of a menstrual period caused by an obstruction to the flow of blood from the uterus. Literally, it means "hidden menstruation," which can be caused by an obstruction in the vagina. Typically there is pain each month that would coincide with the timing of the period.

cryptorchidism The medical term for undescended testicles (literally, it means "hidden testicle") in which one or both testicles fail to descend from the abdomen into the scrotum by age 1. Cryptorchidism is a common childhood disorder that affects about a third of premature babies and 3% of full-term babies.

Incomplete testicle descent isn't just a physical abnormality, since it can lead to infertility and testicular cancer. Normally, the testicle will descend by the time the child is born or by the end of the first year of life. However, if the testes remain in the abdomen, sperm production (and fertility) is usually impaired. If not repaired by age 6, the condition may cause permanent infertility.

If only one testicle has descended, the male will have a low sperm count, whereas if both remain in the abdomen, there is usually no sperm in the semen. Researchers believe that this is because the higher temperature in the abdomen destroys the enzymes and proteins needed for normal sperm production.

There are several types of cryptochidism:

- true undescended testes: positioned within the normal route of descent, they can't be manually lowered into the scrotum
- retractile testes: usually occurs between age 3 and 6 due to hyperactivity of the abdominal muscles that elevate the testes
- ectopic (displaced) testes: found outside the normal route of descent in areas such as the upper groin, floor of the pelvis, penile shaft, or thigh. (Many researchers believe that there is less chance of cancer in ectopic testes than in true undescended testes.)

Cause
Most cryptorchidism cases have no known cause.

Symptoms
Cryptorchidism should be suspected if the testis can't be felt in the scrotum, or the testis is very soft and small.

Treatment
There is controversy among doctors about whether to treat this condition surgically or with hormonal therapy, although most experts rec-

ommend some form of treatment between the child's first and second birthday. In the United States, most doctors prefer to treat one undescended testicle with surgery, placing the testis in the normal position before the second birthday so that it has more of a chance of developing normally and producing sperm cells.

If both testicles are undescended, many specialists prefer a combination of surgery and hormone therapy with HUMAN CHORIONIC GONADOTROPIN (hCG) or GONADOTROPIN-RELEASING HORMONE (Gn-RH) or both. European doctors usually rely on hormone therapy alone as the primary treatment for all patients with undescended testicles.

Unfortunately, if the testes have been injured by failure to descend, this injury usually can't be corrected. Men with undescended testicles are more likely to have hormone abnormalities or abnormal testicular ducts. Some doctors report improvements in sperm quality among men who receive medical therapy with CLOMIPHENE CITRATE (an antiestrogen drug) and human chorionic gonadotropin (hCG).

Patients with low sperm counts may need ASSISTED REPRODUCTIVE TECHNOLOGIES (ART) such as IN VITRO FERTILIZATION (IVF), ARTIFICIAL INSEMINATION using the husband's sperm, artificial insemination using DONOR SPERM (AID), GAMETE INTRAFALLOPILAN TRANSFER (GIFT), or INTRACYTOPLASMIC SPERM INJECTION (ICSI).

cumulative chance of pregnancy The accumulating likelihood of successfully getting pregnant over a period of months. A monthly chance of pregnancy at 20% means there is a 20% chance of getting pregnant by the end of the first month. The next month, there is a 20% of 80% chance of pregnancy (i.e., 16%) by the end of the second month, which would mean a cumulative 36% chance of pregnancy by the end of the second month—and so on.

cumulus oophorus A sticky, cloudlike group of cells that surrounds the egg at OVULATION.

cup insemination One type of ARTIFICIAL INSEMINATION (also known as homologous insemination). In this procedure, the semen is washed, separated to improve movement (motility), and placed in a diaphragmlike cup at the cervix during ovulation.

A couple using washed sperm must be inseminated at a clinic or doctor's office, but in many cases doctors show their patients how to insert the cup properly so that between sperm washes, couples can perform the procedure with fresh, unwashed sperm.

However, the success rates for the cup are low; so far these procedures haven't proved to be any more successful than spontaneous conception for men with a low sperm count.

Cushing's syndrome A condition in which an overproduction of the hormone cortisol leads to high blood pressure and water retention, as well as a number of other symptoms. If the adrenal male hormones (androgens) are also high, this will lead to low sperm production or ovulatory failure. A woman with Cushing's syndrome also may develop male secondary sex characteristics, including abnormal hair growth. Cushing's *disease* is a different condition featuring the same symptoms, but caused by a pituitary tumor.

Sometimes called "hypercortisolism," Cushing's syndrome is relatively rare and most commonly affects adults aged 20 to 50. An estimated 10 to 15 of every million people are affected each year.

Some patients may have high cortisol levels without the effects of Cushing's syndrome. These high cortisol levels may be compensating for the body's resistance to cortisol's effects. This rare syndrome of cortisol resistance is a genetic condition that causes high blood pressure and chronic high levels of male hormones.

Sometimes other conditions may be associated with many of the symptoms of Cushing's syndrome. These include POLYCYSTIC OVARY SYNDROME, which may cause menstrual disturbances, weight gain from adolescence, excess hair growth, and sometimes impaired insulin action and diabetes. Commonly, weight gain, high blood pressure, and abnormal levels of cholesterol and triglycerides in the blood are associated with resistance to insulin action and diabetes; this has been described as the "metabolic syndrome-X." Patients with these disorders don't have abnormally elevated cortisol levels.

Symptoms

Symptoms vary, but most people have heavy upper bodies with a rounded face, increased fat around the neck, and thinning arms and legs. Children tend to be obese with slowed growth rates. Other symptoms appear in the skin, which becomes fragile and thin, bruises easily, and heals poorly. Purplish pink stretch marks may appear on the abdomen, thighs, buttocks, arms, and breasts. The bones are weak, and routine activities such as bending, lifting, or getting up may lead to backaches or rib and spinal-column fractures. Most people have severe fatigue, weak muscles, high blood pressure, and high blood sugar. Irritability, anxiety, and depression are common.

Women usually have excess hair growth on their faces, necks, chests, abdomens, and thighs. Their menstrual periods may become irregular or stop. Men have fertility problems and lessened desire for sex.

Cause

The syndrome occurs when the body is exposed to high levels of cortisol for a long time, such as when a person takes glucocorticoid hormones for asthma, rheumatoid arthritis, lupus, or other inflammatory diseases. It's also possible to develop Cushing's syndrome if the body produces too much cortisol.

The form of the syndrome known as Cushing's *disease* is caused by benign tumors of the pituitary gland, which cause most cases of Cushing's and affects women five times more frequently than men.

Sometimes, a problem with the adrenal glands (usually a tumor) causes Cushing's syndrome by releasing too much cortisol into the blood.

Adrenal cancers are the rarest cause of Cushing's syndrome. Cancer cells produce many adrenal cortical hormones, including cortisol and adrenal androgens. These cancers usually cause very high hormone levels and rapid development of symptoms.

Although most cases of Cushing's syndrome aren't inherited, occasionally a few people develop the syndrome due to an inherited tendency to develop tumors of one or more endocrine glands.

Diagnosis

Cushing's is diagnosed after a medical history, physical, and lab tests. X rays of the adrenal or pituitary glands can help detect tumors. Once Cushing's syndrome has been diagnosed, other tests are used to determine the exact abnormality that leads to excess cortisol production. Scans can find any tumor that may exist.

Treatment

Specific treatment depends on the reason for high cortisol levels, but may include surgery, radiation, chemotherapy, or medication. If the cause is due to long-term use of steroids to treat another disorder, the doctor will gradually reduce the dosage; once control is established, the daily dose of glucocorticoid hormones may be doubled and given on alternate days to lessen side effects.

cycle day The day of a woman's menstrual cycle. The first day (day 1) is when full flow starts before midafternoon.

cystic fibrosis This hereditary disease with a recessive inheritance pattern frequently causes infertility in men. Men with cystic fibrosis may have no sperm because of the congenital absence of the vas deferens, the tube connecting the testicle and EPIDIDYMIS to the ejaculatory duct. This makes it impossible for the sperm to pass through the penis. The infertility that results can be treated by surgically extracting sperm from the testicles prior to IN VITRO FERTILIZATION.

Using TESTICULAR SPERM EXTRACTION, a urologist can obtain enough sperm to allow excellent success with IVF and INTRACYTOPLASMIC SPERM INJECTION (ICSI), but not enough sperm can be retrieved to make INTRAUTERINE INSEMINATION (IU) an effective option.

Because cystic fibrosis is a recessive genetic disorder, abnormal gene contributions from both parents are necessary for the condition to be present. Both copies of the gene are abnormal in men with CF. Although people carrying a single copy of an abnormal gene don't have this condition, when paired with a partner with CF, their offspring have a 50% chance of having the disease.

cytoplasm   The fluidlike material within a cell that contains microscopic structures related to cell function, including the mitrochondria. The egg's cytoplasm into which a sperm cell is injected is part of INTRACYTOPLASMIC SPERM INSERTION.

cytoplasmic transfer   An extension of IN VITRO FERTILIZATION, in which the genetic material from a mother's egg is combined with the cytoplasm of a donor egg. Two methods of cytoplasm transfer were developed, one that transfers a small amount of cytoplasm by tiny needle from the donor to the recipient egg, the other that transfers a larger amount of cytoplasm, which is then fused to the recipient cytoplasm with electricity. This research technique is not clinically advisable at the present time.

Dalkon shield A type of plastic INTRAUTERINE DEVICE (IUD) that was introduced in 1970 and recalled in 1975 because of links to MISCARRIAGE and PELVIC INFLAMMATORY DISEASE (PID), an infection that can cause infertility. Although initial studies found no association with either of these problems, once the court battles started, researchers found very high rates of complications with the Dalkon shield and an unexpected link between all types of intrauterine devices and PID. Modern researchers have criticized both the conclusions of these older studies and the way they were conducted. After reexamining the data, they feel that other factors, such as lifestyle, may play a crucial role in the development of complications among women using an IUD.

Ever since 1909, IUDs have been manufactured in many different shapes and sizes. These simple nickel, bronze, and catgut rings later gave way to FDA-approved plastic devices that looked like S's (Lippes loop, 1964–85), ram's horns (Saf-T-Coil, 1967–83), the number 7 (Copper-7, 1973– 86), and the letter T (Copper T-380A, 1984– , Progestasert, 1976– , Copper-T, 1976–86). A string attached to the bottom of each IUD was intended to dangle from the cervical opening, which was the indication that the IUD was still in place. This string also made removal easier. The Dalkon shield looked like a round bug with one eye and five legs on each side. Its unique tail was made of many fibers wound together and enclosed in a sheath. It was this string that led to its downfall, because experts thought the string was a breeding ground for bacteria and that it drew bacteria

up from the vagina into the uterus and on into the fallopian tubes, causing dangerous infections. Some scientists now believe that the string had nothing to do with the increased rates of infection seen with the Dalkon shield. Although the Dalkon shield came in two sizes (large for women who had given birth, small for those who had never had children) and both sizes had a multifilament string, only the larger size was associated with pregnancy-related deaths.

During the 1960s and 1970s, IUDs thrived. All of them were made of plastic with some barium sulfate added so that they would show up on X rays. The first American IUD, a large device called the Margulies coil, caused a lot of bleeding and cramping and had a hard plastic tail that sexual partners often found uncomfortable. The softer Lippes loop replaced it, followed by the Saf-T-Coil and the short-lived Majzlin spring.

The Dalkon shield was introduced just as the U.S. Senate was investigating the safety of oral contraceptives. It was immediately popular, especially among young women who were worried about the pill's side effects. Not long after A. H. Robins introduced the shield, about 40% of all IUDs were shields.

In 1974, the FDA warned doctors to remove IUDs immediately from any woman who became pregnant, because 12 IUD users had died after miscarriages led to severe infections. Ten were wearing the Dalkon shield at the time, and two wore the Lippes loop. By June 1974, when the FDA requested suspension of further sales, 2.8 million women had purchased the device. Although IUD-related death from miscarriages ceased to be a problem after doctors removed them from pregnant patients, these events sparked an explosion of fear and distrust of all IUDs.

Data connecting the Dalkon shield to miscarriage and death were overwhelming. Doctors reported that Dalkon shield users were twice as likely to be hospitalized as other women, and that those who became pregnant while wearing an IUD (especially the shield) increased their chance of dying by up to 50 times. Although some scientists pointed out weaknesses in the studies, women still avoided the device.

After the Dalkon shield scandal, some researchers began charging that IUDs were also responsible for an increased risk of pelvic inflammatory disease. Initial studies showed that women using other forms of birth control did indeed have a lower rate of PID than did IUD users. Barrier methods blocked bacteria; and the pill, which thickened cervical mucus, made it hard for bacteria to enter.

However, when compared with women using no birth control, IUD users actually have a lower risk of PID—and the greatest risk factor for PID is frequent sex with multiple partners. Since use of IUDs peaked during the sexual revolution of the 1960s and '70s, IUDs mistakenly got the blame that increased sexual freedom deserved.

The Dalkon shield disaster continued to affect sale of all forms of intrauterine devices. Copper IUDs, which were introduced during and shortly after the shield publicity, never became popular in the United States. Total IUD sales declined from 2.2 million to 0.7 million between 1981 and 1988 as lawsuit costs skyrocketed. Although copper IUDs were never proved dangerous, most disappeared from the market by the late 1980s. Only two (the Copper T-380A and the Progestasert) are sold in the United States today.

IUDs remain popular in other parts of the world where the negative reports didn't reach; about 100 million women now use these devices. In fact, they are the most popular form of birth control in such countries as China, Norway, Finland, and Egypt.

But despite the Dalkon experience, other IUDs didn't disappear. Instead, scientists made a second generation of the devices safer and more appealing. Now, American women are once again turning to IUDs for effective long-term birth control. Today, most experts agree that IUDs are an excellent contraceptive choice for most women as long as the devices are inserted under sterile conditions. Women at risk for sexually transmitted disease, however, should probably choose another form of birth control.

IUDs increase a monogamous woman's chances of getting PID only in the first 3 weeks to 3 months after insertion. No women have died after an IUD-related miscarriage since 1977, and IUDs have the lowest failure rate of all reversible contraceptives (less than 1%). Users say they are more satisfied with their method than are women using any other type of birth control; 98% of IUD users report satisfaction, while 92% of pill users and 87% of condom users say they are satisfied.

danazol (Danocrine)   A hormonal drug used to treat ENDOMETRIOSIS that suppresses pituitary production of the hormones LH and FSH and stops MENSTRUATION, allowing the endometrial implants to waste away. Danazol is a weak ANDROGEN; many women who take this drug experience a number of side effects, including weight gain, increased muscle bulk, oily skin, facial hair, muscle cramps, a deepened voice, or enlarged clitoris.

Danazol is less often prescribed compared with Gn-RH agonists such as Lupron (LEUPROLIDE ACETATE).

Danocrine   See DANAZOL.

D-chiro-inositol   An experimental drug (also known as INS-1) that normalizes the body's use of insulin and that seems to be a promising treatment for POLYCYSTIC OVARY SYNDROME (PCOS), the leading cause of female INFERTILITY in the United States. One recent study found that the treatment usually restores women's ovulatory cycles while reversing hormonal imbalances, decreasing total testosterone.

Polycystic ovary syndrome affects up to 6 million American women, who are usually first affected by the endocrine disorder anywhere from puberty through their early 20s. PCOS is the leading cause of menstrual irregularities and infertility due to lack of ovulation.

Until recently, researchers thought PCOS was caused by excess production of male hormones (ANDROGEN), but recent research has shown that insulin resistance plays a central role in a woman's development of the disorder. Women with PCOS are resistant to their own insulin and produce high levels of insulin to counter the resistance. Excess insulin in the bloodstream causes the ovaries to produce higher levels of androgens (such as testosterone), which can disrupt the relationship between the ovaries and the pituitary gland, preventing the ovaries from releasing an egg each month. The excess androgens can also cause acne, male-pattern hair loss, facial and body hair, and, in more severe cases, dark, velvety patches on the skin.

In addition to an overabundance of testosterone, the female hormones are often out of balance. The two hormones secreted by the pituitary gland in the brain, follicle-stimulating hormone (FSH) and luteinizing hormone (LH), may be produced at an abnormal level, perpetuating incomplete follicular development and preventing these women from ovulating regularly.

Although women with PCOS produce enough estrogen, they produce virtually no progesterone. Lack of this hormone can lead to an overgrowth of the uterine lining and increase the risk of endometrial cancer. Signs of the problem include lack of menstruation, high insulin levels, obesity, high blood pressure, and excessive facial hair caused by unusually high TESTOSTERONE levels.

Earlier studies have shown that drugs that treat insulin resistance (the body's failure to respond properly to insulin) can relieve the condition. However, these drugs can have a variety of unwanted side effects. Doctors found that D-chiro-inositol, which occurs naturally in fruits and vegetables, appears effective without causing side effects. There are currently no drugs approved in the United States specifically to treat this condition.

D&C The abbreviation for dilation and curettage, a procedure used to dilate the cervix and scrape out the lining and contents of the uterus. A D&C may be performed to diagnose or treat the cause of abnormal bleeding, or to terminate an unwanted pregnancy. It may be performed for bleeding between periods or after sexual intercourse, heavy menstrual bleeding, investigation of infertility, uterine fibroids, endometrial polyps, early uterine or cervical cancer, thickening of the uterus, an embedded IUD, an elective ABORTION, or following a MISCARRIAGE. This fairly minor surgical procedure may be performed in the hospital or clinic using general or local anesthesia.

Rarely, a woman may need an emergency D&C if she has heavy bleeding that cannot be stopped with tablet treatment. However, a D&C is usually used to make a diagnosis, and is not used as part of treating a bleeding problem.

The Procedure

To perform a D&C, the cervical canal is widened (dilated) using a metal rod; the doctor then inserts a curette (a metal loop on the end of a long thin handle) into the uterus and scrapes the inner layer of the uterus away. Tissue is usually collected for examination.

Risks

A D&C has relatively few risks. It can ease bleeding, and it can be used to diagnose problems, including infection, cancer, infertility, and other diseases. There is a slight risk of damage to the inner lining of the uterus, a dilated cervix that fails to return to normal size, a punctured uterus, laceration of the cervix, or scarring.

After Surgery

It is normal to experience irregular bleeding in the days following the D&C, as well as pelvic cramps and back pain. Pain can usually be managed well with medications. Tampon use is not recommended for a few weeks, and sexual intercourse is not recommended for a few days. A woman should contact her doctor if there is heavy bleeding with large clots, severe lower abdominal pain, bleeding, or high fever. The patient may resume normal activities the same day.

dehydroepiandrosterone sulfate (DHEAS) A male hormone (ANDROGEN) produced primarily by the adrenal gland. When DHEAS levels are too high, it may lead to fertility problems in both men and women.

In women, high DHEAS levels may lead to the formation of male secondary sex characteristics and the suppression of LH and FSH production by the pituitary gland. High levels of DHEAS may be found in women with polycystic ovaries or with a tumor in the pituitary gland, adrenal gland, or ovary.

An "androgen panel" usually includes a measure of the amounts of TESTOSTERONE and DHEAS in the woman's blood. A high level of testosterone but normal level of DHEAS suggests that the ovaries, not the adrenal glands, are the likely source of excess androgens. In a woman, the normal values of DHEAS are 35 to 430 ug/dl.

Depo-Provera (depot-medroxyprogesterone acetate; DMPA) The brand name of a prescription method of reversible birth control using a hormone like PROGESTERONE, one of the hormones that regulates the menstrual cycle. A Depo-Provera shot in the buttock or arm can prevent pregnancy for 12 weeks. It does this by preventing the ovaries from releasing eggs and thickening cervical mucus to keep sperm from joining eggs.

About 99.7% effective against pregnancy, the shot is one of the most effective reversible methods of birth control. Of every 1,000 women who use it, only 3 will become pregnant during the first year.

Protection is immediate if a woman gets the shot during the first 5 days of her period. Otherwise, she should use an additional method of contraception for the first 2 weeks. However, the shot does not protect against sexually transmitted diseases.

Depo-Provera is convenient, long lasting, and doesn't need to be taken daily or put in place before having sex. It doesn't require surgery, contains no estrogen, lessens menstrual cramps and anemia, protects against endometrial and ovarian cancers, and can be used while breastfeeding (6 weeks after delivery).

Side Effects

Irregular bleeding is the most common side effect. Periods become fewer and lighter for most women (most will have no periods after 5 years of getting the shot). After a woman stops taking Depo-Provera, it may take a year for her periods to resume. Some women have longer and heavier periods; others have light spotting and breakthrough bleeding. Less commonly, some women may experience increased appetite and weight gain, headache, sore breasts, nausea, nervousness, dizziness, depression, rashes, or spotty darkening of skin, hair loss, increased facial or body hair, and increased or decreased sex drive. If a woman does develop side effects, they may continue for up to 8 months until the medication is cleared from the body.

Serious side effects include vaginal bleeding that lasts longer and is much heavier than a usual period, major depression, a lump in a breast, sudden and severe abdominal pain, or yellowing of skin or eye.

Women should not take Depo-Provera if they

- are pregnant
- want to get pregnant within 18 months
- have unexplained vaginal bleeding

- have a serious liver disease
- have a known or suspected breast cancer
- have Cushing's syndrome

See also MEDROXYPROGESTERONE ACETATE.

depression and fertility drugs Women taking fertility drugs or pursuing fertility treatments sometimes experience depression, which can be severe. In fact, one Harvard study found that women undergoing fertility treatments showed depression levels equal to those of a woman facing treatment for cancer or AIDS. Fertility drugs may trigger hormonal changes that can worsen a depression.

dermoid A benign ovarian tumor that may contain hair, teeth, and bone fragments. It is also known as a teratoma or germ cell tumor.

DES See DIETHYLSTILBESTROL.

DES Action USA A national, nonprofit consumer organization dedicated to informing the public about DES (DIETHYLSTILBESTROL) and helping DES-exposed individuals. DES Action maintains a National Attorney Referral List of attorneys who handle DES-related cases and offers a quarterly newsletter and many publications on various aspects of DES exposure. Contact: DES Action USA, 610 16th Street, Suite 301, Oakland, CA 94612; phone: (510) 465-4011; website http://www.desaction.org.

DHEAS See DIHYDROEPIANDROSTERONE SULFATE.

diabetes A common condition caused by an insufficient amount of insulin or the inability of cells to efficiently use insulin (insulin resistance). Insulin is necessary to help transport sugar from the blood to the inside of the cells; unless sugar gets into the cells, it can't be used by the body. Excess sugar that remains in the blood is removed by the kidneys, causing elevated sugar levels in the urine—a sign of diabetes. The cause of diabetes is unknown, but heredity and diet are believed to play a role in its development. Diabetes can affect fertility in both women and men by damaging blood vessels and nerves.

Diabetic men may experience IMPOTENCE or retrograde EJACULATION (backward flow of semen into the bladder instead of out the urethra).

About 60% of all men over age 50 who have diabetes may be impotent. This may occur because diabetes can damage the small blood vessels and nerves responsible for creating an erection. Damage to the large vessels also can affect blood flow to the penis.

Retrograde ejaculation linked to diabetes occurs when nerve function at the opening of the bladder is lost; this causes sperm to shoot backward during ejaculation.

Recent research in women has uncovered a link between POLYCYSTIC OVARY SYNDROME and insulin resistance. Scientists have found that lowering insulin levels in women with PCOS helps restore menstrual cycles and lower the abnormally high testosterone levels common to PCOS. In addition, drugs used to treat type II (which reduce insulin resistance) diabetes are also now used successfully in treating PCOS.

Women who are insulin resistant tend to have too much insulin in their bloodstream, which causes the ovaries to produce higher levels of male hormones (such as testosterone), disrupting the relationship between the ovaries and the pituitary gland and preventing ovulation. In addition to an overabundance of testosterone, this insulin resistance often triggers an imbalance in female hormones: Follicle-stimulating hormone (FSH) and luteinizing hormone (LH) may be produced in abnormal amounts, perpetuating incomplete follicular development and preventing these women from ovulating regularly. Signs of PCOS include lack of menstruation, high insulin levels, obesity, high blood pressure, and excessive facial hair caused by unusually high TESTOSTERONE levels.

Earlier studies have shown that drugs that treat insulin resistance can relieve PCOS. However, these drugs can have a variety of unwanted side effects. In a new study, doctors found that a substance called D-CHIRO-IUNOSITOL that occurs naturally in fruits and vegetables appears effective without causing side effects.

Diane-35/Dianette   One type of BIRTH CONTROL PILL that contains estrogen and the progestogen known as cyproterone acetate, used to treat severe acne associated with high levels of androgens in women. It is also an effective oral contraceptive. See also BIRTH CONTROL METHODS.

diaphragm   A type of BIRTH CONTROL METHOD that prevents pregnancy in two ways: First, its dome-shaped rubber disk has a flexible rim that covers the cervix so that sperm can't reach the uterus, while the SPERMICIDE applied to the diaphragm before insertion kills sperm. Available by prescription only, a diaphragm must be sized by a health professional to achieve a proper fit.

The diaphragm protects against pregnancy for 6 hours; after that time (or for repeated intercourse within this period), fresh spermicide must be inserted into the vagina with the diaphragm still in place. It must remain in place for at least 6 hours after the last act of intercourse but no more than 24 hours because of the risk of toxic shock syndrome (TSS), a rare but potentially fatal infection. Used consistently and correctly, the diaphragm carries a failure rate of about 6%, but the typical failure rate is closer to 18%.

Diaphragm fit should be checked at an annual gynecological exam

• whenever the woman gains or loses 10 pounds or more

• after an ABORTION

• after a MISCARRIAGE

• after a full-term pregnancy

diethylstilbestrol (DES)   A man-made ESTROGEN prescribed in the 1950s and 1960s to prevent MISCARRIAGE. Fetuses exposed in the uterus to this drug can develop numerous deformities, including blockage of the vas deferens, abnormal uterus or cervix, miscarriages, and unexplained infertility. DES is no longer prescribed for pregnant women.

dihydrotestosterone (DHT)   The most active male sex hormone (ANDROGEN) produced from TESTOSTERONE, which is the main type of androgen in the blood. Testosterone must be converted into DHT before it can function.

dilation and curettage   See D&C.

directional motility   A term used to describe sperm that can move in a straight line.

dizygotic twins   The medical term for non-identical (fraternal) twins, formed from two fertilized eggs.

Dolly   A lamb that was the first viable offspring cloned from a single cell of an adult mammal.

Most larger animals reproduce sexually, a process that involves two individuals each contributing half of the genetic material to the offspring via sperm and egg. CLONING involves the production of a new, genetically identical individual from a single animal. More than 60 years of research on animals such as sea urchins, frogs, and mice suggested that this might be impossible. But in 1995, a group of scientists at the Roslin Institute in Edinburgh, Scotland, had discovered a way to modify farm animals genetically. A year before Dolly's birth, they cloned Megan and Morag from embryo-derived cells, cultured for several weeks in the laboratory. This breakthrough did not arouse much public interest; Dolly is more famous because she is the first clone of an adult animal.

In the cloning procedure that produced Dolly, researchers removed an unfertilized egg cell from an adult ewe and replaced its nucleus with the nucleus of an adult sheep mammary gland cell. This egg was then implanted in another ewe; Dolly was born on July 5, 1996. This feat demonstrated that with careful handling, the genetic material of cells from adult animals can be introduced into an egg cell, and that normal cell development can occur.

Since then, other research teams have cloned tadpoles and cattle from embryo tissue. Indeed, the same researchers that produced Dolly have raised several other sheep from egg cells whose nuclei had been replaced with nuclei from either fetal or embryonic tissue.

However, experts have noted that most cloned animals either do not survive or develop significant health problems after birth.

dominant follicle The largest follicle of a group that contains the egg that will ovulate.

donor eggs Eggs from a fertile woman that are donated to an infertile woman for use in an ASSISTED REPRODUCTIVE TECHNOLOGY (ART) procedure, including IN VITRO FERTILIZATION and EMBRYO TRANSFER. Donor eggs are used if the woman is older, if she has hormone problems interfering with normal egg production, or genetic problems making her eggs unsuitable for ART.

Donation Process

To get the eggs, a donor is first screened carefully by the health care team. She receives medication to stimulate egg production, and her eggs are retrieved; they are then fertilized in the laboratory with sperm from the recipient's partner and then later transferred to the recipient's uterus in an attempt to achieve a pregnancy.

In "identified donation," donor eggs may either be given by a friend or family member; in an anonymous donation, eggs are obtained from an infertility program. Some women have advertised for egg donors, but there are organizations, psychologists, and social workers who can help find donors. Some programs have their own donors.

The cost depends on how the couple finds the donor, but donors are usually paid something to compensate them for risk and time involved. The amount of compensation generally varies from $1,000 to $5,000, in addition to a fee charged by the agent finding the donor (this also may vary from $1,000 to $5,000). The entire process is confidential. If the eggs are obtained from a clinic, donors and recipients never meet.

A woman who donates her eggs must be healthy and between 21 and 34 years old. She must be covered by health insurance and must have both her ovaries. The screening procedure includes interviews, written questionnaires, psychological evaluations, nursing consultations, blood screening, and a meeting with a REPRODUCTIVE ENDOCRINOLOGIST.

If a donor is selected, she must receive hormone injections each day for 10 to 12 days to induce her ovaries to produce several eggs instead of the more typical one egg. Also, she must undergo ultrasound exams and blood tests (hCG) to monitor the eggs' development. Once her eggs have matured, another injection is given to trigger egg maturation. While the risks are minimal to the donor, there is the slight chance of OVARIAN HYPERSTIMULATION SYNDROME (OHSS), together with a low risk of infection during retrieval.

A doctor coordinates the donor's cycle with the cycle of the recipient. As the donor starts her medication, the recipient starts taking estrogen to develop the uterine lining. On the day the donor's eggs are retrieved, a sperm specimen is taken from the partner to fertilize the eggs; generally, the recipient begins taking progesterone on that day. Usually 2 days later, the embryos are transferred to the recipient's uterus.

After the embryos have been transferred, the woman keeps taking estrogen and daily progesterone. Ten to 14 days later, a pregnancy test is done. If it is positive, the woman needs to continue the estrogen and progesterone for about two more months. At that time the baby's placenta will take over, and no more medication is necessary.

The first successful pregnancy using donated eggs was reported in 1984 in Australia, when eggs were taken from a fertile donor, fertilized, and placed into the uterus of a woman with ovarian failure. At first, this procedure had been used primarily for young women with premature ovarian failure. More recently, egg donation has been used successfully in women who are still menstruating but whose ovaries don't respond well to FERTILITY DRUGS. In addition, women who have had multiple IVF cycles and failed to achieve a pregnancy may be candidates for egg donation, since they may have faulty eggs.

Experienced programs report clinical pregnancy rates of 35% to 50% per egg donation cycle. About 15% to 20% of these pregnancies will miscarry. Approximately 25% will be multiple births. These success rates are better than pregnancy rates in IVF cycles using a woman's own eggs.

donor insemination (DI) A type of ARTIFICIAL INSEMINATION using sperm not from the male partner or husband. It may be needed if there are abnormal semen characteristics and if the woman is proved to be fertile.

Causes for MALE FACTOR INFERTILITY could include lack of sperm, abnormally shaped sperm, previous VASECTOMY, radiation or chemotherapy treatment, or diseases (such as mumps or CYSTIC FIBROSIS). Donor insemination also may be considered if the husband is a carrier of a genetic disorder, such as Huntington's disease, Tay-Sachs disease, hemophilia, or chromosomal problems. In addition, DI may be used if the mother is Rh sensitized and the male is Rh positive. Finally,

single women or lesbian couples may also request elective donor insemination.

Insemination is scheduled as close as possible to the woman's OVULATION; if she ovulates irregularly, the doctor may prescribe drugs to induce ovulation. Inseminations are usually performed once or twice a month, depending on how regular the woman's menstrual cycle may be.

The simple procedure takes only a few moments. For intracervical insemination (ICI), the doctor injects the semen into the cervical opening using a syringe. A plastic-coated cap may be placed into the vagina to keep the sperm near the cervix; it can be removed between 4 to 6 hours after insemination. In INTRAUTERINE INSEMINATION, the doctor inserts washed sperm directly into the uterus.

The success rate for donor insemination depends on several factors, the most important being the woman's age (women over age 35 have a lesser chance of a successful pregnancy). Success rate is higher if the woman has had one successful pregnancy already.

In general, if the insemination is performed each month, the overall chance of pregnancy using frozen sperm is about 10% each cycle. However, other factors (such as age) affect success rates. There is also a 2% to 4% chance of birth defects in any birth, including babies born as the result of donor insemination. The risk of birth defects after donor insemination is the same as the natural abnormality rate.

donor sperm Donor semen specimens are commonly used in infertility treatment, either for single women, couples facing MALE FACTOR INFERTILITY or a genetic abnormality, or for lesbian couples. More than 30,000 babies are born each year as a result of donor insemination technology.

SPERM BANKS are the laboratories where semen samples are frozen. Frozen semen for donor insemination may be bought from commercial semen banks that ship specimens from a selected donor to various parts of the country.

Screening

Today, semen is always frozen and stored for adequate screening to make sure that the samples aren't contaminated with viruses such as HIV, the virus that causes AIDS. Prior to the emergence of AIDS, fresh semen was often used for donor insemination. To guard against AIDS, the AMERICAN SOCIETY FOR REPRODUCTIVE MEDICINE recommends that all sperm be frozen for at least 6 months before insemination. The donor is screened for HIV and other infectious diseases at the time of semen donation and then tested again 6 months later, so that any infection that was undiagnosed the first time would be found on the second test. It may take from 3 to 5 months for the virus to show up in the blood. While this doesn't completely eliminate the risk of HIV-infected semen, it makes the risk very small.

Sperm banks may vary in the extent of screening for HIV and other infectious and genetic diseases. The AMERICAN SOCIETY OF REPRODUCTIVE MEDICINE, the U.S. Centers for Disease Control, and the U.S. Food and Drug Administration have recommended that only frozen, quarantined, not fresh, semen be used for artificial insemination. The AMERICAN ASSOCIATION OF TISSUE BANKS provides stringent professional standards for the collection, testing, storage, and tracking of semen and performs on-site inspections in order to accredit sperm banks.

People interested in donor sperm can obtain a list of sperm banks that meet certain criteria and allow inspections by the American Association of Tissue Banks, 1350 Beverly Road, Ste. 220-A, McLean, VA 22011; phone: (703) 827-9582; website http://www.aatb.org.

Sperm banks should have a thorough medical history of the donor and his family. Donors should be fertile and less than 40 years old. Donors should be required to be tested for a range of common diseases, including Rh factor, hepatitis B and C, and other sexually transmitted diseases. A limit of 10 pregnancies per donor reduces the chance of offspring intermarriage.

Many donor sperm recipients like to match certain characteristics of their male partner with the donor, and sperm banks often have this information about physical traits. Some provide detailed information about the donor's personal habits, hobbies, talents, and personal characteristics. Of course, there is no guarantee that any of these traits will be passed on to the offspring. It is important that the sperm bank keep a permanent confidential record of the donor's health and genetic-screening information.

douching and infertility   Women who are trying to get pregnant should not douche, since those who do are less likely to get pregnant. In one study by the National Institute of Environmental Health Sciences, women between 18 and 24 who douche had a 50% drop in their monthly fertility; women between 25 to 29 had a 30% decrease. Those who douched more than once a week had the lowest pregnancy rate. After a year of trying to get pregnant, 27% of women who douched did not conceive, compared with 10% of those who didn't douche or douched only rarely.

Douching may be toxic to sperm or adversely affect cervical mucus.

doxycycline   A tetracycline derivative that kills many of the bacteria infecting the reproductive tract. Many doctors routinely treat with this or other antibiotics before some infertility treatments.

duration of infertility   An important variable influencing the chance of getting pregnant naturally. The longer the duration of infertility, the more likely that the cause is a significant one.

echinacea and infertility   See HERBS AND INFERTILITY.

ectopic pregnancy   Also called a tubal pregnancy, this is a condition in which the embryo implants outside of the uterus, usually in the fallopian tube, although it can also occur in the ovary or abdominal cavity. If such a pregnancy is allowed to continue, it may eventually rupture the fallopian tube and cause life-threatening hemorrhage. Such a pregnancy can never be sustained and often leads to decreased or complete loss of function in the affected tube.

The Centers for Disease Control (CDC) discovered that between 1970 and 1987, the rate of ectopic pregnancies during this 17-year period jumped almost 4-fold (from 4.5 per 1,000 pregnancies to 16.8 per 1,000 pregnancies). During this same time period, the fatality rate from ectopic pregnancies dropped almost 90% (from 35.5 per 1,000 to 3.8 per 1,000). Despite the sharp drop in the fatality rate, ectopic pregnancies are still the second leading cause of maternal death in the United States. The reason for the increase in ectopic pregnancy during this time period is not clear. Some experts suspect that better diagnosis and more sexually transmitted diseases (which damage fallopian tube transport of embryos into the uterus) are both responsible for a significant portion of the increased number of cases.

Ectopic ("out of place") pregnancy occurs once in every 100 pregnancies, but some women are at slightly higher risk, including those who

- use an intrauterine device (IUD)
- have used the "morning after" pill
- use the progestin only or "mini" pill
- have tubal damage caused by infection
- have had tubal surgery (such as tubal ligation or sterilization reversal)
- are undergoing IVF and GIFT
- have had a previous ectopic pregnancy

Symptoms

At first an ectopic pregnancy may seem just like a normal pregnancy, beginning with a missed menstrual period and symptoms such as sore breasts and nausea. However, there is often abnormal vaginal bleeding that may occur around the time of (or a little later than) the expected period and that may be mistaken for a period. Pain on the side where the embryo has implanted is common; the pain may be associated with a feeling of lightheadedness or a desire to go to the bathroom. If the tube ruptures, this usually causes severe abdominal pain and fainting.

Diagnosis

Early diagnosis and treatment is important and may even allow the tube to be saved. Women who are at increased risk may be advised to have an ultrasound scan in early pregnancy, particularly if they have any vaginal bleeding.

Pregnancy must be confirmed by a pregnancy blood test; if negative, the test virtually excludes any risk of a significant ectopic pregnancy. If the test is positive, an ultrasound scan can usually establish whether the pregnancy is in the uterus. Sometimes a pregnancy sac may be seen outside the uterus, which confirms the diagnosis.

However, identifying an ectopic pregnancy may be very difficult, and LAPAROSCOPY is often the only way of confirming the diagnosis if no pregnancy can be seen in the uterus. In this technique, a thin telescope-like instrument is inserted near the navel, which allows the gynecologist to see the pelvic organs. A pregnancy in the fallopian tube can be easily seen this way.

Treatment

Ectopic pregnancies were first described in the 11th century and for a long time were always fatal for the mother. Since then, several developments in the management of ectopic pregnancies have led to remarkable success in saving the mother's life. Further developments recently have resulted in a shift in focus from saving the mother's life to saving the woman's fertility.

Traditionally, tubal pregnancy has been treated by removing the tube involved. However, newer and more sensitive tests mean that doctors can make a diagnosis early enough that the tube can often be saved. It may be possible to remove the pregnancy using a laparoscope, thus avoiding major surgery.

Chemical methods of treating unruptured ectopic pregnancies are also now becoming available, including the use of methotrexate to dissolve the pregnancy without causing major damage to the fallopian tubes. Conceiving naturally after a history of an ectopic pregnancy increases the risk of another such pregnancy. Studies suggest that women can remain fertile after taking methotrexate to resolve an ectopic pregnancy. In the 80% of women who got pregnant after methotrexate treatment, 87% of the pregnancies were located in the uterus and 13% were ectopic.

ectopic pregnancy rate   The percentage of ECTOPIC PREGNANCY among total clinical pregnancies. The normal rate is less than 1% and is increased if there are predisposing conditions such as abnormalities of the FALLOPIAN TUBES, assisted conception, and so on.

egg   The female reproductive cell, also called an ovum. See also DONOR EGGS; EGG RECOVERY/RETRIEVAL.

egg aspiration   See EGG RECOVERY/RETRIEVAL.

egg donation   See DONOR EGGS.

egg recovery/retrieval   A procedure used to collect eggs from a woman's follicles for use in IN VITRO FERTILIZATION (IVF), usually performed with ultrasound-directed needle aspiration during IVF.

Blood testing and ultrasound are used to check the maturity of the follicles before the eggs are retrieved. Medications are then adjusted according to the stage of development of the follicles; hCG is given to complete egg maturity. It may also be used to retrieve eggs for GIFT, ZIFT, and TET.

Laparoscopy

For this procedure, a light, general anesthesia is given. The doctor inserts a laparoscope through a small incision underneath the navel, and uses two small puncture sites to place a needle and manipulate instruments. The doctor then aspirates the eggs from a mature follicle. The operation requires absorbable stitches.

Ultrasound-Directed Needle Aspiration

The alternative to laparoscopy is ultrasound-directed needle aspiration, which avoids surgery and is performed under a local anesthetic. Typically, the needle is inserted through the top of the vagina or the back of the bladder into the ovary.

ejaculation disorders   Because of the complexity of the ejaculation process, there are many problems that may occur that could impact a man's fertility. These include ejaculating too early (premature ejaculation), taking too long to ejaculate (delayed ejaculation), failing to ejaculate at all (ANEJACULATION), or ejaculating in the wrong direction (retrograde ejaculation).

Some severe ejaculatory dysfunctions can be emotionally crippling. Because these problems are complex, they require treatment by experts with a special interest and experience in treating these conditions. Despite this, some cases might not respond well to treatment.

Premature Ejaculation

This very common condition may affect as many as 75% of all men at some point in their lives.

Not all cases of PE are alike, however. Some men ejaculate when just thinking about sex; others seem to be able to last longer, but not long enough to satisfy their partners. According to the American Psychiatric Association's Diagnostic and Statistical Manual of Mental Disorders (DSM-IV), premature ejaculation is a "persistent or recurrent ejaculation with minimal stimulation before, during, or shortly after penetration and before the person wishes it."

Physical (nonpsychological) causes of PE include injury to the nervous system, pelvic fractures, prostate problems, urethritis, diabetes, heart disease, genitourinary disease, polycythemia, or polyneuritis. There are a range of possible treatment options for PE, but the most popular involves antidepressant drugs (the selective serotonin reuptake inhibitors) such as Prozac. (See also DIABETES and INFERTILITY.)

Delayed Ejaculation

This condition is in many ways the exact opposite of premature ejaculation—a persistent difficulty in ejaculating despite sexual desire, erection, and stimulation. While it may seem as if this condition could help the partner achieve orgasm, in fact many times a man with this problem constantly worries about when he is going to finish. His partner may have already attained orgasm and stopped lubricating, making sex painful.

Occasionally, delayed ejaculation evolves into the more serious ejaculatory incompetence, in which a man can never ejaculate inside his part-

ner's vagina. This poses additional problems when the couple wants to have a baby.

A very common reason for delayed ejaculation is linked to masturbation. Many men exert much more pressure with their hands than they are likely to experience during sex; this trains them to respond sexually to strong pressure. Many men can learn to reach orgasm with a partner if they masturbate slowly and with much less pressure than usual. Some men get into the habit of thinking about how difficult it's been in the past to reach orgasm during sex, which slows down arousal and makes orgasm more elusive. Other factors that can contribute to delayed ejaculation include obsessive-compulsive disorders, marital conflict, and chronic substance abuse (alcohol and drugs). Delayed ejaculation is often related to anger or resentment toward women, an oppressive upbringing, a lack of emotional involvement with the partner, or fears of commitment.

In addition, many physical causes can contribute to delayed ejaculation, such as many neurological and endocrine illnesses, diabetes, cancer, prostate problems, psychiatric drugs, blood pressure medications, and surgery. Physical and psychological factors often coexist. All these conditions will require special intervention.

Delayed ejaculation can be treated with positive reinforcement associated with masturbation. Of course, any physical causes also must be treated.

Retrograde Ejaculation

A male fertility problem in which sperm travels backward into the bladder during ejaculation instead of out the opening of the penis. It is caused by failure in the sphincter muscle at the base of the bladder, previous bladder surgery, or by medications for high blood pressure. This problem can be diagnosed by a urinalysis to look for sperm, performed right after ejaculation. Sometimes part of the semen is ejaculated normally, and part ends up in the bladder. (See also MALE FACTOR INFERTILITY.)

Patients with retrograde ejaculation usually achieve orgasm normally and feel the sensation of having ejaculated. However, little or no seminal fluid emerges from the penis. Instead, the patient often notices that urine passed after sexual intercourse is cloudy with semen.

DIABETES is a very common cause of retrograde ejaculation due to nerve damage that impairs the nerve supply to the bladder. Nearly one of three diabetics will have some degree of retrograde ejaculation. Other causes of retrograde ejaculation are spinal cord lesions and injuries and surgery on the spine, bladder, neck, or prostate. Many medications that affect the neurological control of the bladder neck also may cause retrograde ejaculation.

Retrograde ejaculation may not respond to treatment. Drugs such as imipramine, ephedrine, and phenylpropanolamine may not be effective. Since sexual function is usually normal, treatment is not necessary if fertility is not a concern.

For men who want to father children retrograde ejaculation is a problem. However, these men can be successfully treated by retrieving sperm from the urinary bladder, followed by assisted reproduction.

Anejaculation

This condition, which is characterized by the inability to ejaculate, can be caused by a psychological or physical problem. Psychological anejaculation is usually not accompanied by orgasm. Situational anejaculation means that a man can ejaculate in some situations but not in others. For instance, a man may be able to ejaculate and attain orgasm with one partner but not with another. This usually occurs when there is a psychological conflict or a relationship difficulty with one partner. Or he may be able to ejaculate quite normally during masturbation but not during sex. It can also occur in stressful situations, as when a man is asked to collect a sample of semen in a laboratory during an infertility workup. In total anejaculation, the man is never able to ejaculate when awake. Deep-rooted psychological conflicts are usually the cause. Such men, however, usually have normal emissions during night sleep. Treatment depends on the cause and includes psychosexual counseling, drugs such as ephedrine and imipramine, vibrator therapy, and electroejaculation (a procedure in which an electrical current is applied to the ejaculatory organs to stimulate ejaculation).

Physical anejaculation, which includes retrograde ejaculation, can occur as the result of obstruction. Obstructions to the ejaculatory pathway require surgery.

electroejaculation   A process that can be used to stimulate ejaculation in men who have been paralyzed below the waist or who cannot ejaculate normally. Using a device known as an electroejaculator, a specially designed electric probe is inserted into the rectum next to the prostate. The current stimulates the nerves and contracts the pelvic muscles, resulting in an ejaculation. The semen specimen is collected and processed in the lab; if the specimen is of very good quality, it can be used for INTRAUTERINE INSEMINATION (IUI). If there are few sperm or if the sperm have low motility, the specimen can be used with IN VITRO FERTILIZATION with INTRACYTOPLASMIC SPERM INJECTION (ICSI) to establish a pregnancy.

Electroejaculation must be performed under general anesthesia in patients who have sensation in the abdominal and perirectal regions. Anesthesia isn't required for men with spinal cord injuries who have no sensation.

Before the procedure, the patient should have a complete urologic evaluation to detect and treat any urinary tract infections.

electromagnetic fields   Low-frequency electromagnetic fields similar to those emitted from power lines can stunt the development of parts of the ovaries in mice, according to one study by Italian scientists.

Humans are exposed to low doses of electromagnetic fields in the home by appliances such as refrigerators, washing machines, and other electrical devices, and by power lines.

However, no effects of electromagnetic fields on the human ovary has ever been demonstrated.

embryo   A term that describes the time from fertilization of the egg until the eighth week of pregnancy.

embryo banks   Similar to a SPERM BANK, an embryo bank offers long-term storage of embryos. At most embryo banks, the service of frozen embryo storage is only provided to legally married couples. In this case, both parties usually must sign for storage, release, or destruction of embryos. The ultimate use of the embryos is limited to the woman whose name appears on the storage contract.

embryo freezing   See   CRYOPRESERVATION; EMBRYO STORAGE.

embryo storage   Today it is possible to freeze one or more embryos quickly and store them in liquid nitrogen at very low temperatures. Many ASSISTED REPRODUCTIVE TECHNOLOGY (ART) centers now have the ability to preserve for future use embryos that haven't been used in a particular ART cycle. This process, called embryo CRYOPRESERVATION, allows patients to reduce the risk of a multiple birth, to have future replacement cycles at much lower cost if pregnancy doesn't occur, and to allow more pregnancies and children without additional IVF or ICSI cycles.

Techniques such as IN VITRO FERTILIZATION (IVF) and INTRACYTOPLASMIC SPERM INJECTION (ICSI) usually produce between 5 and 12 viable embryos during each treatment cycle. It's not unusual for some couples to end up with 20 or more embryos after an ART procedure. Usually, couples chose to replace three or four embryos in the woman's uterus and freeze the rest for possible future use. But if a couple is successful

on the first or second attempt at ART, this means that there may be spare embryos created. They are then faced with the decision about what to do with the extra embryos.

A minority are donated for research, and a small percentage are contributed anonymously for use by people without the physical capability (or, sometimes, the money) to attempt in vitro fertilization on their own.

A single in vitro fertilization cycle at a typical clinic costs about $5,600 if no supplementary procedures are used and may pass $8,000 if they are. Insurance firms in only eight states pay nearly all the costs of reproductive procedures; in other states, the corresponding prices range from $8,000 to double that amount. Implantation of a frozen embryo, by contrast, costs as little as $1,200 anywhere, although the process does not guarantee either a pregnancy or a live birth.

Once they are frozen and stored, the embryos can be viable for a long time. However, the storage of large numbers of frozen embryos also raises important ethical and moral questions. More and more medical clinics nationwide are using these frozen embryos left over from in vitro fertilization treatments in what has essentially become a new form of adoption. Infertile patients who provided neither the eggs nor the sperm used to produce them are receiving this surplus of embryos, raising provocative questions about family relationships and genetic disclosure.

Child-welfare specialists and medical ethicists worry that unscrupulous practitioners could sell frozen embryos, a practice that may or may not be legal because state statutes prohibit the sale of human beings but don't address the question of whether fertilized eggs fall into that category. Even well-intentioned clinicians could inadvertently push poor patients into "donating" their frozen embryos in exchange for fertility treatments, which can cost tens of thousands of dollars.

No governmental or medical group tracks how many embryos are stored in cryogenic states by the more than 300 clinics in the United States that offer in vitro fertilization, but experts estimate that the count has doubled (to about 200,000) between 1998 and 2000.

Most clinics abide by guidelines for embryo donation issued by the AMERICAN SOCIETY FOR REPRODUCTIVE IMMUNOLOGY in 1998. Among other things, these call for screening to determine whether the donated embryos might carry any diseases, for recipients to release donors from any liability, and for donors to relinquish all their rights to the embryos and to any children they might produce. Following these guidelines is voluntary, however, and there is no way to find out if a clinic is complying with the guidelines.

In some countries, freezing of embryos is restricted or banned (for example, Germany and Switzerland will only allow freezing of the zygote—that is, before the first cell division of the fertilized egg).

embryo transfer   Placing an egg that has been fertilized outside the womb into a woman's uterus or (rarely) into the fallopian tube after IN VITRO FERTILIZATION.

emergency contraception   A type of contraception (also called postcoital contraception) that can prevent pregnancy after unprotected sex. There are two types of emergency contraception: administration of two types of hormonal EMERGENCY CONTRACEPTIVE PILLS (incorrectly termed the "morning after pill") or insertion of a copper-releasing INTRAUTERINE DEVICE (IUD). Emergency contraception has been available for more than 25 years and could prevent 1.7 million unintended pregnancies and 800,000 abortions each year.

ECPs are taken in two doses, the first within 72 hours of unprotected sex and the second 12 hours later. Because they have a 3-day window of effectiveness and require multiple doses of pills, the popular term "morning-after pill" is not really correct.

An IUD can be inserted to prevent pregnancy up to 5 days after unprotected intercourse. More than 8,400 copper-bearing IUDs have been inserted postcoitally since 1976, with only eight pregnancies occurring—a rate of fewer than one in 1,000, reducing the risk of pregnancy by more than 99%.

Who Should Not Use EC
Almost every woman who needs emergency contraception can safely use ECPs—even some women who can't regularly use oral contraceptives. The ECPs should not be used by women who are already pregnant, not because they are harmful but because they can't terminate established pregnancies.

A woman should not use an IUD for emergency contraception if she is already pregnant; has a sexually transmitted infection such as HIV, chlamydia, or gonorrhea; has a history of pelvic inflammatory disease; or has a variety of other conditions that affect her reproductive system. IUDs are usually not recommended for women who wish to bear children in the future because of the slightly increased risk for PID, which can cause infertility.

How They Work
Emergency contraceptive pills act by delaying or inhibiting ovulation, or altering the transport of sperm or egg. They also may alter the endometrium, interfering with implantation. They cannot be used to abort an established pregnancy.

The IUD used as a regular method of contraception affects the sperm and egg so that fertilization does not occur. Experts believe that postcoital emergency contraceptive insertion of an IUD probably also interferes with implantation.

Side Effects
Side effects of IUD insertion may include abdominal discomfort, vaginal bleeding or spotting, and infection. Possible side effects of IUD use include heavy menstrual flow, cramping, infection, infertility, and uterine puncture.

Side effects of ECPs may include nausea and vomiting.

STDs

Neither ECPs nor IUDs prevent the spread of sexually transmitted infections, including HIV. Many women who need emergency contraception are at risk of these infections. For those at risk of sexually transmitted infections, ECPs are likely to be a safer choice than IUD insertion, since bacteria from a preexisting infection can be introduced into the sterile uterine cavity during IUD insertion. Untreated, such infections can lead to pelvic inflammatory disease. HIV infection can also increase the risk of pelvic inflammatory disease associated with an IUD.

emergency contraceptive pills (ECPs) A type of emergency contraceptive pill that can prevent pregnancy after unprotected sex in cases of unanticipated sexual activity, contraceptive failure, or rape. Mistakenly known as the "morning after pill," ECPs actually involve more than one pill, and they don't need to be taken on the morning after unprotected sex. Moreover, they should not be confused with the so-called abortion pill (MIFEPRISTONE) because ECPs can't terminate an established pregnancy.

ECPs have been prescribed for several decades, usually in the case of sexual assault. However, by the end of the 1990s, ECPs were widely recognized as a safe and effective method for all women at risk for unintended pregnancy.

The most common way to use ECP is called the Yuzpe regimen, named for Canadian professor A. Albert Yuzpe, who, in 1974, published the first studies demonstrating the safety and efficacy of ECPs. The Yuzpe regimen consists of giving two doses of combined oral contraceptive pills that contain the hormones estrogen and progestin. The first dose is taken within 72 hours after unprotected sex, the second dose 12 hours later.

Before the U.S. Food and Drug Administration's approval, the Yuzpe regimen had been approved by the drug regulatory agencies of the

United Kingdom, Germany, Sweden, Switzerland, and New Zealand. Another type of ECP, which contains a single progestin (levonorgestrel), first became available in Eastern Europe. Pharmaceutical companies have since introduced such products in other countries, including the United States, where the progestin-only ECP is known as PLAN B.

Before September 1998, no ECP product had been approved, labeled, and marketed in this country, and emergency hormonal contraception was available only through "off-label" use of oral contraceptive pills. Off-label use of approved medications is a common (and legal) practice, and some hospital emergency rooms, family planning clinics, and university health centers began providing women with emergency contraception this way. However, despite decades of safe and effective use of ECPs around the world, the off-label status of ECPs concerned some providers in the United States who were concerned about legal liability. There was no commercial advertising of emergency contraception, and most women knew nothing about it. In reproductive health circles, emergency contraception became known as "the nation's best-kept secret."

In February 1997, the FDA issued an official notice in the Federal Register, declaring common regimens of emergency contraception to be safe and effective. The FDA also said it would accept applications to manufacture and market ECPs without requiring expensive new drug trials, because the safety and efficacy of emergency contraception had already been demonstrated.

The FDA approved in 1998 the application of Gynetics, Inc., of Belle Mead, NJ, to market America's first dedicated ECP product, the PREVEN Emergency Contraceptive Kit. PREVEN consists of Yuzpe regimen ECPs, a pregnancy test, and instructions. The approval of PREVEN, however, did not mean the end of off-label use of oral contraceptive pills like ECPs. Some providers continue to prescribe oral contraceptive pills for emergency use, and for some women, the ECP dosage becomes the beginning of daily, non-emergency oral contraceptive use. The launch of PREVEN represented the first commercial ECP advertising to American women.

In July 1999, the FDA approved the first progestin-only ECP available in the United States. Produced by the Women's Capital Corporation of Bellevue, WA, Plan B contains only one hormone, the progestin levonorgestrel. A World Health Organization–supported study has found that the levonorgestrel regimen is more effective and has fewer side effects than the Yuzpe regimen.

Effectiveness

The Yuzpe regimen of combined estrogen and progestin ECPs reduces the risk of pregnancy by roughly 75%. Not every woman at risk of pregnancy actually becomes pregnant. On average, only 8 of 100 women will become pregnant after having unprotected sex during the second or third week of their menstrual cycles. If they take ECPs, only 2 of those 100 women will become pregnant; therefore, ECPs cut the risk of pregnancy by about 75%, preventing 6 of 8 likely pregnancies.

When used correctly, progestin-only ECPs were found to reduce the risk of pregnancy by 89% in a World Health Organization–supported study involving almost 2,000 women in 21 clinics around the world. When taken within 24 hours of unprotected intercourse, they were found to reduce the risk of pregnancy by 95%.

The amount of time between unprotected sex and the point in a woman's cycle at which she had sex influence the effectiveness of emergency contraception. The earlier ECPs are taken after unprotected sex, the more effective they are, and the closer a woman is to ovulation at the time of unprotected sex, the less likely that ECP will succeed. ECPs aren't as effective as consistent use of "before sex" methods such as the pill, the IUD, or contraceptive implants or injections, and they don't protect against sexually transmitted diseases.

Side Effects

Nausea and vomiting are far less common using progestin-only ECPs than using the Yuzpe regimen. In a recent World Health Organization–supported study using levonorgestrel, nausea occurred in 23.1% of cases, and vomiting in 5.6%. Other side effects were also less common.

emotions and infertility   Infertility can be an emotional roller coaster with dramatic highs and lows. Many couples experience anger that infertility seems to rule their lives, frustration that treatments can't guarantee a baby, and anxiety over the treatment procedures. A couple may experience an entire range of emotions at different times, such as after test results, during new treatments, holidays, or when friends announce their own pregnancies.

One of the most stressful parts of dealing with infertility is going through cycles of treatment, when it's normal for couples to feel frustrated and exhausted. Couples often feel that sex during treatment cycles is less than spontaneous and exciting, but this is a common experience. At times, psychological counseling and support may be needed.

empty sella syndrome   A condition that occurs when spinal fluid leaks into the bony chamber housing the pituitary gland. The pressure of the fluid compresses the pituitary gland and may interfere with its ability to secrete LH and FSH; this may result in higher prolactin levels.

Endocrine Society, The   With more than 10,000 members from 80 countries, the Endocrine Society is the world's largest and most active organization devoted to the research, study, and clinical practice of endocrinology. Together, the scientists, educators, clinicians, nurses, and students who make up the organization's membership represent all basic, applied, and clinical interests in endocrinology.

Since its inception in 1916, the Endocrine Society has worked to promote excellence in research, education, and the clinical practice of endocrinology. Contact: The Endocrine Society, 4350 East West Highway, Suite 500, Bethesda, MD; 20814-4410; phone: (301) 941-0200; website http://www.endo-society.org.

endocrine system   All tissues and major endocrine glands that secrete hormones including the thyroid, pancreas, parathyroid, pineal, adrenal, ovaries, testes, and pituitary. Many other organs also secrete hormones, including the kidney, heart, stomach, hypothalamus, brain, bone, and placenta. Hormones are body chemicals that profoundly affect every known physiological function. All aspects of reproduction are regulated by hormones.

Hormones set off and regulate reproduction, growth, development, and response to stress and the environment. They provide energy and nutrients important in cell function, and inhibit tumor growth and infection. These natural chemicals increase the body's efficiency and regulate activity levels, appetite and thirst, digestion, blood circulation, salt and water balance, and the excretion of metabolic wastes. Some promote storage of fuel after eating, and others access the reserves during exercise. Insulin and some other hormones are absolutely essential for sustaining human life. They also influence mood, perception, libido, learning, memory, and behavior. See also ENDOCRINOLOGY; ENDOCRINOLOGIST.

endocrinologist   A professional who specializes in diagnosis and treatment of problems related to hormones or endocrine gland abnormalities. Endocrinologists are involved in either the research, study, or clinical application of this vast area of human health. A wide spectrum of professionals make up the field of endocrinology, including physicians, biochemists, physiologists, geneticists, educators, immunologists, pharmacologists, molecular and cellular biologists, veterinarians, neuroendocrinologists, nurses, and technicians.

Endocrinologists conduct research and provide treatment for a wide range of functions and disorders of the human body, including infertility, metabolism, glandular cancers, birth control, short stature, growth, genetic dysfunction, diabetes, heart disease, and hormonal imbalances.

Clinical and research endocrinologists work in a variety of settings, including private practice, industry, education, and the government. Clinical endocrinologists are physicians who complete an internship and residency program specializing in endocrinology.

endocrinology   All of the disciplines concerned with circulating and locally acting hormones and their roles in health and disease. Endocrinology is unique in its impact on all aspects of human health, including a wide range of regulatory functions and disorders of the human body. See also ENDOCRINE SYSTEM; ENDOCRINOLOGIST.

endometrial atrophy   Thinning of the lining of the uterus, usually due to lack of the hormone ESTROGEN.

endometrial biopsy   A removal of a small piece of the uterine lining for microscopic study. It can be used to check for LUTEAL PHASE DEFECT (to see if the lining of the uterus is ready to allow implantation of an embryo), to confirm OVULATION, and also to rule out benign and malignant disorders of the uterine lining.

The biopsy is usually performed late in the cycle, 1 to 2 days before a menstrual period is expected. A couple should not have sex, or they should use barrier contraception during the cycle in which the biopsy is performed.

endometrial cavity   The space inside the uterus.

endometrial hyperplasia Overgrowth or thickening of the lining of the uterus usually caused by prolonged action of estrogen unopposed by PROGESTERONE, typically as the result of POLYCYSTIC OVARY SYNDROME. This condition is especially dangerous because it can lead to uterine cancer if left untreated.

Unless the lining of the uterus sheds regularly, tissues and glands will build up and may later become a breeding ground for abnormal cells. Any woman of childbearing age who has missed more than two consecutive periods but is not pregnant needs to investigate the reason.

During adolescence and in the years before menopause, women may have many cycles without ovulation during which there is continuous unopposed estrogen activity. Polycystic ovary syndrome is another condition in which women don't ovulate and have unopposed estrogen. Similarly, hormone replacement therapy with estrogen without progesterone may lead to endometrial hyperplasia.

Types

Some cases of hyperplasia are more advanced than others. *Mild hyperplasia,* known as cystic glandular hyperplasia or cystic endometrial hyperplasia, is characterized by an excess of tissue with normal endometrial cells. This kind of hyperplasia is always caused by too much estrogen and rarely develops into cancer.

When mild hyperplasia isn't treated, it may lead to *adenomatous hyperplasia without atypical cells.* This benign condition refers to a buildup of of glandular cells (the glandular endometrial cells are growing but are still noncancerous). This kind of hyperplasia rarely develops into cancer.

Atypical adenomatous hyperplasia (also called severe hyperplasia or carcinoma in situ—CIS) means that either a small area on the endometrium or the entire lining consists of cells that are abnormal. The cells seem to be more aggressive but may still be harmless. It still isn't malignant, but more women with severe hyperplasia may go on to develop uterine cancer.

Risk

Women who are 25 to 50 pounds overweight are three times as likely to develop hyperplasia. Women who are more than 50 pounds overweight are nine times as likely to develop hyperplasia. Women at higher risk also include those who have always had irregular periods or who have DIABETES. Other potential causes of excess estrogen include environmental toxins; certain herbs (such as ginseng); hormone-fed meats and poultry; certain cosmetics made from estrogen; and hormonal contraceptives that contain estrogen.

A postmenopausal woman with an intact uterus on unopposed estrogen replacement therapy (ERT) is also at risk for developing hyperplasia. An estrogen/progesterone combination therapy can reverse as much as 96.8 percent of all postmenopausal hyperplasia cases.

Diagnosis

This diagnosis can only be made by the pathologist who examines a sample of tissue removed from the thickened endometrium by a sampling procedure such as ENDOMETRIAL BIOPSY, D&C, or HYSTEROSCOPY.

Treatment

In younger women particularly, severe hyperplasia can be reversed with hormonal therapy. Adding progesterone by taking a progestin or resuming ovulation (spontaneously or with medications) can eliminate hyperplasia. If this doesn't work, a D&C is the next logical step. A hysterectomy is not necessary unless the hyperplasia persists after the lining is removed. If severe hyperplasia persists and keeps redeveloping despite HRT and a repeat D&C, then a hysterectomy may be required.

endometrial polyp An overgrowth of endometrium tissue that forms grapelike structures within the uterus. These polyps may not cause any symptoms but sometimes may lead to abnormal bleeding. The problem can often be diagnosed at a HYSTEROSALPINGOGRAM or HYSTEROSCOPY.

endometriomas   See CHOCOLATE CYST.

endometriosis   A chronic condition in which some of the normal endometrial tissue is found outside the uterus—most often in the pelvic area involving the ovaries. Less often, it may be found in the lung, arm, thigh, and other locations. Endometriosis may also interfere with ovulation and with the implantation of the embryo. It affects 5.5 million women and girls in the United States and Canada, and millions more worldwide.

This misplaced tissue responds to the menstrual cycle in the same way that the tissue of the uterine lining does: Each month the tissue builds up, breaks down, and sheds. Since the blood and tissue shed from endometrial growths has no way of leaving the body, this leads to internal bleeding, breakdown of the blood and tissue from the lesions, and inflammation, causing pain, infertility, scar tissue, and bowel problems.

Common sites for endometriosis growths include the ovaries, the fallopian tubes, the ligaments that support the uterus, and, sometimes, the bladder, bowel, or vagina. It can occur in menstruating women of all ages, including teenagers.

While the connection between less severe forms of endometriosis and infertility is not clearly understood, early detection may result in successful control and preservation of fertility. Endometriosis runs in families, so a woman should tell the doctor if her mother or sisters had symptoms or were diagnosed with the disease.

Cause

The cause of endometriosis is unknown. Some experts believe that during menstruation, some of the menstrual tissue flows backward through the fallopian tubes, and then implants in the abdomen and grows. Since all women experience some menstrual tissue backflow, experts believe that an immune system problem or a hormonal problem allows this tissue to grow in the women who develop endometriosis.

Another theory suggests that endometrial tissue moves from the uterus to other parts of the body through the lymphatic or blood systems. Some experts believe that heredity may play a role and that the disease may be carried in the genes in certain families or that some families may have predisposing factors to endometriosis.

Yet another theory suggests that remnants of embryonic tissue may later develop into endometriosis or that some adult tissues retain the ability they had in the embryo stage to transform reproductive tissue in certain circumstances.

Research by the ENDOMETRIOSIS ASSOCIATION revealed a startling link between the toxic chemical dioxin (TCCD) exposure and the development of endometriosis. Dioxin is a toxic chemical by-product of pesticide manufacturing, bleached pulp and paper products, and medical and municipal waste incineration. The EA discovered a colony of rhesus monkeys that had developed endometriosis after exposure to dioxin. In this research, 79% of the monkeys exposed to dioxin developed endometriosis, and the more dioxin exposure, the more severe the endometriosis.

Symptoms

Increased estrogen levels cause endometriosis tissue to grow and bleed, which causes irritation, swelling, painful menstrual cramps that may worsen with time, diarrhea or painful bowel movements (especially around the menstrual period), and painful sexual intercourse.

Diagnosis

The condition may not cause any symptoms. The diagnosis in most cases must be confirmed with LAPAROSCOPY, a minor surgical procedure in which the surgeon can view the inside of the abdomen through a tiny lighted tube that is inserted through one or more small abdominal incisions. A laparoscopy usually shows the location, size, and extent of the growths that can help doctor and patient make better treatment choices.

Treatment

Although there is no cure for endometriosis, a variety of treatment options exist (short of hysterectomy) that can ease pain, shrink or slow endometrial growths, restore fertility, and prevent or delay recurrence.

Doctors may prescribe over-the-counter pain relievers such as aspirin and Tylenol, as well as prostaglandin inhibitors such as ibuprofen, naproxen sodium, indomethecin, and tolfenamic acid. In some cases, prescription drugs may be required.

Hormonal treatment is designed to stop ovulation for as long as possible and may include BIRTH CONTROL PILLS, PROGESTERONE drugs, a TESTOSTERONE derivative (DANAZOL), and GNRH AGONISTS (GONADOTROPIN-RELEASING HORMONE drugs). Side effects may be a problem for some women.

Surgery may be needed to remove or destroy the growths and relieve pain. Surgery also may allow pregnancy to occur in some cases. Conservative surgery can involve laparoscopy or laparotomy (a more extensive procedure with a full incision and longer recovery period). Hormonal therapy may be prescribed along with surgery.

More radical surgery may be necessary in severe cases; a HYSTERECTOMY removes all growths and may include removal of ovaries.

Endometriosis Association, The   A nonprofit, self-help organization dedicated to providing information and support to patients with ENDOMETRIOSIS. The group provides information about the disease, and conducts and promotes research related to endometriosis.

The Endometriosis Association was the first organization in the world created for those with endometriosis. As an independent self-help organization of women with endometriosis, doctors, and others interested in the disease, it is a recognized authority in its field, whose goal is to work toward finding a cure for the disease as well as providing education, support, and research.

Founded in Milwaukee, WI, in 1980 by Mary Lou Ballweg and Carolyn Keith, it is now a worldwide organization with a network of chapters, groups, and sponsors in 66 countries throughout the world. Information is available in 25 different languages. The group offers a wide range of literature, fact sheets, videotapes, and audiotapes.

As part of its research program, the association has established a special program at Dartmouth Medical School and has funded and assisted a number of researchers in various parts of the world. It also maintains a large research registry and continues work on the relationship between dioxin and endometriosis, a relationship the association discovered. The association has recently joined with Vanderbilt University School of Medicine to create a dedicated research facility to address the cause of endometriosis. Among other research projects supported by the association are a study of dioxin-exposed young women in Seveso, Italy; publicity and help obtaining patients and families for a genetic study at Oxford University, England; support for research on a noninvasive dignostic technique by a U.S. researcher; and small grants and tissue samples for a number of researchers studying dioxin and related toxins and endometriosis. For more information, contact the Endometriosis Association International Headquarters at 8585 North 76th Place, Milwaukee, WI 53223 USA; phone (414) 355-2200 or (800) 992-3636; Internet http://www.endometriosisassn.org.

endometritis   Infection or inflammation of the uterine lining. Endometritis may occur after childbirth, ABORTION, or INTRAUTERINE DEVICE (IUD) insertion. Other risk factors include a history of SALPINGITIS, CERVICITIS, or other pelvic infections, including SEXUALLY TRANSMITTED DISEASES.

It's possible to prevent endometritis by using safer sexual practices and by early diagnosis and adequate treatment of sexually transmitted diseases. The risk is reduced by careful, sterile techniques used by doctors performing deliveries, abortions, IUD insertions, and other gynecological procedures.

Symptoms

General discomfort, uneasiness, malaise, fever from 100° to 104°F, lower abdominal or pelvic pain, abnormal vaginal bleeding or discharge, discomfort with bowel movement, or constipation.

Diagnosis

Tests may include blood tests, culture, an endometrial biopsy, or a laparoscopy.

Treatment

More complicated cases (those occurring after childbirth or those involving more widespread or well-established infection) may require hospitalization and antibiotics. Rest and fluids are important. It is essential to treat sexual partner(s) and have the patient use condoms throughout the course of treatment.

Prognosis

Most cases of endometritis are curable with antibiotics. Untreated endometritis can progress to more serious infection and result in complications with pelvic organs, reproduction, and general health.

environmental estrogens and infertility   Environmental estrogens are chemicals in the environment that act like the female sex hormone ESTROGEN (ESTRADIOL). These estrogenlike chemicals may occur naturally in nature in plants and in the human diet. Others are man-made and may be found in plastics or insecticides such as PCBs, DDT, dioxins, and furans. Another man-made chemical that mimics estrogen is DIETHYLSTILBESTROL (DES), which has been used in the past to prevent MISCARRIAGE and to promote growth in livestock and poultry.

It is important to understand the effects of these compounds, because they may remain in the body for a long time and mimic the action of natural hormones, which are the chemical messengers of the body's endocrine system, triggering or blocking a response to the body's natural hormones.

The natural hormonal balance maintains normal body activities by binding to receptor molecules in cell tissues like the breast, uterus, prostate, brain, and skin. There the receptor acts as the translator of the hormone in the cell. When synthetic compounds mimic these hormones, they also bind to the receptor. Some foreign chemicals interact with the estrogen receptor and produce estrogenlike effects on the development of the brain, male and female reproductive organs, and breasts, causing a variety of disorders, including overgrowth of the vaginal lining, premature breast development, feminization of male offspring, and infertility.

Infertility strikes one out of every 25 men, and between 30% to 40% of these men have abnormal sperm (either the sperm look abnormal, don't move properly, are dead, or occur in very low numbers). More and more evidence suggests that MALE FACTOR INFERTILITY is rising as a result, at least in part, of environmental toxins. There has been a decline in the quality of human semen since 1973, according to one 1995 report published in the *New England Journal of Medicine.* Environmental estrogens also have been linked to rising cases of reproductive cancer in both men and women, and in ENDOMETRIOSIS and FIBROIDS in women.

Much more information is needed to understand the adverse effects of these compounds and how they affect daily life, especially in children and the elderly. For instance, contamination of food with the man-made estrogen DES has been associated with premature breast development in young boys and girls. Exposure to estrogen during sexual development has been associated with feminization of the male reproductive system in animals; estrogens contained in plants can decrease reproduction in wild and domestic animals that eat them.

Research continues to examine environmental factors and mechanisms for a wide range of conditions that affect the human endocrine system, including infertility, aging, cancer, AIDS, asthma, and birth defects. More research is needed to evaluate the possible public-health effects of known environmental estrogens and the potential estrogenic activities of other chemicals.

environmental factors and infertility   Exposure to some types of chemicals and environmental toxins may affect a person's ability to conceive. For reasons that are "largely unknown," according to the National Toxicology Program and the National Institute of Environmental Health Science (NIEHS):

- between 5% and 10% of couples who want to have children can't
- about half of all pregnancies aren't successfully completed, and NIEHS research has shown that many fertilized fetuses disappear before the prospective mother is even aware she is pregnant
- some 3% to 5% of newborns suffer from major birth defects
- a decline in human sperm counts over recent decades has been reported

In part because of these concerns, NIEHS and the National Toxicology Program established the Center for the Evaluation of Risks to Human Reproduction to convene experts to evaluate data indicating that a chemical or mixtures of chemicals could impair human reproduction and development.

The testicles are the most sensitive to environmental agents in a man's body; pesticides, radiation, and industrial solvents are all capable of affecting sperm production by interfering with hormone production or sperm formation. Because the cells in the testicles make new sperm each day, they are especially vulnerable to toxic substances (such as radiation and cancer drugs) that primarily affect rapidly dividing cells.

There is considerable controversy over which substances may harm fertility, but several sub-stances are currently regulated because they have been shown to affect a couple's ability to have a child. They include:

Lead
Exposure to lead has been shown to affect fertility in humans, including people who work with paints or varnish, or people who manufacture autos.

Dibromochloropropane (DBCP)
Handling toxins found in pesticides such as DBCP may cause ovarian problems that could lead to early menopause.

Ethylene oxide
Exposure to this chemical used in sterilization of surgical instruments and manufacturing pesticides may cause birth defects in early pregnancy and has the potential to trigger early miscarriages.

Methoxychlor
Recent rat studies suggest that exposure to breakdown products of this pesticide used to preserve fruits and vegetables significantly lowered testosterone levels.

Radiation and Chemotherapy
Exposure to these medical treatments has been shown to affect sperm production and contribute to ovarian problems. See also CENTER FOR THE EVALUATION OF RISKS TO HUMAN REPRODUCTION; CHEMICALS AND INFERTILITY.

epididymal sperm aspiration (ESA)   A technique in which a surgeon removes sperm from the epididymas to be used for INTRACYTOPLASMIC SPERM INJECTION (ICSI) at the time of IN VITRO FERTILIZATION (IVF).

epididymal obstruction   An obstruction of the tiny tubular structure called the EPIDIDYMIS attached to the testicle where sperm mature and are stored. Such an obstruction can block the passage of sperm to the penis that leads to lower sperm counts and impaired fertility. Normally, however, the other epididymis (if not also obstructed) should be able to produce enough sperm cells.

Cause

Epididymal obstruction may be caused by a number of different problems, including

- birth defects (the lack of a VAS DEFERENS and part of the epididymis)
- infection or inflammation: history of EPI-DIDYMITIS (tuberculosis or chlamydia)
- accidental injury: from prior surgery such as hydrocele repair or surgery for undescended testes, testis biopsy, or after a VASECTOMY

Treatment

The microsurgical treatment for epididymis obstruction is called a vasoepididymostomy, a specialized procedure for the treatment of male infertility. Surgeons must have experience to be able to properly perform this procedure on the vas deferens and epididymis.

epididymis   A coiled, tubular organ attached to and lying on the testicle that stores the sperm before ejaculation. Within this organ the developing sperm mature, eventually leaving through the VAS DEFERENS. Sperm that have not passed through the epididymis fertilize an egg very poorly, if at all.

After they pass through this organ, sperm are more ready to fertilize an egg. This is because in the epididymis, sperm go through certain maturational steps not yet well understood. Scientists are studying certain proteins produced in the epididymis that may have an effect on sperm.

epididymitis   An inflammation of the EPI-DIDYMIS (the first part of the duct draining each testis) that may cause infertility if the infection spreads to the testicles. Epididymitis is typically caused by bacterial organisms associated with urinary tract infections, SEXUALLY TRANSMITTED DISEASES (such as chlamydia and gonorrhea), infec-

tion of the prostate, or following removal of the prostate. Sexually active men who don't practice safe sex are at higher risk, as are men who have recently had surgery or have a history of structural problems involving the genitourinary tract.

Symptoms

Epididymitis may begin with a mild fever and chills and a heavy sensation in the testicle, which becomes increasingly sensitive to pressure. There may be lower abdominal discomfort or pelvic discomfort, and urination may cause burning or pain. Sometimes there may be a discharge from the urethra, blood in the semen, or pain on ejaculation.

Diagnosis

A physical examination together with urinalysis and culture, chlamydia and gonorrhea tests, complete blood count, and blood chemistry.

Treatment

Antibiotics together with bed rest, elevation of the scrotum, and ice packs applied to the area. Epididymitis usually responds to appropriate antibiotic therapy without any damage to sexual or reproductive abilities, but recurrence is fairly common and sometimes may develop into a chronic problem.

epididymovasostomy   The reversal of a VASECTOMY; reconnecting the vas deferens to the epididymis because of an obstruction in the vas deferens. The vas deferens is responsible for directing and propelling the sperm into the urethra.

Normally, a vasectomy is reversed by reconnecting the two severed ends of the vas deferens. This procedure is called a VASOVASOSTOMY. However, in some cases the surgeon finds that one part of the vas deferens is still blocked at another point. In this case, the one end of the vas deferens is connected directly to the epididymis, bypassing the other vas deferens.

The surgeon's skill is extremely important in performing this procedure. The complex surgery is performed under a general anesthetic, although a regional anesthetic (spinal or epidural) can also be used.

CRYOPRESERVATION of sperm (sperm banking) is often performed at the time of vasectomy reversal if whole, moving sperm are found. Cryopreservation is performed just in case there are low sperm counts after surgery, requiring ICSI and IVF in the future.

The typical pregnancy rate with this procedure is about 45%—lower than with a standard vasovasostomy, which ranges between 50% and 75%.

epispadias A rare malformation of the penis present at birth, in which the urethral opening is located on the top surface anywhere along the shaft. The foreskin is not completely formed, and the shaft curves upward. If the condition is severe (the urinary opening is close to the body), reconstructive surgery is usually advised immediately, because the rest of the bladder may be involved and the child may have complete urinary incontinence. Epispadias occurs only once in every 120,000 male births. A pediatric urologist should be consulted in any case of epispadias. Rarely, girls may be born with the female version of this condition.

Epispadias in boys is found in one of three forms:

- urethra open on top of the head of the penis
- entire urethra open the full length of the penis
- entire urethra open with the bladder opening on the abdominal wall

Males with this condition have normal sperm production. However, if the problem is untreated, ejaculated sperm can't be deposited directly into the cervix. This is corrected through plastic surgery, which constructs a new opening at the tip of the penis and closes up the old opening.

Treatment

Surgery usually can repair the damage so that urine flows correctly and that the penis looks normal. However, persistent urinary incontinence can occur in some people even after surgery. See also HYPOSPADIA.

erectile dysfunction (ED) The persistent or repeated inability for at least three months of getting or keeping an erection that's firm enough for sexual satisfaction. Experts estimate that 30 million men in the United States suffer from ED, popularly known as impotence, but 95% of those cases can be treated.

Erectile dysfunction is a more precise term than impotence, which some associate with being sterile or lacking vigor or power. ED is also defined by the degree to which it bothers the man and his partner. Occasional ED is not uncommon and perfectly normal, but a persistent problem is usually caused by psychological factors. However, medical tests should be done to rule out any physical problem in the case of chronic ED. Although ED is not an inevitable consequence of aging, its incidence increases with age because the condition is often a side effect of other medical problems that come with age, such as vascular disease or DIABETES.

Normal function

The penis contains two chambers filled with spongy tissue, smooth muscles, fibrous tissues, veins, and arteries. The urethra, which is the channel for urine and ejaculate, runs along the underside of the chambers.

Erection begins as impulses from the brain and local nerves relax the muscles of the penis so that blood flows in, filling the open spaces and making the penis expand. Erection is reversed when muscles in the penis contract, stopping the inflow of blood and opening outflow channels.

Since an erection requires a sequence of events, ED can occur when there is a problem with any of the events. Disease-related damage to arteries, smooth muscles, and fibrous tissues is the most common cause of impotence; diabetes, kidney problems, alcoholism, multiple sclerosis, atherosclerosis, and vascular disease account for about 70% of ED.

In addition, surgery can injure nerves and arteries near the penis, and injury to the penis, spinal cord, prostate, bladder, and pelvis can lead to ED by damaging nerves, smooth muscles, arteries, and fibrous tissues. Many common medicines also can lead to ED, including high blood pressure drugs, antihistamines, antidepressants, tranquilizers, appetite suppressants, and the ulcer drug cimetidine.

Experts believe that 10% to 20% of ED is caused by psychological factors such as stress, anxiety, guilt, depression, low self-esteem, and fear of sexual failure. Other possible causes of impotence are smoking, which affects blood flow in veins and arteries, and hormonal abnormalities, such as insufficient testosterone.

Diagnosis

The doctor will begin with a medical and sexual history to understand the nature of the problem, and look for diseases that might have caused the problem. Lab tests for systemic diseases related to ED include blood counts, urinalysis, lipid profile, and measurements of creatinine and liver enzymes. For cases of low sexual desire, testosterone measurements can reveal information about any hormone problems. Monitoring erections that occur during sleep can help rule out certain psychological causes of ED. Since healthy men have involuntary erections during sleep, a lack of nocturnal erections suggests the cause of ED is probably physical, not psychological. Tests of nocturnal erections are not completely reliable, however. Scientists have not standardized such tests and have not determined when they should be applied for best results.

The following specialists may play a role in the diagnosis and treatment of erectile dysfunction:

- UROLOGISTS: These specialists most commonly treat ED, especially those with physical causes. Urologists can diagnose and treat ED and evaluate the nerves, arteries and veins that control the erection process. They also prescribe medications and perform surgery to correct erection problems.

- Psychologists and psychiatrists: These specialists treat psychological causes of ED, such as depression, anxiety, and relationship problems.

- ENDOCRINOLOGISTS: an appropriate choice if ED is due to testosterone deficiency, a thyroid disorder, or another hormonal prblem.

Treatment

Treatments for ED depend on the underlying cause. Medication-related ED will be treated by cutting back on any harmful drugs. Psychological factors respond well to therapy or behavior modification. Underlying medical conditions should be treated to restore erectile function. If these treatments aren't effective, there are several other options.

Drugs for treating impotence can be taken orally, injected directly into the penis, or inserted into the urethra at the tip of the penis. Sildenafil citrate (Viagra) was the first oral pill to treat ED. Approved in 1998, Viagra is taken an hour before sex and works by enhancing the effects of nitric oxide, a chemical that relaxes smooth muscles in the penis during sexual stimulation, boosting blood flow. While Viagra improves the response to sexual stimulation, it doesn't trigger an automatic erection as injected drugs do.

Oral testosterone can reduce impotence in some men with low levels of natural testosterone. Patients also have claimed effectiveness of other oral drugs, including yohimbine hydrochloride, dopamine and serotonin agonists, and trazodone, but no scientific studies have proved the effectiveness of these drugs in relieving ED.

Many men gain potency by injecting drugs into the penis, causing it to become engorged with blood. Drugs such as papaverine hydrochloride, phentolamine, and alprostadil (Caverject) widen blood vessels. However, these drugs may create unwanted side effects, including persistent erection (known as priapism) and scarring. Nitroglycerin, a muscle relaxant, sometimes can enhance erection when rubbed on the surface of the penis.

A system for inserting a pellet of alprostadil into the urethra is marketed as MUSE. The system uses a pre-filled applicator to deliver the pellet about an inch deep into the urethra at the tip of the penis. An erection will begin within 8 to 10 minutes and may last 30 to 60 minutes. The most common side effects of the preparation are aching in the penis, testicles, and area between the penis and rectum; warmth or burning sensation in the urethra; redness of the penis due to increased blood flow; and minor urethral bleeding or spotting.

Mechanical vacuum devices cause an erection by creating a partial vacuum around the penis, which draws blood into the penis, engorging and expanding it. The penis is placed into a plastic cylinder, and a pump draws air out of the cylinder. An elastic band is placed around the base of the penis, to maintain the erection after the cylinder is removed and during intercourse by preventing blood from flowing back into the body. A variation of the vacuum device is a semi-rigid rubber sheath placed on the penis that remains there during sex.

If the above treatments aren't successful, surgery may be used to implant a device to cause the penis to become erect, to reconstruct arteries to boost blood flow to the penis, or to block off veins that allow blood to leak from the penile tissues. Implanted devices can restore erection in many men with ED, but they carry risks of breaking down and infection, although mechanical problems have diminished in recent years because of technological advances. Malleable implants usually consist of paired rods, which are inserted surgically into the twin chambers running the length of the penis. The user manually adjusts the position of the penis and, therefore, the rods. Adjustment does not affect the width or length of the penis.

Inflatable implants consist of paired cylinders surgically inserted inside the penis that can be expanded using pressurized fluid. Tubes connect the cylinders to a fluid reservoir and pump, which also are surgically implanted. The patient inflates the cylinders by pressing on the small pump, located under the skin in the scrotum. Inflatable implants can expand the length and width of the penis somewhat. They also leave the penis in a more natural state when not inflated.

Surgery to repair arteries can reduce ED caused by obstructions that block the flow of blood to the penis. The best candidates for such surgery are young men with blocked artery due to an injury to the crotch or pelvic fracture. The procedure is less successful in older men with widespread blockage.

Surgery to veins that allow blood to leave the penis usually involves an opposite procedure—intentional blockage. Blocking off veins can reduce the leakage of blood that diminishes rigidity of the penis during erection. However, experts have raised questions about this procedure's long-term effectiveness.

An oral form of the drug phentolamine may soon be available as another choice for a noninvasive ED treatment. Other treatments in the experimental stages include reconstruction surgery for damaged veins and arteries in the penis. Whether or not this method proves to be safe and effective, ongoing improvements in traditional methods should continue to create more successful and widespread treatment of impotence.

Prevention

Recent research has found that exercise can help prevent the onset of ED, according to the Massachusetts Male Aging Study. Men who burned 200 calories or more a day in physical activity (a level that can be met with as little as two miles or brisk walking) cut their risk in half. The researchers also found that the more exercise, the lower the chances that men would develop impotence.

The findings make physiological sense because regular aerobic exercise fights vascular disease, including fat clogs that narrow the arteries. Such clogs could block blood flow through arteries that engorge the penis, so exercise should help to keep those arteries healthy and clear.

Estrace   A brand name for ESTRADIOL.

Estraderm   A brand name for ESTRADIOL.

estradiol   The principal and most powerful natural ESTROGEN produced by the ovary and released during OVULATION. Estradiol (E2) is responsible for the formation of the female secondary sex characteristics; it also supports the growth of the follicle and the development of the uterine lining.

Eggs contain follicles that contain cells designed to produce estradiol and release it into the blood. Since the more follicles, the more estradiol, measuring the estradiol level helps measure how many follicles are actively developing. The longer they continue to develop, the longer the estradiol level continues. As they develop, the level continues to rise. This rise can further indicate that the egg within the follicles is reaching its maturity.

Tests for Estradiol

The level of estradiol is measured in almost every blood sample taken during the monitoring of almost every type of assisted pregnancy. It is arguably the most informative of the three tests. The blood test to monitor estradiol is called E2—Rapid Assay. Women on FERTILITY DRUGS may have E2 measured to determine the ovarian response.

Blood tests of estradiol can be used together with ultrasound scans to help indicate how (and if) the ovaries are responding to stimulation. While exact figures aren't possible (estradiol levels vary from one person to the next) as a rough guide, a level in the range of 150 to 500 pg/ml is generally considered reasonable for the eighth day of a stimulated cycle. An approximate doubling of this level every 48 hours is considered a sign of continued good follicle development.

estrogen   One of the two principal female sex hormones (the other is PROGESTERONE) responsible for triggering growth of the female reproductive system—including the vagina, cervix, uterus, and the fallopian tubes—and the growth of the breasts. In the first half of the menstrual cycle (prior to ovulation), this hormone stimulates the uterine wall to become richly supplied with blood. Estrogen also boosts the amount and thins the consistency of cervical mucus, about day 14 of the menstrual cycle. Estrogen production drops off during the second phase of the menstrual cycle. As estrogen levels drop, the top layer of the uterine lining begins to slough off, flowing from the body as menstrual discharge.

The primary estrogen is ESTRADIOL, which is produced by the developing follicle in the ovary as well as the CORPUS LUTEUM (the empty follicle after the egg has emerged), the placenta, and the body's fat tissues.

After MENOPAUSE, the most prevalent estrogen is the weaker one (ESTRONE), produced by the conversion of ANDROSTENEDIONE by the body's fat.

estrone   A weak form of ESTROGEN that is converted in the uterus to the stronger hormone ESTRADIOL. It is the main estrogen in the blood after MENOPAUSE.

ethinyl estradiol   An oral form of ESTRADIOL often found in BIRTH CONTROL PILLS.

extracorporeal fertilization   See IN VITRO FERTILIZATION.

exercise and infertility   Proper exercise is an important part of maintaining good health and has no effect on reproduction, but excessive exercise can interfere with sperm and egg production by decreasing the brain messages to testes and ovaries.

A normal exercise program will not affect fertility for most couples. While it's impossible to know just how much exercise is too much for any one person, it's generally believed that running more than 10 miles a week is considered too much when trying to conceive. The best way to treat fertility problems caused by too much exercise is to decrease or modify the amount of exercise.

fallopian tubes Hollow ducts through which eggs travel to the UTERUS once released from the FOLLICLE. SPERM normally meet the egg in the fallopian tube, the site at which FERTILIZATION usually occurs. The fallopian tubes play a crucial role in reproduction. This complex organ is capable of picking up a newly released egg, providing nutrients and movement for it, and then transporting sperm up to the egg. Once the sperm arrives, the fallopian tubes sustain an environment for fertilization and then transport the fertilized egg into the uterus.

Fallopian Tube Infertility

Fallopian tube disease accounts for about 20% of INFERTILITY cases. One cause of infertility is a blocked or damaged fallopian tube, which interferes with the egg and sperm meeting, or with proper embryo implantation after fertilization. Blocked tubes can be caused by PELVIC INFLAMMATORY DISEASE or an infection as a result of an IUD or bacteria, such as CHLAMYDIA or GONORRHEA. Other causes may include ENDOMETRIOSIS, TUBAL LIGATION (sterilization), abnormalities present since birth, or lower abdominal surgery. There may be no symptoms at all to indicate a problem with the fallopian tubes, which may only be discovered during an infertility exam.

To test whether or not the fallopian tubes are open, the doctor performs a HYSTEROSALPINGOGRAM (a special X ray of the uterus and fallopian tubes). This diagnostic test can detect any birth defects involving the uterus and fallopian tubes, fibrous masses in the uterus, and adhesions (fibrous bands that connect normally unconnected structures) in the uterus or pelvis.

For reasons not clearly understood, fertility appears to be slightly improved after a normal hysterosalpingogram is performed. Therefore, the doctor may wait to see if a woman becomes pregnant after this test has been performed before ordering additional tests of fallopian tube function.

If the hysterosalpingogram shows a problem such as scars in the uterus, the doctor will examine the uterus with a hysteroscope (a viewing tube inserted through the cervix into the uterus). The hysteroscope may be manipulated to break adhesions during the procedure, which can then boost chances for pregnancy.

If more information is needed, the doctor can insert a LAPAROSCOPE (a small viewing tube) through a small incision in the abdomen. This procedure, typically performed with general anesthesia, allows the doctor to see the uterus, fallopian tubes, and ovaries. The laparoscope also may be used to remove abnormal tissue if the woman has ENDOMETRIOSIS or to break adhesions in the pelvic cavity.

Drugs can be used to treat endometriosis, and antibiotics can treat infections. Surgery can try to repair a damaged fallopian tube caused by ECTOPIC PREGNANCY, tubal ligation, or infection, but it results in a low rate of normal pregnancies and a high rate of ectopic pregnancies. For these reasons, surgery isn't recommended often. See also FALLOPOSCOPY.

falloposcopy A procedure in which a doctor can look inside the FALLOPIAN TUBE from the direction of the UTERUS with a very small flexible, fiber optic instrument. The scope is passed through the cervix and uterus into the tubes, which allows a doctor to diagnose the health of the tube lining.

This type of examination can help decide whether tubal corrective surgery or IN VITRO FERTILIZATION would be the better treatment for tubal infertility. Falloposcopy is an outpatient procedure that requires no incision and only light anesthesia. Obstruction of the uterine end of the tube also can often be corrected through the falloposcope. However, this test isn't common or part of a routine fertility examination.

family planning   See NATURAL FAMILY PLANNING.

FASIAR   The abbreviation for "follicle aspiration, sperm injection, and assisted follicular rupture," an experimental technique to treat INFERTILITY.

In this technique, after inducing OVULATION the doctor punctures the FOLLICLE and retrieves the eggs and fluid in a syringe that also contains SPERM. The mixture is then reinjected near the ruptured follicle. The procedure can be done in the physician's office. However, the technique has not been proven successful, and is rarely performed.

fecundability   The ability to become pregnant.

fecundity rate   The ability of a woman to become pregnant during any given month. It is described as a percentage (such as 25% per month).

female condom   A type of barrier BIRTH CONTROL designed for women. Less likely to slip or burst than the male version, the female condom is a lubricated polyurethane sheath with a closed flexible ring at one end and a larger open ring at the other. The closed ring is inserted into the vagina, fitting over the cervix, leaving the open end hanging outside the vagina where it partially covers the labia.

Female condoms were approved by the FDA in 1993 and are sold under the brand names Femidom and Reality. They must be removed carefully after sex, and a fresh condom must be inserted for each subsequent act of sexual intercourse. If these rules are followed, the female condom seems to be as effective as the diaphragm or cervical cap. A female condom should not be used together with a male condom because they may not both stay in place.

female factor infertility   A woman may be infertile because some parts of her reproductive system aren't functioning properly due to disease, infections, problems with hormone production, or problems present from birth.

In women, five key hormones serve as chemical messengers to manage the reproductive system. The hypothalamus first releases GONADOTROPIN-RELEASING HORMONE (Gn-RH) which in turn stimulates the pituitary gland to produce FOLLICLE-STIMULATING HORMONE (FSH) and LUTEINIZING HORMONE (LH). ESTROGEN and PROGESTERONE, secreted by the OVARIES, complete the hormonal interplay necessary for conception.

Blocked tubes account for about 35% of all female infertility problems, and irregular or abnormal ovulation accounts for about a quarter of all female infertility cases. ENDOMETRIOSIS is found in another 35% of infertile women who have LAPAROSCOPY as part of their infertility workup.

Female infertility factors can interfere with reproduction in a number of ways:

- OVULATION may not occur.
- The UTERUS may not be properly prepared to receive the developing embryo, either because of congenital problems, surgical scarring, or fibroids and polyps.
- FALLOPIAN TUBES may be blocked, diseased, or scarred with adhesions from previous surgery, previous infections, or ECTOPIC PREGNANCY.

- There may not be adequate CERVICAL MUCUS for the sperm's survival.
- abnormalities of the cervix.

A cause can be found in about 80% of infertility cases, but despite extensive tests, for about 20% of couples the cause remains elusive. There are a number of factors that could cause a woman to be infertile, including age, weight, exercise, lifestyle, job or environmental toxicity, emotions, and disease.

Age

Between 1982 and 1988 there was an increase of 37% in childless women between the ages of 35 to 44. The number of infertile women is expected to reach 6.3 million in the year 2000 and may rise to 7.7 million in 2025. A woman's age (or, more precisely, the age of her eggs) plays a major role in fertility.

At age 25, the chance of getting pregnant within the first 6 months of trying is 75%; at age 40, it falls to 22%. This decrease in fertility appears to be due to a higher rate of chromosome and genetic damage to the eggs as time passes.

Weight and Excess Exercise

Although most of a woman's estrogen is produced in her ovaries, 30% is produced by fat cells. Because a normal hormonal balance is essential for conception, extreme weight levels can contribute to infertility. Body fat levels that are 10% to 15% above normal can produce too much estrogen, which will interfere with the reproductive cycle. Body fat levels 10% to 15% below normal can completely shut down the reproductive process. Women with eating disorders such as anorexia or bulimia, or those who are on very low-calorie diets, are at risk, especially if their periods are irregular. Strict vegetarians might also have problems if they lack important nutrients like vitamin B12, zinc, iron, and folic acid. Any woman who exercises intensely (such as marathon runners or dancers) may risk an abnormal menstrual cycle and infertility.

Lifestyle

Smoking, caffeine, and alcohol all can contribute to infertility. Women who smoke a pack a day or more, and those who started smoking before age 18, are at higher risk for infertility. Caffeine has been linked to infertility, and even moderate alcohol intake (as few as five drinks a week) can impair conception and have adverse effects on the developing fetus. Regular vaginal douching may reduce fertility by raising the risk for ectopic pregnancies and PELVIC INFLAMMATORY DISEASE. Unhealthy sexual practices (such as having multiple partners, and not using condoms), increase the risk of sexually transmitted diseases that can lead to infertility. See also CAFFEINE AND INFERTILITY.

Job/Environmental Risks

A woman's job can affect her fertility, particularly if she is exposed to chemicals, toxic substances, high temperatures or radiation. Of particular concern are environmental chemicals such as certain pesticides, aldrin, dieldrin, PCPs, dioxins, and furans, with estrogenlike effects. Although tests of single chemicals containing estrogen have produced mixed results, a study showed that the effects of combinations of these drugs can be very harmful. For example, studies have suggested an increased risk for infertility in women farm workers probably due to exposure to pesticides and in health care workers who give chemotherapy. See ENVIRONMENTAL FACTORS.

Studies on the effects of electromagnetic wave emissions, including those from computer monitors (VDTs), have been inconclusive. Nearly all monitors now comply with guidelines that reduce emissions; laptop computers are completely safe because they use liquid crystal display monitors. In any case, women should avoid the side and back of computers where wave emission is strongest and sit as far from the front of the screen as possible.

Emotions

Depression is very common in women who are trying to become pregnant, and depression may have a direct effect on hormones that regulate reproduction. However, the link between infertility and depression or anxiety has not been satisfactorily demonstrated.

Ovarian Failure

Certain conditions affect the ovaries themselves. Some women may experience premature ovarian failure because of adrenal or thyroid problems. Treatments for cancer can destroy follicles and cause ovarian failure. Sometimes the reasons for ovarian failure are unknown and may even be temporary. Some cases of unexplained infertility may result from early loss of ovarian function, which causes hormonal alterations so subtle that they are not picked up using routine laboratory tests. Women with a rare genetic disorder called TURNER'S SYNDROME don't develop functional ovaries.

Ovulation and Hormonal Disorders

Given the intricate interaction of the five hormones necessary for ovulation, it's not surprising that about 33% of infertility cases can be traced to problems with ovulation or hormones. This may result in the failure of the ovarian follicle to rupture, an empty follicle, or entrapment of the egg so that it isn't released. Even slight irregularities in the hormonal system can result in ovulation disorder.

In women who aren't pregnant or nursing, high levels of prolactin (a hormone that stimulates breast milk production) can inhibit ovulation and may reflect the presence of a pituitary tumor. Some drugs, including oral contraceptives and antidepressants can also boost levels of prolactin. Milk flow not related to pregnancy or nursing (galactorrhea) is a telltale symptom of high prolactin levels.

Immune System Abnormalities

In some cases, women have antibodies to sperm—substances in the immune system that recognize sperm as foreign proteins and attack them. If a woman's immune system attacks her own cells (autoimmunity), this may lead to premature ovarian failure if the antibodies are directed toward the ovary. Certain autoimmune disorders, such Hashimoto's hypothyroidism, are associated with infertility and miscarriage.

Implantation Failure

LUTEAL PHASE DEFECT is a general term referring to problems in the corpus luteum that interfere with the adequate production of progesterone. Because progesterone is necessary for thickening and preparing the uterine lining, this will mean that the egg can't implant in the uterine lining successfully. Between 25% and 60% of women who experience recurrent spontaneous abortions have a luteal phase defect. However, experts question the validity of the luteal phase defects.

Surgical Problems

Bands of scar tissue that grow together after surgery (called surgical ADHESIONS) can restrict the movement of ovaries, fallopian tubes, or the uterus, and may cause infertility. Laparoscopic surgery is less likely to cause adhesions than standard surgery.

While abortion performed under sterile conditions is very safe and carries few risks, a woman who has frequent abortions may experience problems with fertility: The cervix can weaken and be unable to sustain a pregnancy, or scar tissue can form inside resulting in a closed uterus (Asherman's syndrome).

Medications

Among the medications that can cause temporary infertility are many used to treat chronic disorders, as well as antidepressants, hormones, antibiotics, pain killers, anticancer drugs, and radiation.

Disease

A number of diseases can result in infertility among women, including PELVIC INFLAMMATORY DISEASE, ENDOMETRIOSIS, POLYCYSTIC OVARY SYNDROME, and OVARIAN CYSTS.

Pelvic Inflammatory Disease

One major cause of infertility is pelvic inflammatory disease (PID), which covers a variety of infections that can affect the uterus, fallopian tubes, ovaries, appendix, parts of the intestine, or the entire pelvic area. The sites of infection most often linked to infertility are the fallopian tubes—a condition known as salpingitis.

Although PID can be a complication of abortions, use of an IUD, or a ruptured appendix, many infections are caused by sexually transmitted diseases. Chlamydia trachomatis is an infectious organism that causes 75% of salpingitis cases. Gonorrhea is responsible for most of the remaining cases. Severe or frequent attacks of PID can eventually cause scarring, abscess formation, and tubal damage that result in infertility. The severity of the infection, not the number of the infections, appears to determine the risk for infertility. About 20% of women who develop symptoms of PID become infertile. PID also significantly increases the risk of ectopic pregnancy. However, most women with PID don't have symptoms, indicating that the disease may be silent or misdiagnosed.

Endometriosis

About a third of women with infertility have ENDOMETRIOSIS. This disorder develops when fragments of the endometrial lining are implanted in other areas of the pelvis. This occurs in retrograde menstruation, when the menstrual tissue flows backward from the uterus to the tubes, implanting on pelvic organs such as ovaries. These endometrial implants develop into cysts, which respond to hormonal changes, slowly increasing in size with each menstrual cycle and eventually causing ovarian scarring and inflammation. Endometrial implants in the ovaries or fallopian tubes are particularly likely to cause infertility, even if the endometriosis is mild. Severe endometriosis accounts for 6% of infertility cases.

Polycystic Ovary Syndrome

POLYCYSTIC OVARY SYNDROME (PCOS) is the major cause of infertility in American women. In PCOS, the ovary produces high amounts of hormones commonly found in higher amounts in men (testosterone). LH levels are high and FSH levels are low, and the follicles are unable to produce a mature egg. Instead, they swell with fluid and form small cysts. The high levels of androgens may cause facial hair and acne. Lack of a menstrual period and infrequent menstruation are quite common. Without ovulation, progesterone is no longer produced. If left untreated for many years, this imbalance also increases the risk for endometrial cancer.

The cause of PCOS is still unknown, although many women with PCOS have high levels of insulin that the body can't use efficiently—a condition known as insulin resistance. Such high levels of insulin may increase androgen production in the ovaries of certain women.

Polycystic ovary syndrome should not be confused with an ovarian cyst, which is a small, fluid-filled sac that grows in the ovary. This type of cyst usually goes away within two or three menstrual periods and does not cause infertility.

Fibroid Tumors

Benign fibroid tumors in the uterus are extremely common in women in their 30s. These overgrowths (leiomyoma) occur in the smooth muscle cells of the uterus. They rarely cause infertility unless they interfere with the uterine lining, block the fallopian tubes, or change the position of the cervix, thus preventing sperm from reaching the uterus. Fibroids respond to estrogen, such as when a woman is pregnant or takes the birth control pill. The predisposition to have fibroids can be hereditary.

Other Medical Causes of Infertility

There are a number of medical conditions that can impair fertility, including a ruptured appendix, diabetes, kidney disease and thyroid disorders. Ectopic pregnancies can destroy the fallopian tubes and increase the risk for infertility. An earlier diagnosis of ectopic pregnancy reduces the potential for tubal damage.

Diagnosis

The first step in an infertility examination is a complete medical history and physical exam, including details of sexual history, menstrual history, family history, drug, alcohol, and caffeine consumption, and a profile of the patient's general medical and emotional health. The male partner should also be interviewed and examined. The basic infertility evaluation includes

- hormone levels (such as FSH)
- thyroid function tests
- prolactin blood levels
- confirmation of normal ovulation
- X ray of uterus and fallopian tubes (HYSTEROSALPINGOGRAM)
- Sometimes a LAPAROSCOPY is indicated (insertion of a thin lighted device into the abdomen to look at the uterus, ovaries, and fallopian tubes to exclude causes such as endometriosis and scarring that may not be revealed by HSG).
- semen analysis.

(See also MALE FACTOR INFERTILITY.)

ferning A pattern of dried cervical mucus viewed on a slide that indicates the mucus has been thinned and prepared by ESTROGEN for the passage of SPERM. If the sample doesn't show the fern pattern, the mucus will be hostile to sperm.

ferning test See SPINNBARKEIT TEST.

fertile time The period in a woman's monthly menstrual cycle when she is most likely to get pregnant.

Conception is possible during OVULATION, when an egg is available for FERTILIZATION. However, it's not necessary to have sex precisely at the moment of ovulation; there are actually about 4 days during which sexual intercourse is most likely to result in pregnancy.

A woman's most fertile time is about 12 to 15 days before the beginning of the next menstrual period. In a typical 28-day menstrual cycle, therefore, cycle days 12 to 15 would be the most likely days to get pregnant. At this time, the woman is most likely to ovulate (release the egg). Ovulation is triggered by a burst of the hormone LH from the pituitary gland. Ovulation occurs 36–48 hours after the initiation of the LH surge in the blood.

Urine LH test kits are sensitive to LH in the urine (which occurs 12 hours after it is detected in the blood). Since ovulation will occur about 24 hours after LH appears in the urine, sex should take place within 12–24 hours after the surge is detected. Since sperm lasts 48–72 hours within the female reproductive tract, sex shortly after the detection of LH allows for plenty of overlap between sex and ovulation.

Even with no fertility problems, it may still take several months to conceive. In fact, a couple without fertility problems has only a 25% chance of getting pregnant each month, although this percentage varies with age. In order to time intercourse for a woman's most fertile time, she should monitor the menstrual cycle and predict ovulation.

fertilin A newly identified SPERM protein that is involved in sperm movement and which helps the sperm to bind to an egg to begin fertilization.

fertility cap Also known as a conception or CERVICAL CAP, this is a new do-it-yourself fertility device recently approved in the United States. Although it requires a doctor's prescription, it can be used without a doctor's intervention. It appeals to couples who experience problems in getting pregnant but who are reluctant to seek help at a FERTILITY CLINIC. It is designed to help with INFERTILITY related to low SPERM counts, reduced sperm motility (movement), or hostile vaginal environment.

The fertility cap is used at the end of CONDOM-protected intercourse. The sperm is emptied from the condom into the cap, which is then applied inside the vagina. The device can remain in place for up to three days, giving women a higher chance of getting pregnant.

For more serious infertility problems, women will usually undergo more complicated treatments.

It is expected that the fertility cap will be marketed as one component in a "conception kit" by the small British firm Veos. The kit will contain an ovulation predictor, a conception cap, a condom, and a pregnancy test. The conception kit provides a couple with the means to effect sperm concentration at a biologically appropriate time.

fertility clinic   A program of fertility specialists offering a range of fertility services, usually including ASSISTED REPRODUCTIVE TECHNOLOGIES (ART). Information and reports on fertility clinics across the country are available from the AMERICAN SOCIETY FOR REPRODUCTIVE MEDICINE and the Society for Reproductive Technology.

Most INFERTILITY service providers will explain their record in helping couples, but often success rates are calculated differently, making it confusing to select among the more than 300 programs offering these advanced services. In addition, a particular infertility service may have a lower success rate than others, but specialize in more difficult cases. Or a service may have a very good overall success rate but not be the best one to treat a particular problem. Infertility experts emphasize that a couple's chance for success depends on many factors, such as age and cause of infertility.

Selecting the best medical practice for fertility treatment can often be a confusing experience for couples faced with infertility. It is difficult to interpret all of the various statistics quoted by fertility programs because of a lack of a standard inclusion criteria among the different programs.

The Society for Assisted Reproductive Technologies (SART) publishes clinic-specific data on 310 of the 330 programs across the United States. SART focuses on high-tech clinical issues, and since 1993, they have been gathering and publishing information on ART programs in the United States and Canada. Any program that is a SART member and performs more than 40 treatment cycles a year must report its results to the registry.

This comprehensive report provides valuable information about a program, including, among other matters, number of cycles, pregnancy rates by age, with or without male factor, miscarriage rates, and average patient age. An analysis of these data will reveal trends or patterns that will provide insight as to the quality, stability, and experience of the programs being considered, especially if evaluated over time.

Clinics should provide documentation on statistics, as well as a breakdown by age and diagnosis. When comparing infertility services, ask how the success rates are calculated.

Because some services cite only national statistics when discussing success rates, couples should be wary of claims not based on a provider's own experience. The quoted success rate should match the couple's particular profile, such as age and cause of infertility. Couples should ask about the staff's medical training, how long the service has existed, and how many patients have been treated. To get an idea of a program's strengths and weaknesses, a couple should interview former or current patients. Consumers should evaluate how each infertility service tabulates its success rate and consider how meaningful these figures are.

Fertility clinics offering assisted reproductive techniques are not regulated by the government, and abuses have been reported, including lack of informed consent, unauthorized use of embryos, and failure to routinely screen donors for disease. Fortunately, abuses are rare. Couples should request the clinic's TAKE-HOME BABY RATE (not just their pregnancy success rate) for other couples with similar infertility problems. For examples, some clinics exclude high-risk women (such as those who are older or fail to produce a lot of eggs), which inflates their success rates.

Advanced fertility procedures and medications are expensive and often not covered by insurance. Several states, including Massachusetts and Illinois, have laws mandating insurance coverage for infertility. Couples should be cautious about offers of rebates in the event of failure; the clinics offering them are often significantly more expensive than those that don't. See also FERTILITY CLINIC REPORT.

fertility clinic report   A consumer report listing the pregnancy success rates of fertility clinics, published by the U.S. Centers for Disease Control and Prevention (CDC). The report provides statistical information about ASSISTED REPRODUCTIVE TECHNOLOGY (ART).

The annual reports are required by the FERTILITY CLINIC SUCCESS RATE AND CERTIFICATION ACT OF 1992 authored by Sen. Ron Wyden (D-Oreg.). They are prepared jointly by the CDC, The Society for Assisted Reproductive Technology (an affiliate of the AMERICAN SOCIETY OF REPRODUCTIVE MEDICINE), and the consumer organization RESOLVE. The reports answer two questions that infertile couples frequently ask:

- What are the chances of having a child using assisted reproductive technology?
- Where can patients go for this treatment?

The national report presents overall success rates and shows how they are influenced by certain patient and treatment characteristics. For example, it can give couples a good idea of what their average chances are of having a child by using ART. The reports include information on how many cycles of ART were carried out that resulted in live births; the live birth rate per cycle for fresh, nondonor eggs; and what percentage of all live births resulting from ART were multiple births.

A woman's chances of getting pregnant and having a live birth by using ART is related to a clinic staff's expertise, the quality of its lab, and a variety of factors outside the clinic's control. Factors outside a clinic's control covered in this report include the woman's age, the cause of the infertility, and the number of children that the woman has already had. Other factors that may also be important in affecting success rates for

which data were not available include the length of time that infertility has been a problem and the number of previous unsuccessful ART attempts. Given the number of factors not included in the national registry, the statistics should not be used to compare programs. A program with the highest success rate may not be a "better" program, mainly due to patient selection.

The report is published in separate volumes based on geographic region. Each volume contains a national summary that uses the information from all the reporting fertility clinics to provide an in-depth national picture of ART, fertility clinic reports that provide ART success rates for U.S. clinics, an appendix with a glossary of terms used in the national and clinic reports, an explanation of how the age-standardized rates were calculated, and the names and addresses of the reporting clinics in the geographic region.

The CDC emphasizes that before beginning treatment, consumers may want to examine financial, psychological, and medical issues, as well as a clinic's location, counseling and support services, and staff rapport.

A copy of the full report for each year is available by contacting RESOLVE at 1-888-299-1585. People with questions about ART may also contact RESOLVE.

Fertility Clinic Success Rate and Certification Act of 1992 (P.L. 102-493)   A law written by Sen. Ron Wyden (D-Oreg.) that requires the government (through the Centers for Disease Control) to report pregnancy success rates of fertility clinics, to provide comparable information about the effectiveness of infertility services, and to certify embryo labs.

The report provides information that will help patients and health care providers make informed decisions about assisted reproductive technology (ART). The law also includes standards states can use to inspect and certify labs used in fertility clinics that provide assisted reproductive technology (ART) such as IN VITRO FERTILIZATION. See also FERTILITY CLINIC REPORT.

fertility drugs A group of drugs given to women to improve fertility. Some women can't get pregnant because they don't secrete enough hormones at the right time during the cycle and, as a result, don't ovulate. Fertility drugs, which are the mainstay of treatment for INFERTILITY, can help these women.

The treatment success with fertility drugs varies with age. Doctors have known for some time that advancing age adversely affects the health of a woman's eggs.

Fertility drugs are given for two main reasons: To help women ovulate who don't do so on their own, or to produce multiple eggs for the purpose of INTRAUTERINE INSEMINATION or IN VITRO FERTIL-IZATION. Fertility drugs are also used to treat some men with MALE FACTOR INFERTILITY.

Drugs used to treat infertility include clomiphene, FOLLICLE-STIMULATING HORMONES, human menopausal hormones, and HUMAN CHORIONIC GONADOTROPINS. Other drugs, often used in combination with other medications, include BROMOCRIPTINE, GnRH AGONISTS AND GnRH ANTAG-ONISTS.

Clomiphene

The most common medication given to stimulate and induce OVULATION, it's also the oldest and least expensive. CLOMIPHENE CITRATE (Clomid, Sero-phene) is a synthetic drug that blocks ESTROGEN receptors in the hypothalamus, tricking it into thinking there is an estrogen deficiency. As a result, the hypothalamus tells the pituitary to release more LH and FSH. As FSH levels rise, it stimulates the development of a follicle, which then secretes estrogen on its own. When treatment stops, the hypothalamus notices the high estrogen levels and tells the pituitary to start the LH surge to trigger the release of a mature egg. Clomiphene is a good first-choice drug when a woman's reproductive organs are working but just need a bit of a boost. In women whose only fertility problem is irregular or no ovulation, about 80% will ovulate; about 50% of these women will become pregnant within 6 months of clomiphene treatments. About 3% of women on

clomiphene have a multiple pregnancy (usually twins).

If a woman responds to clomiphene and develops a mature follicle but has no LH surge by cycle day 15, then a hormone (hCG) can be injected to stimulate egg maturation and egg release. A woman tends to ovulate about 36 hours after an LH surge or the hCG injection.

It's important to monitor women taking clomiphene to determine when ovulation occurs, either by using BASAL BODY TEMPERATURE CHARTS or with an ovulation predictor kit. Blood tests and ultrasounds also may be used. There are potential side effects with this drug; in a few patients their cervical mucus becomes hostile, interfering with the sperm's ability to swim from the vagina through the uterus and into the fal-lopian tubes. Other side effects may include hot flashes, upset stomach, headaches, visual distur-bances, mood swings, and breast tenderness.

Some women don't ovulate with clomiphene; others ovulate but don't become pregnant. If clomiphene fails, a woman will often respond to FSH in the form of injectable GONADOTROPINS. There are two types of these gonadotropins: one contains FSH and LH, the other contains mostly FSH with just a bit of LH. These injectable drugs give the doctor control over the amount and length of time of FSH stimulation.

The doctor will closely monitor a woman hav-ing injected gonadotropins, since the potential for overstimulation (hyperstimulation) or understimulation exists.

Human Chorionic Gonadotropin

This fertility drug (Profasi or Pregnyl) is chemi-cally similar to LH and will produce an LH surge, triggering ovulation. This is given either after other medications mature the egg, or in unmed-icated cycles, to time ovulation. Since most women undergoing induced ovulation won't release an egg spontaneously, the hCG is needed to trigger the release.

Side effects include bloating, fluid retention, mild nausea, or headaches. A more serious side effect is OVARIAN HYPERSTIMULATIN SYNDROME, in which the ovaries get too big and can trigger a range of serious symptoms.

Human Menopausal Gonadotropins

These drugs (Pergonal, Humegon, Repronex) are given to stimulate the ovaries directly to produce more than one egg in a cycle. This is the most potent drug available; it is given if clomiphene hasn't worked. HMG will raise levels of FSH and keep them high, and is especially helpful if a woman has problems with low FSH. Because this drug is very strong, follicle development is closely monitored by both ultrasound and estrogen blood tests. Once one or two follicles develop and estrogen levels are correct, an injection of hCG is given to trigger ovulation. If too many eggs have developed, the hCG injection is withheld.

Because hCG is so strong, there is a higher risk of multiple pregnancy, as well as a higher risk for ECTOPIC PREGNANCY, spontaneous abortions, and premature delivery.

Follicle-Stimulating Hormones

These drugs stimulate follicle growth directly and include Metrodin, Follistim, Gonal-F, and Fertinex. These are usually given when clomiphene hasn't worked. They are especially useful with women who have PCOs and high LH levels, because the drugs have very little LH. Ovulation usually occurs within a week of FSH treatment. Women undergoing FSH treatment will be closely monitored by ultrasound and blood tests, and given an hCG injection to stimulate egg release.

Bromocriptine (Parlodel)

This fertility drug is used to reduce the prolactin secreted from the pituitary in those women with high prolactin levels. Prolactin interferes with the release of LH and FSH. Although this treatment is successful in bringing down prolactin levels, clomiphene or hMG may also need to be given.

Gonadotropin-Releasing Hormone (Gn-RH)

This drug (Factrel or Lutrepulse) can replace missing Gn-RH and will stimulate the pituitary to release FSH and LH. It is given to women who have not ovulated while taking clomiphene or hMG, and is especially helpful for those women with PCOs or defects of the luteal phase. Because only a few follicles develop with this drug, there is not much chance of a multiple pregnancy.

Gn-RH Agonists

Known as Lupron (LEUPROLIDE ACETATE), Synarel (NAFARELIN ACETATE), or Zoladex (GOSERELIN ACE-TATE), these drugs trigger the release of LH and FSH from the pituitary, suppressing normal ovarian function to allow precise ovulation induction. By stopping the production of Gn-RH, they allow the doctor to prescribe the exact amount of FSH or LH necessary. Gn-RH agonists are especially helpful for those women undergoing ART procedures. These drugs also can be given to shrink fibroids and cysts and to treat ENDOMETRIOSIS.

Success Rates

Almost all women given injectable gonadotropins will ovulate, but not all women will conceive. Unfortunately, not every woman who ovulates will get pregnant.

Most pregnancies that occur do so in the first three ovulatory treatment cycles. If a woman doesn't conceive during the first six treatment cycles, her chances of getting pregnant are diminished. The cumulative pregnancy rate after several ovulatory cycles on clomiphene is less than 50%. As with any treatment, the ovulation rates may be lower depending on the individual's age, the presence of other factors, and the precise reason a woman is being treated.

Side Effects

When used in low doses for a short time, clomiphene and HCG rarely cause side effects. However, fertility drugs may cause hot flashes, breast tenderness or swelling, heavy menstrual periods, bleeding between menstrual periods, nausea or vomiting, dizziness, lightheadedness, irritability, nervousness, restlessness, headache, tiredness, sleep problems, or depression. These problems usually go away as the body adjusts to the drug and do not require medical treatment unless they continue or they interfere with normal activities. Other side effects are possible. Anyone who has unusual symptoms after taking infertility drugs should get in touch with a doctor.

Infertility drugs may make some medical conditions worse, including endometriosis, uterine fibroids, unusual vaginal bleeding, ovarian cysts, enlarged ovaries, inflamed veins caused by blood clots, liver disease, and depression.

Depression

Women who take fertility drugs may experience depression, which can sometimes be quite severe. One recent Harvard University study found that women undergoing fertility treatments showed depression levels equal to a woman facing treatment for cancer or AIDS. In the first place, the condition of infertility itself can be a depressing condition for many couples. In addition, fertility drugs trigger hormonal changes that can cause depression by interfering with estrogen (a natural antidepressant). Women with severe symptoms should discuss their feelings with their physician.

Drug Interactions

Infertility drugs may interact with other medications so that the effects of one or both of the drugs may change, or the risk of side effects may be higher.

fertility monitor   A simple home device that predicts ovulation by measuring two hormones (ESTROGEN and LUTEINIZING HORMONE) in urine to determine a woman's fertility status every day of the cycle. A woman performs 10 tests each cycle, although women with long or irregular cycles may need to do 20 tests. It provides more information than a simpler OVULATION TEST KIT designed to test women with regular cycles by tracking just one hormone (LH) in the urine. While considerably more expensive, it may be more accurate and simpler to use than the one-hormone ovulation test.

fertility nurse specialist   A nurse with special training in caring for people undergoing INFERTILITY treatments.

fertility specialist   A doctor who specializes in the diagnosis and treatment of INFERTILITY. While any doctor who treats infertility problems could be called a "fertility specialist," this term does not accurately describe a licensed medical specialty. A doctor can't become a board-certified fertility specialist because, so far, there is no postgraduate board-certification course in the country. Because there is no such certification, this means that any doctor (or even a person with a Ph.D. degree, not an M.D.) can be called a "fertility specialist," whether or not the person is qualified to treat fertility problems.

Although physicians who are board certified in family practice, internal medicine, general obstetrics and gynecology (ob-gyn), or urology receive some training in the diagnosis and treatment of infertility, they may lack the additional training and experience of physicians who specialize in reproductive medicine.

A male "infertility specialist" can be a UROLOGIST or an ANDROLOGIST (an M.D. or Ph.D. who specializes in male fertility and in ASSISTED REPRODUCTIVE TECHNOLOGIES). Many urologists are also andrologists.

A REPRODUCTIVE ENDOCRINOLOGIST is an obstetrician-gynecologist who specializes in reproductive endocrinology and who is qualified to manage female fertility. The AMERICAN COLLEGE OF OBSTETRICIANS AND GYNECOLOGISTS certifies this subspecialty for ob-gyns who receive extra training in infertility and endocrinology (the study of hormones).

Any person or couple who decides to undergo assisted reproductive technology also may need an embryologist, a Ph.D.-level scientist who specializes in embryo transfers. A couple should see a fertility specialist if they

- need microsurgery, or treatment for ENDOMETRIOSIS or tubal damage

- have a history of three or more miscarriages
- have irregular menstrual cycles with evidence of irregular ovulation
- have a poor semen analysis with low count or motility or poor morphology
- are women over age 35 years
- are women with a previous history of pelvic infection
- are a couple whose basic fertility tests came back normal but who haven't been able to conceive after two years

fertility testing   There are a range of tests and diagnostic procedures a doctor can perform to determine if and why a couple is infertile. Infertility treatment should not start until all these tests have been performed and all possible treatable problems have been ruled out. These tests may include

- blood tests to check hormone levels in the woman (thyroid, prolactin, and androgen levels)
- SEMEN ANALYSIS
- POSTCOITAL TEST (this test is less frequently performed today)
- X ray to evaluate if a woman's FALLOPIAN TUBES are open (HYSTEROSALPINGOGRAM)
- ENDOMETRIAL BIOPSY to check the quality of the uterine lining (this test is not routinely performed)
- LAPAROSCOPY (out-patient surgery to check for ENDOMETRIOSIS or pelvic scarring)

The first step in testing a woman is to discover whether or not she is producing an egg each month. This can be done by using a home OVULATION TEST KIT or by undergoing ultrasound or blood tests in the doctor's office. The results determine whether additional tests are needed.

In many cases, a doctor will need to determine whether or not a woman's fallopian tubes are open. This may be done with an X ray exam called an HYSTEROSALPINGOGRAM, which can reveal whether the tubes are open, as well as define the shape of the uterus. The tubes also can be examined by LAPAROSCOPY. With this technique, a doctor can use a miniature light-transmitting telescope called a LAPAROSCOPE to look into the abdomen and inspect the female organs for disease.

The first test for male infertility is an analysis of his SEMEN. Usually the man is asked to bring a sample of his semen into the laboratory for examination. Semen analysis includes a check of the sperm shape and appearance (morphology), a measurement of the volume and pH, and an analysis of the sperm count and movement characteristics.

If there is any question about the findings, additional tests may be conducted or the husband may be referred to a urologist (a doctor who specializes in matters involving the urinary tract, testes, and related reproductive organs).

fertilization   Penetration of the egg by the SPERM cell. For fertilization to take place, several processes must take place successfully at exactly the right time.

The sperm must swim through a woman's cervix, through the uterus, and into the FALLOPIAN TUBE to meet the egg, where fertilization occurs. The fertilized egg (called an EMBRYO) then continues to travel down the fallopian tube into the uterus, where it will then attach itself into the uterine wall (implantation). In nature, fertilization occurs inside the fallopian tube (in vivo) but it also may occur in a petri dish (in vitro). See also IN VITRO FERTILIZATION.

Fertinex   The brand name for UROFOLLITROPIN.

fetal reduction   A technique that reduces the number of fetuses in a multifetal pregnancy to reduce the risks of a high-order multiple pregnancy. This procedure is usually considered with three or more fetuses. In a reduction, the number of fetuses is often reduced to two, although in some circumstances they may be reduced to one.

The reduction (also called selective abortion) is usually performed between 9 and 12 weeks of gestation. The procedure is most successful when performed early in the pregnancy. It is done on an outpatient basis by inserting a needle guided by ultrasound either through the abdomen or vagina to destroy the fetus.

While there is also a risk of loss of the remaining fetuses from miscarriage, this risk is minimized when an experienced physician performs the procedure. The incidence of miscarriage associated with this procedure is 4% to 5%. Premature labor occurs in about 75% of pregnancies following reduction, but miscarriage of the remaining fetuses or maternal infection rarely occur.

The choice to continue a pregnancy fraught with risk, as well as to experience a fetal reduction, can be extremely stressful. Couples who have invested time, money, and energy in pursuing pregnancy are often unprepared to make this decision. Professional counseling before undergoing the procedure is a good idea. Both partners need to be comfortable with their decision and may need emotional support prior to and immediately following the procedure. See also MULTIFETAL REDUCTION.

fetus A term used to describe an unborn child during the period of gestation, from the period of time when the EMBRYO is fully formed at around 8 weeks, until birth.

fibroids and infertility Fibroids (also called myomas or leiomyomas) are benign tumors of the uterine muscle and connective tissue. They more commonly occur in women as they get older, although they can appear during a woman's 20s.

Fibroids can grow almost anywhere around the UTERUS—on the outside, within the wall, or protruding within the cavity. However, the closer the fibroid is to the interior of the uterus, the more likely that the fibroid will interfere with reproduction and disturb menstrual bleed-

ing. Even small tumors located in the uterine cavity may cause heavy bleeding, prolonged periods, bleeding between periods, anemia, pain, infertility, or miscarriage. Fibroids located in the uterine wall and those that protrude outside the uterine wall may reach a large size before causing symptoms, and are less likely to cause infertility.

It is generally accepted that fibroids may occasionally cause INFERTILITY, recurrent pregnancy losses, and premature delivery. In one uncontrolled study of 94 infertile women with sizeable uterine fibroids and no other apparent cause for infertility, 59.5% of these women conceived after surgical removal of fibroids (myomectomy), most within a short time. The miscarriage rate among women with fibroids is about 40%. Following myomectomy, 80% of patients with a history of repeated miscarriages will have a successful pregnancy. However, while nearly 30% of all women have fibroids at some time in their lives, only about 9% of infertility cases are caused by fibroids alone.

Fibroids begin somewhere in the uterus as a single cell that grows the wrong way, but experts still don't know for sure why this happens. Scientists do know that estrogen is necessary for a fibroid to grow, and that fibroids can get larger during pregnancy because of the increase in hormones.

It is important to remember that most women with fibroids have no problem conceiving. Fibroids may cause problems in becoming pregnant if they are near the opening of both of the fallopian tubes or they distort the shape of the uterine cavity.

fimbria Fingerlike projections at the end of the fallopian tube nearest the OVARY. When stimulated by the fluid released from the follicles during ovulation, the fingerlike ends grasp the egg and sweep it into the tube.

fimbriectomy A type of STERILIZATION procedure in which the fingerlike end (fimbriae) of each FALLOPIAN TUBE is removed surgically. Unlike other sterilization techniques, this procedure can't be reversed. The absence of the fimbriae make it unlikely that the egg can be recovered, and failure rates are very low.

fimbrial end   The outside end of the FALLOPIAN TUBE that touches the surface of the OVARY, from which it picks up the egg from the ruptured follicle.

fimbriolysis   Microsurgical technique to separate a damaged outside end of the FALLOPIAN TUBE (the fimbriae) that has become stuck together. The surgery requires special skills using either a LAPAROTOMY or LAPAROSCOPY. A laparoscopy is less invasive, and patients can leave the hospital sooner. Laparotomy is performed when the amount of damage can't adequately be treated by laparoscopy.

fimbrioplasty   A surgical procedure that reconstructs the fingerlike projections at the end of the FALLOPIAN TUBE and allows the fimbriae to function properly.

follicle   A fluid-filled sac in the OVARY that contains the eggs. A woman is born with a fixed number of eggs or follicles (between 1 and 2 million), which drops to about 300,000 by puberty. Afterward, one egg is released monthly. For every egg that is released, about 1,000 wither in the ovary (called atresia). The eggs remain microscopic until they begin to grow a few weeks before the cycle begins. The follicles also produce ESTROGEN.

follicle aspiration   The procedure for harvesting eggs. See EGG RECOVERY/RETRIEVAL.

follicle cells   Cells in the FOLLICLE that surround the egg. The follicle grows when the cells increase in number.

follicle, primary   The first growth stage of the FOLLICLE in which the egg is surrounded by a single layer of follicle cells.

follicle-stimulating hormone (FSH)   A reproductive hormone (also called a GONADOTROPIN) secreted by the pituitary gland. FSH stimulates SPERM production in a man; in a woman, FSH stimulates the growth of the ovarian FOLLICLE and the production of eggs.

An FSH assay measures the quantity of FSH in the blood; high levels of FSH indicate a problem with a man's testicles or a woman's ovaries. The reason for this is that poor egg or sperm production has a negative feedback effect on the pituitary and causes FSH levels to rise in an attempt to further stimulate the OVARY or TESTICLE. Abnormal FSH levels may be seen in hypopituitarism, KLINEFELTER'S SYNDROME, POLYCYSTIC OVARY SYNDROME, TURNER'S SYNDROME, or ovarian failure.

follicular fluid   The fluid inside the follicle that cushions and nourishes the egg. When released during OVULATION, the fluid stimulates fingerlike projections at the end of the FALLOPIAN TUBE to grasp the OVARY and sweep the egg into the fallopian tube.

follicular phase   The portion of a woman's cycle before OVULATION during which a FOLLICLE grows and high levels of ESTROGEN cause the lining of the UTERUS to grow. Normally, this phase lasts between 12 and 14 days.

folliculogenesis   The process in which follicles grow.

follistatin   A protein hormone found in the FOLLICULAR FLUID that controls FOLLICLE growth.

follitropin (Follistim)   A new drug that stimulates the development of multiple follicles in women who don't ovulate naturally, and in those participating in an ART program. Unlike other drugs containing FSH (FOLLICLE-STIMULAT-ING HORMONE), it is not made from the urine of postmenopausal women but from recombinant FSH technology. Similar in structure and activity to a woman's own FSH, it has led to successful ovulation in 85% of the women by the third cycle of treatment.

The drug works like natural FSH produced in a woman's own body, binding to the surface of the follicle and triggering the maturation of the egg. After follicular growth, OVULATION is induced with the administration of CHORIONIC GONADO-TROPIN (trade name PREGNYL or Profasi). This drug is given as the follicles reach the right size (about 15–20 mm). HCG acts like LUTEINIZING HORMONE to induce egg maturation and ultimately to release the mature egg from the follicle.

The woman's progress is monitored through blood tests and ultrasound scans. The blood tests monitor the amount of estrogen in the blood, which is released as the follicles develop in re-sponse to follitropin.

If a woman is undergoing OVULATION INDUC-TION, she will be asked to have sex after the hCG injection. If a woman is undergoing IVF, her doc-tor will remove the mature eggs 34 to 36 hours after administering hCG. If a woman is having the GIFT (GAMETE INTRAFALLOPIAN TRANSFER), the mature eggs and sperm will be transferred to her fallopian tubes. For IN VITRO FERTILIZATION (IVF), the eggs will be fertilized in the lab and the embryo transferred into the woman's body later.

Side Effects

Minor problems include vaginal bleeding, abdominal pain, and pain or bruising at the injection site. A few patients experience ovarian cysts, enlargement of the ovaries, and body rash.

In addition, ECTOPIC PREGNANCY, MISCAR-RIAGES, and OVARIAN HYPERSTIMULATION SYN-DROME were reported in 3% to 11% of the cases. These rates are similar to those of women under-going treatment with other FSH-containing drugs.

FSH   See FOLLICLE-STIMULATING HORMONE.

galactorrhea   Milk production in the breasts in women who aren't nursing or who have never been pregnant. It may be caused by disease in the breast or wall of the chest, or by a pituitary tumor.

gamete   Generic term for a sperm or egg.

gamete intrafallopian transfer (GIFT)   A technique developed in 1984 to assist conception, in which the female GAMETE (egg) and the male gamete (sperm) are brought together by retrieving eggs from the OVARY, placing them with SPERM into a catheter, and immediately delivering them into the FALLOPIAN TUBE for FERTILIZATION. They are usually introduced into the fallopian tube during a LAPAROSCOPY. If it is fertilized, the embryo then travels into the UTERUS for implantation. If a woman has healthy fallopian tubes, this procedure may be used instead of IN VITRO FERTILIZATION (in which eggs are removed from the ovary, fertilized by sperm in the lab, cultured into early embryos, and then transferred to the uterus).

GIFT is a good way to induce pregnancy for those who have been infertile for a long time, or for women with normal fallopian tubes and for whom other conventional methods of treatment have failed. This method is used in the hope that it will result in better, stronger, and faster-growing embryos compared to in vitro fertilization. Some experts believe that this occurs because these embryos reach the uterus at the right time and in the correct direction after they have been fertilized.

GIFT is more expensive than IVF but carries more risk because it usually requires laparoscopic surgery with general anesthesia, as opposed to in vitro fertilization (IVF), which calls only for a local or intravenous sedation. Therefore, GIFT is considered less desirable than IVF. GIFT takes place in an operating room (IVF may be performed in a procedure room).

The procedure begins with hormone injections to induce follicular development. Thirty-six hours after the injection, the doctor removes the eggs and usually places up to five eggs and sperm into each fallopian tube, depending on the woman's age, prior fertility history, and number of eggs recovered. Fertilization takes place in the fallopian tube, as it would in natural conception, and the embryos then move down into the uterus.

There is a higher rate of both pregnancy and multiple pregnancy with this technique. The pregnancy rate for GIFT has been reported to be higher than for IVF, with 28.1% deliveries per retrieval for GIFT vs. 18.6% deliveries per retrieval for IVF. However, this difference may not reflect a better technique but rather more stringent patient selection. For this reason, GIFT is much less often recommended compared to IVF.

ganirelix acetate   (Antagon)   An injectable drug used to inhibit premature OVULATION in women undergoing fertility procedures. Approved in 1999, ganirelix is specifically indicated for the prevention of premature LUTEINIZING HORMONE (LH) SURGE in women undergoing controlled OVARIAN STIMULATION. Ganirelix is unique because it is the first in a new class of medications known as the GONADOTROPIN-RELEASING HORMONE (Gn-RH) ANTAGONISTS to be released in the United States. Gn-RH is produced in a part of the brain called the hypothalamus and is responsible for controlling the pituitary gland's production and release of LH and FOLLICLE-STIMULATING HORMONE (FSH). Throughout a woman's menstrual cycle, the amount of Gn-RH released from the hypothalamus gland fluctuates. About halfway through each cycle, a large amount of Gn-RH is released, which triggers the LH surge, a rapid rise in the production and release of LH. This LH surge triggers ovulation. Gn-RH antagonists instantly prevent Gn-RH from acting on the pituitary to release FSH and LH. By preventing LH release, ovulation cannot occur.

When used as part of an infertility treatment regimen such as IN VITRO FERTILIZATION (IVF), ganirelix works to prevent ovulation. This allows the doctor to have better control of egg development and not have it shortened by premature ovulation.

Until now, the only available therapy for the prevention of premature LH surges were the GN-RH AGONISTS (Lupron, Synarel, Zoladex), products very similar in structure and action to natural Gn-RH. The end result of the administration of Gn-RH agonists is the same as ganirelix, but in order to achieve the same effect women must administer the Gn-RH agonists for a longer period of time (approximately 14 days). Unlike the antagonists that instantly inhibit LH production, Gn-RH agonists initially stimulate the release of LH and FSH, before they have their desired effect to prevent LH release. Because ganirelix immediately blocks the effect of Gn-RH it can be administered for a much shorter time. In clinical trials, the average duration of time of administration of ganirelix was 5.4 days.

Side Effects

The most frequent side effects of Antagon are abdominal pain, headache, nausea, vaginal bleeding, and injection site reactions.

gender selection   A medical process in which a couple chooses the sex of their unborn child. The idea of preselecting the sex of a child had been the dream of ancient civilizations of China, Egypt, and Greece, which developed countless myths, potions, and poultices in their quest. This desire continues into the present, as eager couples try unproven techniques such as dietary change, the time and frequency of intercourse, and delay or promote orgasm to conceive either a male or female infant.

The sperm that carries an X chromosome determines a female, and one carrying a Y chromosome determines a male. Methods have been developed to separate the X from Y chromosome bearing sperm.

While many people are interested in sex selection procedures, the subject is controversial, and in some countries it is still illegal. Critics of sex selection are concerned that more couples will choose a boy, especially if they are planning to have only one child. In one study of U.S. couples who would use gender selection, 81% of women and 94% of men reported a preference for first-born sons. On the other hand, many times couples who are interested in gender selection already have at least one child of a certain sex and simply want to balance their family by choosing the gender of their next child.

One of the most common ways to select a specific gender is by the Microsort method, an expensive, high-tech approach that separates the X-sperm from the Y for artificial insemination. Normal semen contains an equal mix of X-bearing and Y-bearing sperm. The desired sperm is then implanted in the woman, or the eggs are fertilized outside of the womb and then implanted. Not all REPRODUCTIVE ENDOCRINOLOGISTS perform this procedure, however. The likelihood of success is 50% to 90% for a female and 50% to 70% for a male. The lack of better statistics has made the procedure less attractive than it might otherwise be.

The Microsort method makes use of the one well-known difference between X and Y sperm, which is the amount of DNA each contain.

Because it contains less DNA, the Y-sperm is slightly smaller and lighter than the X. By filtering the seminal fluid and then forcing it through a long, thin tube, the sperm are forced to line up one by one. At the end of the tube, a mechanism steers X-bearing sperm in one direction and Y-bearing sperm in a different direction. Costs of this method are about $2,500 per separation and insemination.

Embryo Selection

With today's technology, gender selection can focus not just at the sperm level but by preselecting male or female embryos as well. Embryo preselection is performed in conjunction with IN VITRO FERTILIZATION (IVF). Once the embryo has grown to 8–10 cells, it's possible to remove one of the cells to test for the presence or absence of a Y chromosome. It is then possible to introduce embryos of one particular gender.

There are several drawbacks to the procedure. Only half of the original embryos will contain the desired sex, so many embryos can't be used with this method. The cost is also quite high (about $20,000 per attempt). However, if a pregnancy results, the correct sex will occur close to 100% of the time.

Ethics

There could be several reasons why a couple may choose embryo selection. Certain genetic diseases are more common in boys, such as hemophilia, Duchenne muscular dystrophy (the most common and severe form of the muscular dystrophies), Lesch-Nyhan syndrome, and X-linked mental retardation. Couples who are facing such a situation may choose gender selection to guarantee a female so as to avoid the genetic disease. Other couples facing multiple pregnancy who decide to choose a reduction also choose to select a particular gender at that time.

Gender selection based solely on couple preference is more controversial. Some question whether it's appropriate to try to artificially choose one sex over another simply because the parents prefer to have a boy or girl.

germ cell The precursor of other cells. In a man, the germ cell is the testicular cell that divides to produce immature SPERM cells; in a woman it is the ovarian cell that divides to form the egg.

germ cell aplasia An inherited condition in which the TESTICLES have no germ cells and thus are unable to produce sperm. Since men with this condition have normal LEYDIG CELLS (the testicular cell that produces TESTOSTERONE) they will develop normal male sexual characteristics.

Cause

The condition may be caused by prolonged exposure to toxins such as chemotherapy, and also to radiation. The sperm-forming germ cells of the testis are very sensitive to radiation, probably due to their high rate of cell division. The higher the dose of radiation, the greater the chance of damage and the less chance of repair. Sperm cell damage is reversible at single exposures below 600 rads, but permanent infertility is likely after exposure beyond that limit. After exposure to 200 to 300 rads (the dose usually prescribed for Hodgkin's disease patients) it may take up to three years for sperm production to fully recover; at 400 to 600 rads, recovery time may take about five years.

Patients who want to preserve fertility should try to guard the testes from radiation when radiation is applied to the pelvis and abdomen. If the radiation field is close to the testicles, a testicular shield can minimize radiation exposure.

Chemotherapy is also a cause of germ cell aplasia. It is especially noticeable after treatment with chemotherapy drugs known as alkylating agents, such as nitrogen mustards (chlorambucil, cyclophosphamide), nitrosoureas (CCNU, BCNU, MNU), methanesulfonic acid compounds (MMS, EMS, busulfan), ethylenimines (TEM, TEPA), and hydrazines (procarbazine). Other chemotherapy drugs that may kill germ cells include doxorubicin, vinca alkaloids (vinblastine, vincristine), antimetabolites (cytosine arabinoside, methotrexate), antitumor antibiotics, and cis-Platin.

Since many modern chemotherapy treatment protocols call for combinations of drugs, the risk of toxicity may be even greater. For example, multiagent regimens such as "MOPP" (nitrogen mustard, vincristine, procarbazine, and prednisone) cause permanent sterility in about 90% of male patients treated for Hodgkin's disease.

Treating children with chemotherapy presents particular problems. Before puberty, the germ cell tissues of the testes seem to be more resistant to small doses of chemotherapy than they are to adults. Yet during adolescence, severe germ cell toxicity may occur after the same drug doses. For example, researchers have observed germ cell aplasia among adolescent boys who received MOPP chemotherapy for Hodgkin's disease. By contrast, prepubertal boys don't show this problem.

Treatment

There is no treatment for this disorder; couples who want to have children may choose DONOR INSEMINATION or ADOPTION.

While semen CRYOPRESERVATION (freezing of semen) won't treat germ cell aplasia, it may offer an alternative to infertility among adolescent boys and men who must receive chemotherapy or radiation. Semen cryopreservation may be used together with ARTIFICIAL INSEMINATION or IN VITRO FERTILIZATION techniques to conceive children. However, some cancer patients have underlying defects in sperm production. Semen from these patients may be of poor quality and not suited for freezing and preservation.

gestation The medical term for pregnancy.

gestational surrogacy A type of surrogacy (also known as gestational care) in which a SURROGATE MOTHER is implanted with the genetic offspring of another couple and then turns the baby over to them at birth. In this case, a woman is implanted with embryos from an infertile couple who have undergone IN VITRO FERTILIZATION and hired her to carry their baby to term. After the surrogate receives the embryo, she carries the baby to term, gives birth, and then gives the baby to the baby's genetic parents.

The technique is usually performed when a woman has an absent or abnormal UTERUS and is unable to carry a pregnancy to term. With this technique, a woman must be able to produce viable eggs, which are retrieved and then fertilized with her partner's SPERM. The resulting embryos are then placed into the uterus of the carrier (or surrogate).

However, the surrogate is at risk for potential psychological problems inherent in carrying a pregnancy for another couple and then giving up the baby. There may also be legal issues as a result of a gestational surrogate who does not want to part with the baby. Extensive psychological assessment is necessary to determine whether the gestational carrier is emotionally prepared to undertake such an arrangement. There are many ethical considerations concerning gestational care that the couple need to discuss with a doctor or clinical staff.

GIFT See GAMETE INTRAFALLOPIAN TRANSFER.

Gn-RH See GONADOTROPIN-RELEASING HORMONE.

Gn-RH agonist Medications that enable doctors to block the pituitary secretion of LH and FSH that are required for OVULATION. The drugs suppress LH and FSH after a few days of administration and in fact increase LH and FSH initially. By suppressing normal ovarian function in this way, the doctor can then induce FOLLICLE development with great precision.

Gn-RH medication is begun a month before the IN VITRO FERTILIZATION cycle. These drugs have been especially helpful for women who are undergoing IVF. Long-acting forms of these drugs given monthly are sometimes given to women with ENDOMETRIOSIS, and fibroids.

Gn-RH agonists include buserlin, GOSERELIN, LEUPROLIDE ACETATE, nafarelin, and triptorelin.

Side Effects

Gn-RH agonists if given alone will suppress FSH and LH and reduce the ovarian production of eggs and ESTROGEN. Low estrogen levels are characteristic of MENOPAUSE. Side effects are typical of those seen during menopause, including hot flashes, headaches, mood swings, vaginal dryness, painful intercourse, reduced breast size, and bone loss.

Gn-RH analogs   Synthetic versions of the natural hormone Gn-RH (GONADOTROPIN-RELEASING HORMONE) that are much more potent than the natural hormone. They are called "analogs" because they are structurally similar to the native Gn-RH. The two types of Gn-RH analogs are GN-RH ANTAGONISTS and GN-RH AGONISTS. Antagonists instantly suppress LH and FSH and Gn-RH agonists take a few days to suppress the pituitary.

The most common Gn-RH analog which is an agonist in the United States is Lupron (LEUPRO-LIDE ACETATE).

Gn-RH antagonist   A newer medication that stops the pituitary gland from releasing FOLLICLE-STIMULATING HORMONE (FSH) and LUTEINIZING HORMONE (LH). They can be administered toward the end of stimulation and will block LH and hence, OVULATION. This has many advantages, by giving the doctor more control over the cycle. Antagonists require fewer injections than the agonists (Lupron).

However, antagonists only recently have been available and doctors are still gaining experience with their use. Theoretically, antagonists may be a better choice over agonists, but the role of the medications is evolving. See also GN-RH ANTAGONISTS.

gonad   The gender-neutral term for the ovaries and testicles. In men, the testicles make sperm and testosterone; in women, the ovaries produce eggs and estrogen.

gonadotropin   The hormones that stimulate the growth of the FOLLICLE—FOLLICLE-STIMULATING HORMONE, or FSH, and LUTEINIZING HORMONE (LH).

The rate of birth defects after gonadotropin use is no higher than in the general population (2% to 3%); furthermore, children born after gonadotropin use are developmentally no different from their peers.

Many types of gonadotropins exist:

- hMG (HUMAN MENOPAUSAL GONADOTROPIN) (brand names Pergonal, Humegon, or Repronex)
- FSH (follicle-stimulating hormone) (brand name METRODIN, Fertinex)
- hCG (HUMAN CHORIONIC GONADOTROPIN; brand name Profasi or PREGNYL)

During the use of these drugs careful monitoring is required to minimize the risk of side effects, which may include

- *ovarian hyperstimulation syndrome (OHSS)*   Occurring in 1% to 5% of cycles, the risk of OHSS is higher in women with POLYCYSTIC OVARY SYNDROME. It is usually mild and associated with minimal bloating and abdominal discomfort. When severe, OHSS can cause blood clots, kidney damage, ovarian twisting, and fluid buildup in chest and abdomen. In severe cases, hospitalization is necessary; however, the condition lasts only a week or so.
- *multiple gestation*   Up to 20% of pregnancies resulting from the administration of gonadotropins are multiple, in contrast to a rate of 1% to 2% in the general population. While most of these pregnancies are twins, a significant percentage are triplets or higher, which are associated with more problems for both mother and children. (See also MULTIPLE BIRTHS AND FERTILITY DRUGS.)
- ECTOPIC PREGNANCY   While ectopic pregnancy occurs 1% to 2% of the time, with gonadotropin administration the rate is slightly increased (1% to 3%).

- *ovarian twisting*   Known medically as adnexal torsion, this occurs less than 1% of the time. In this condition, the stimulated ovary can twist, cutting off its own blood supply. Surgery is required to untwist or remove it.

- *ovarian cancer*   The risk of ovarian cancer in women seems in part related to the number of times a woman ovulates. Infertility increases this risk, and the use of birth control pills decreases it. There are controversial data that associate ovulation stimulation drugs like gonadotropins to the risk of future ovarian cancer. While research is underway to help clarify this issue, the careful use of gonadotropins is still warranted, especially considering that pregnancy and breast-feeding reduce cancer risk. (See also OVARIAN CANCER AND FERTILITY DRUGS.)

gonadotropin-releasing   hormone (Gn-RH)
Secreted by the hypothalamus about every 90 minutes, Gn-RH stimulates the pituitary to secrete LH and FSH. If a woman's hypothalamus does not produce the pulsating bursts of Gn-RH that trigger release of LH and FSH, she won't release LH or FSH and therefore won't ovulate.

Women who don't ovulate can sometimes be treated with Gn-RH. Because Gn-RH is released in intervals, treatment must be infused as a pulse with a battery-powered pump into the veins or under the skin. Ovulation occurs from 50% to 90% of the time, and conception rates after 6 months are similar to other ovulation induction treatments.

Women with underdeveloped ovaries because of a lack of production of adequate amounts of LH or FSH, delayed puberty, or POLYCYSTIC OVARY SYNDROME (PCOS) may also respond to Gn-RH.

Unlike FSH medications such as Follistin or Gonal-F (which produce many follicles), Gn-RH–induced cycles usually trigger the development of one follicle. Treatment with Gn-RH costs about as much as treatment with Pergonal.

Risks
There is a slight risk of infection from the injection, and when it is given intravenously there is a rare risk of infection in the bloodstream. Risk of multiple births is rare, and there is much less chance of OVARIAN HYPERSTIMULATION SYNDROME than with other treatments.

Gonal F   A highly pure form of FSH (FOLLICLE-STIMULATING HORMONE), the hormone that is primarily responsible for stimulating the development of follicles containing eggs. When given as a fertility drug, Gonal F can stimulate follicular development.

It is the first recombinant drug to be approved for the treatment of infertility. In recombinant technology, DNA is removed from one organism and recombined with that of a different organism. The resulting DNA strand is called recombinant DNA. Drugs produced this way are called "recombinant."

Gonal F is designed to cause follicles to grow and is now available to be used to produce eggs for women who don't ovulate on their own, those who need multiple eggs for IN VITRO FERTILIZATION, and for other ASSISTED REPRODUCTIVE TECHNOLOGIES.

As a purer form of hormone with a more predictable effect on the body, it can take the place of the HUMAN MENOPAUSAL GONADOTROPINS (hMG) Pergonal, Humegon, or Fertinex or the human follicle-stimulating hormone (hFSH) METRODIN.

A significant benefit for patients is that these newer forms of FSH medications produced by recombinent DNA technology can be given as a subcutaneous injection using a smaller needle and can make it easier for the patient to inject herself. In addition, the new drug has fewer contaminants with less possibility of local reactions from the injection.

Studies comparing Gonal F with Metrodin show it is effective, although the newer medication is slightly more expensive. Gonal F contains 75 IU of FSH. When given to premenopausal women, this hormone stimulates the formation and maturation of follicles, followed by egg production. For actual ovulation to occur, a separate injection of HCG is needed to provide the surge of LH, which triggers the release of the ripened eggs.

Each regimen of gonadotropins is tailored specifically to the needs of each patient and usually involves 7 to 12 days of injections. When a combination of rising estradiol levels and ultrasounds indicate that the follicles are the right size, an injection of hCG is given. At the appropriate time, sex, insemination, or egg retrieval is planned.

Side Effects

Complications are related to hyperstimulation of the ovary and include the possibility of multiple gestation and subsequent risk of premature delivery. Hyperstimulation temporarily enlarges the ovary, causing low abdominal pain, pressure, weight gain, and swelling (usually 5 to 8 days after the HCG injection). These symptoms usually fade away on their own after menstruation, although occasionally a woman may need to be hospitalized for observation and fluids. The risk of hyperstimulation is small when the patient is carefully monitored. There also may be local soreness or redness at the injection site.

The incidence of multiple gestation appears to be between 15% to 20%. Most of these multiple births are twins (75%).

Some studies suggest a slight increase in ovarian cancer in women who have taken fertility drugs, but these studies are controversial.

Success Rate

Medical studies indicate that between 70% and 100% of women ovulate after Gonal F/Follistim treatment. The conception rate is reported to be between 15% and 50%. The 25% rate of miscarriage is somewhat higher than the 15% miscarriage rate seen in the general population.

gonorrhea A sexually transmitted infection caused by bacteria *Neisseria gonococcus* that can cause tubal damage in men and women, leading to infertility; it is a particularly serious problem for women. The bacteria are transmitted through unprotected vaginal, anal, and (less often) oral sex.

Gonorrhea can spread to the UTERUS and FALLOPIAN TUBES, causing PELVIC INFLAMMATORY DISEASES (PID). PID affects at least one in six women with gonorrhea and frequently leads to infertility. In men, gonorrhea can infect the body structure where sperm are stored (EPIDIDYMIS). This infection, called EPIDIDYMITIS, also leads to infertility.

Symptoms

Women may experience abnormal vaginal discharge, bleeding between periods, and/or lower abdominal pain. Men's symptoms include a discharge from the urethra and/or pain during urination.

Symptoms can develop from 1 day to 2 weeks after exposure; however, 50% to 80% of women and 5% of men with genital gonorrhea don't experience any symptoms. Both men and women can have gonococcal infections of the throat and rectum; most of these infections are without symptoms.

Diagnosis

A doctor can make a diagnosis almost immediately by identifying the bacterium (gonococcus) under a microscope. In more than 90% of infected men, gonorrhea can be diagnosed using a sample of discharge from the penis. But only 60% of infected women can be diagnosed using a sample of the discharge from the cervix. If no bacteria are seen under the microscope, the discharge is sent to the laboratory for culture.

If a doctor suspects an infection of the throat or rectum, samples from these areas are sent for culture. Although a blood test for gonorrhea isn't available, a doctor may take a sample of blood to determine whether the person also has syphilis or human immunodeficiency virus (HIV) infection. Some people have more than one sexually transmitted disease.

Treatment

Doctors usually treat gonorrhea with a single injection of ceftriaxone into a muscle or with oral antibiotics (usually doxycycline). If gonorrhea has spread through the bloodstream, the person usually is hospitalized and given intravenous antibiotics. Because many people who have gonorrhea are also infected with chlamydia (which is hard to diagnose), patients are given a weeklong course of doxycycline or tetracycline or a single dose of azithromycin, another long-acting antibiotic.

If symptoms recur or persist at the end of treatment, doctors may obtain specimens for culture to make sure the person is cured. In men, symptoms of urethritis may recur (post-gonococcal urethritis). This condition, usually caused by chlamydia and other organisms that don't respond to treatment with ceftriaxone, occurs particularly in people who do not follow the treatment plan as prescribed.

goserelin (Zoladex)   A Gn-RH agonist commonly used to treat ENDOMETRIOSIS and fibroids.

granulosa cells   The cells within the ovarian FOLLICLE that make ESTROGEN and PROGESTERONE during the OVULATION cycle.

hamster penetration assay (HPA) The medical name for the "hamster test," this is a test of the ability of human SPERM to penetrate a hamster egg that has been stripped of its outer membrane. It is also called the sperm penetration assay (SPA), the sperm-oocyte interaction test, or zona-free hamster egg test.

A normal SEMEN ANALYSIS can't conclusively predict if sperm can penetrate an egg, so in this "test tube" experiment, semen are combined in a dish with hamster eggs, which are anatomically similar to human eggs. Later, the eggs are checked for penetration by the sperm. A penetration rate of greater than 10% is good evidence of the fertile potential of the sperm, whereas a penetration rate of less than 10% may indicate less-than-adequate fertility.

The hamster test is sometimes offered to test the sperm of healthy men

- with unexplained INFERTILITY
- with very low SPERM COUNTS
- as a screen for those entering an IN VITRO FERTILIZATION or assisted reproduction programs

The reliability of this test depends on many variables. In general, a positive result is fairly predictive, but some false negative results have occurred. Moreover, the failure to penetrate a hamster egg does not always mean that the sperm cannot penetrate a human egg.

hatching The embryo breaking out of its shell of the egg (called the ZONA PELLUCIDA), a step necessary before implantation.

hCG See HUMAN CHORIONIC GONADOTROPINS.

heat and infertility Sperm production is best at or slightly below the core body temperature, which is why the SCROTUM is located outside the body. This is why men who are trying to conceive should avoid hot tubs, saunas, and steam rooms.

One study in California showed that men who use hot tubs have lower SPERM counts, but when the heat is avoided for several months, sperm production returns to normal. This makes sense, since sperm production typically takes about 3 months.

Although there is no conclusive evidence, researchers believe that tight underwear and clothing may increase scrotal temperatures and impair sperm production.

hemizona assay A laboratory test of the ability of sperm to bind to the egg shell (ZONA PELLUCIDA). The test involves splitting the egg in half; then one half is tested against the husband's sperm and the other half against sperm from a known fertile man (which acts as a control).

Ethically, this test is acceptable since the microsurgical splitting of the egg prevents any inadvertent fertilization. The major problem with this test is the limited availability of human eggs.

herbs and infertility Taking certain herbal medications could interfere with efforts to achieve pregnancy, whether the herbs are taken by a man or a woman. Specifically, experts believe that the herbs echinacea, gingko biloba, and St. John's wort have a negative effect on sperm production and the capacity to fertilize an egg. In lab studies, these three herbs all interfered with the ability of sperm to penetrate the egg, which is a required first step before fertilization can take place.

Other herbs that some experts believe may negatively affect fertility include black cohosh, ginseng, and kava kava. For this reason, a couple trying to have a baby should tell their doctor about all medications they take—including herbal remedies, over-the-counter medications, and prescription drugs.

heredity and infertility   In addition to a variety of inherited diseases that cause infertility, certain genetic factors may interfere with fertility as well.

Most research in this area has focused on problems of the Y chromosome; specifically, that certain missing parts on this chromosome could explain some cases of infertility. Normal men carry both an X and a Y chromosome, whereas women have two X chromosomes. Researchers have discovered that about 20% of male infertility can be traced either to the loss of a large part of the male Y chromosome or to an abnormal part of the Y chromosome that interferes with sperm production and causes infertility.

Experts hope that identifying genetic abnormalities in men might one day enable researchers to develop gene therapy as a treatment for some types of infertility.

In addition to looking within the Y chromosome for causes of infertility, researchers are searching for clues on the autosomes (any of the sex-neutral chromosomes). Human cells each have 22 pairs of autosomes; missing bits of some of these autosomes also have been linked to infertility.

heterotopic pregnancy   A normal pregnancy that occurs at the same time as an ECTOPIC PREGNANCY.

hMG   See HUMAN MENOPAUSAL GONADOTROPIN.

HMOs and infertility treatment   See INSURANCE COVERAGE FOR FERTILITY TREATMENT.

hormone   A chemical substance that travels via the bloodstream and carries a signal from one part of the body to another. The study of hormones is called ENDOCRINOLOGY. All of the hormone systems of the body are known collectively as the endocrine system.

hormonal birth control   Given in the form of injections, pills, or implants, hormones can be used as a type of BIRTH CONTROL to interfere with normal OVULATION, conception, and implantation very effectively. As with most medications, this type of birth control also can cause a range of side effects, including headaches, acne, weight changes, excess hair or hair loss, nausea and vomiting, depression, and menstrual irregularities.

Despite these problems, for many women the benefits of hormonal methods (simplicity and effectiveness) make them a popular choice. Implants and injections in particular can be a good choice since they are ESTROGEN-free and they are easy to use.

The Pill

Oral contraceptives have been on the market for more than 35 years and are the most popular form of reversible birth control in the United States. The pill works by suppressing ovulation (the monthly release of an egg from the ovaries) as a result of the combined actions of the hormones within the pill (ESTROGEN and progestin). If taken daily as directed, there is an extremely low chance of becoming pregnant. But the pill's effectiveness may be reduced if a woman takes certain other medications (such as some antibiotics) at the same time. If a woman forgets a pill, she should use a backup method of birth control for the next 2 days to be sure she's protected against pregnancy.

BIRTH CONTROL PILLS also can affect other medications or lab test results. The estrogen and progestin in birth control pills can affect liver function. If taken together with other drugs that are metabolized by the liver, there may be higher blood levels of the birth control pill, causing more toxic side effects. These effects might be strongest in pills with large amounts of progestin.

Older versions of the pill contained high doses of estrogen that made this type of contraception dangerous for women over age 35; newer, safer forms are now highly effective and safe for most nonsmoking women up to age 45. Still, the long-term effect of taking these pills is not clear, because not enough women have taken them for that long.

Besides preventing pregnancy, the pill offers significant health benefits of which many women may not be aware. The pill can make menstrual periods more regular, and protects against both PELVIC INFLAMMATORY DISEASE and ovarian and endometrial cancers.

While birth control pills are safe for most women (safer than delivering a baby), they do carry some risks for some women. Especially in women who smoke, the pill may contribute to high blood pressure, blood clots, and blockage of the arteries. One of the biggest questions has been whether the pill increases the risk of breast cancer in past and current pill users. An international study published in the September 1996 journal *Contraception* concluded that women's risk of breast cancer 10 years after going off birth control pills was no higher than that of women who had never used the pill. During pill use and for the first 10 years after stopping the pill, women's risk of breast cancer was only slightly higher in pill users than non–pill users.

Most health experts advise some women not to take the pill:

- women who smoke—especially those over age 35
- women with a history of blood clots
- women with a personal history of breast or endometrial cancer
- women with heart disease
- women over age 45

Some women object to the pill not because of health concerns but because of side effects, which include nausea, headache, breast tenderness, weight gain, irregular bleeding, and depression. While the problems may subside after a few months, some women experience continued problems.

Another type of oral contraceptive called the MINIPILL is taken daily, but contains only the hormone progestin with no estrogen. These pills work by reducing and thickening cervical mucus to prevent sperm from reaching the egg. They also keep the uterine lining from thickening, which prevents a fertilized egg from implanting in the uterus.

Because they lack estrogen, these pills are slightly less effective than combined oral contraceptives. Women who take the minipill late (even by as few as 3 hours) have a higher chance of pregnancy.

Minipills can decrease menstrual bleeding and cramps, as well as carry the risk of endometrial and ovarian cancer and PELVIC INFLAMMATORY DISEASE. Because they contain no estrogen, minipills don't carry the risk of blood clots associated with estrogen in combined pills. They are a good option for women who can't take estrogen because they are breast-feeding or because estrogen-containing products cause them to have severe headaches or high blood pressure. Side effects of minipills include irregular menstrual cycles, weight gain, and breast tenderness.

Emergency Contraceptive Pills (ECPs)

These pills can prevent pregnancy after unprotected sex in cases of unanticipated sexual activity, contraceptive failure, or rape. Mistakenly known as the "morning after pill," EMERGENCY CONTRACEPTIVE PILLS actually involve more than one pill, they don't need to be taken on the "morning after," and they should not be confused with the so-called "abortion pill" (MIFEPRI-STONE) because ECPs can't terminate an established pregnancy.

By the end of the 1990s, ECPs were widely recognized as a safe and effective method for all women at risk for unintended pregnancy. The most common regimen consists of giving two doses of combined oral contraceptive pills that contain the hormones estrogen and progestin. The first dose is taken within 72 hours after unprotected sex, the second dose 12 hours later.

Another type of ECP, which contains a single progestin (levonorgestrel), first became available in Eastern Europe. Pharmaceutical companies have since introduced such products in other countries, including the United States, where the progestin-only ECP is known as PLAN B.

The FDA approved in 1998 the application of Gynetics, Inc., of Belle Mead, NJ, to market America's first dedicated ECP product, the PRE-VEN Emergency Contraceptive Kit. Some providers continue to prescribe oral contraceptive pills for emergency use, and for some women, the ECP dosage becomes the beginning of daily, non-emergency oral contraceptive use. The launch of PREVEN represented the first commercial ECP advertising to American women.

In July 1999, the FDA approved the first progestin-only ECP available in the United States. Produced by the Women's Capital Corporation of Bellevue, WA, Plan B contains only one hormone, the progestin levonorgestrel. A World Health Organization–supported study has found that the levonorgestrel regimen is more effective and has fewer side effects than the Yuzpe regimen.

When used correctly, progestin-only ECPs were found to reduce the risk of pregnancy by 89% in a World Health Organization–supported study involving almost 2,000 women in 21 clinics around the world. When taken within 24 hours of unprotected intercourse, they were found to reduce the risk of pregnancy by 95%.

The amount of time since unprotected sex and the point in a woman's cycle at which she had sex influence the effectiveness of emergency contraception. The earlier ECPs are taken after unprotected sex, the more effective they are, and the closer a woman is to ovulation at the time of unprotected sex, the less likely that ECP will succeed. ECPs aren't as effective as consistent use of "before sex" methods such as the pill, the IUD, or contraceptive implants or injections, and they don't protect against sexually transmitted diseases.

Contraceptive Implants

One of the newest types of birth control options are contraceptive implants (such as NORPLANT)— small, matchstick-sized tubes containing a progestin or levonorgestrel—inserted just under the skin of a woman's arm. Once in place, the implants release a small amount of hormone each day for 5 years, blocking ovulation and thickening cervical mucus. Implants are a very effective method of contraception. Once the implants are removed, a woman can become pregnant again.

The implants can be inserted during an office visit. First the doctor numbs the skin with local anesthetic and then imbeds the tubes under the skin of the upper arm. They must be surgically removed when contraception is no longer desired.

Some women may experience inflammation or infection at the site of the implant. Other side effects include menstrual cycle changes, weight gain, and breast tenderness. Another important but less obvious change may be loss of bone mass.

While implants are very effective, they can cause all of the side effects typically related to hormonal types of birth control. Some serious symptoms include

- arm pain
- pus or bleeding at the insertion site (it could be an infection)
- expulsion of the implant
- delayed menstrual periods after a long time of regular periods

Women should not use implants if they

- are (or might be) pregnant
- have unexplained unusual vaginal bleeding
- take antiseizure drugs
- take the antibiotic rifampin
- have blood clots
- have had pulmonary embolism (blood clots in the lungs)

Several new types of implants are currently being developed. They include a single capsule called Implanon, designed to work for 2 or 3 years, that contains a more potent progestin called 3-ketodesogestrel. The Norplant II is the second generation of Norplant that only requires two implants. Finally, biodegradable implants are being developed that contain progestin and are implanted under the skin of the arm or hip. The hormone is released gradually into the body for 12 to 18 months.

Birth Control Injections

Some women don't like the idea of having tubes inserted into their arms; they prefer hormone injections. These injections, which are considered to be safe and effective, involve a long-acting type of progesterone that is injected every 3 months. The method uses a progestin, which is normally injected into the buttocks.

The injections work by preventing ovulation; when taken as scheduled it's more than 99% effective and completely reversible once the hormone is eliminated from the body. The first injection should be scheduled within 5 days of the start of a menstrual period to get full protection from pregnancy right from the beginning.

Women should not have the injections if they are (or might be) pregnant or if they have unexplained unusual vaginal bleeding any time in the preceding 3 months.

After taking the injections for several cycles, a woman actually has a bit more protection (a few weeks longer than 3 months); this provides a "safety period" until the next shot. However,

once a woman has gotten the injection, there is no way to become fertile again until it wears off about 3 months later.

Because the injections aren't metabolized in the liver, some of the side effects from pills are avoided. However, the injections may cause

- abdominal discomfort
- nervousness
- decreased sex drive
- depression
- acne
- dizziness
- weight gain
- menstrual cycle disruption
- bleeding and spotting

Serious symptoms include excessive weight gain, heavy bleeding, severe headaches, depression, frequent urination, and severe lower abdominal pain (rare).

HOST   See HYPO-OSMOTIC SWELLING TEST.

host uterus   This term refers to a woman who carries another couple's EMBRYO to term and returns the baby to the genetic parents immediately after birth. Another term for "host uterus" is surrogate gestational mother. See also SURROGATE MOTHER.

hot tubs and infertility   See HEAT AND INFERTILITY.

hPG   See HUMAN PITUITARY GONADOTROPIN.

HSG   See HYSTEROSALPINOGOGRAM.

Huhner's test   See POSTCOITAL TEST.

human chorionic gonadotropin (hCG)   A hormone produced by the placenta in early pregnancy that keeps the corpus luteum producing progesterone. It is also used as a fertility drug (trade names: Profasi, Pregnyl) to stimulate OVULATION.

Derived from the urine of pregnant women, the drug is chemically similar to luteinizing hormone and mimics the effect of LH which normally induces the release of the egg (ovulation). It is cheaper and easier, and works for a longer period of time than does LH. It is also used in men to stimulate testosterone production.

Side Effects
Possible hyperstimulation of the ovaries and multiple births, redness or tenderness at the injection site, and lower abdominal tenderness.

human menopausal gonadotropin (hMG) Human menopausal GONADOTROPINS (hMG) are naturally occurring hormones excreted in the urine of postmenopausal women that can be used to stimulate OVULATION in women who don't ovulate and who don't respond to fertility drugs. It is recovered from the urine of postmenopausal women and contains equal amounts of FSH and LH.

The hormones are marketed as Pergonal, Humegon, or Repronex, and are given to stimulate the ovaries directly as a way to produce several eggs in one cycle. When given to premenopausal women, these hormones stimulate ovarian follicle growth and maturation. For ovulation to occur, a separate injection of hCG is needed to release the ripened egg(s). The hormones may cause the OVARY to produce several follicles, which can then be harvested for use in GAMETE INTRAFALLOPIAN TRANSFER (GIFT) or IN VITRO FERTILIZATION (IVF).

The strongest fertility drug available, it is often given if CLOMIPHENE CITRATE has not worked. It is most often used in ovulating women to increase the number of eggs produced or in women who do not ovulate at all to stimulate follicle growth. It also may be used with men to stimulate sperm production.

An ampule of hMG typically contains 75 IU of follicle-stimulating hormone (FSH) and 75 IU of luteinizing hormone (LH). Metrodin contains 75 units of FSH alone.

Each treatment regimen is tailored to the individual patient and is usually given for 7 to 12 days. When a combination of rising estradiol levels and ultrasound indicate that follicle number and size are adequate, an injection of hCG is given. At the appropriate time, sex, insemination or IVF egg retrieval is planned.

The doctor will watch the development of the ovarian FOLLICLES by measuring the amount of ESTROGEN in the blood and by checking the size of the follicles with ultrasound examinations.

Side Effects
Most significant complications and side effects resulting from hMG are related to hyperstimulation of the ovary and also include multiple gestations and possible premature delivery or pregnancy loss. Hyperstimulation causes a temporary swelling of the ovary, leading to low abdominal pain, pressure, weight gain, and swelling, usually 5 to 8 days after the hCG is given.

Symptoms usually go away on their own shortly after menstruation if the treatment failed, although an occasional patient may need to be hospitalized for observation and fluids. Treatment consists of bed rest and pain medication. There also may be local soreness or redness at the injection site(s). If pregnancy occurs, the course of ovarian hyperstimulation may be protracted. In addition, these drugs have been associated with the possibility of a slight increase in developing ovarian cancer, although this is controversial.

Success Rate
Medical studies indicate that between 70% and 100% of women ovulate after using Pergonal and/or Metrodin. The conception rate is reported to be between 15% to 50%, with a 25% incidence of miscarriage (somewhat higher than the 15% miscarriage rate seen in the general population). The chance of multiple gestations appears to be between 20% to 40%. Most of these multi-

ple births are twins (75%), but triplets or more babies are also possible. However, between 60% to 80% of the pregnancies resulting from hMG involve single births. See OVARIAN HYPERSTIMULATION SYNDROME.

human pituitary gonadotropin (hPG) A mixture of FOLLICLE-STIMULATING HORMONE (FSH) and LUTEINIZING HORMONE (LH) extracted from the pituitary gland during an autopsy. It was never used routinely in the United States and since 1986 has not been used anywhere in the world due to the risk of transmitting Creutzfeldt-Jakob disease via tainted brain tissue.

Humegon (hMG) The brand name for HUMAN MENOPAUSAL GONADOTROPIN (hMG).

hyaluronidase An enzyme in the SPERM membrane released during FERTILIZATION so that the sperm can separate the granulosa cells from the egg.

hydrosalpinx Closure of the outer end of the FALLOPIAN TUBE, which becomes distended and results in a fluid-filled sac.

hydrotubation Injection of fluid, often into the FALLOPIAN TUBES, to determine if they are open.

hyperandrogenism Excessive production of androgens in women, often a cause of excessive hairiness and also associated with POLYCYSTIC OVARY SYNDROME (PCOS).

hyperplasia without atypical cells This benign condition refers to a buildup of glandular cells (the glandular endometrial cells are growing but are still noncancerous). This kind of hyperplasia rarely develops into cancer.

Atypical adenomatous hyperplasia (also called severe hyperplasia or carcinoma in situ—CIS) means that either a small area on the endometrium or the entire lining consists of cells that are abnormal. The cells seem to be more aggressive but may still be harmless. It still isn't malignant, but more women with severe hyperplasia may go on to develop uterine cancer.

Risk
Women who are 25 to 50 pounds overweight are three times as likely to develop hyperplasia. Women who are more than 50 pounds overweight are nine times as likely to develop hyperplasia. Women at higher risk also include those who have always had irregular periods or who have diabetes. Other potential causes of excess estrogen include environmental toxins, certain herbs (such as ginseng), hormone-fed meats and poultry, certain cosmetics made from estrogen, and hormonal contraceptives that contain estrogen.

A postmenopausal woman with an intact uterus on unopposed estrogen replacement therapy (ERT) is also at risk for developing hyperplasia. An estrogen/progesterone combination therapy can reverse as much as 96.8% of all postmenopausal hyperplasia cases.

Diagnosis
This diagnosis can only be made by the pathologist who examines a sample of tissue removed from the thickened endometrium by a sampling procedure such as ENDOMETRIAL BIOPSY, D&C, or HYSTEROSCOPY.

Treatment
In younger women particularly, severe hyperplasia can be reversed with hormonal therapy. Adding progesterone by taking a progestin or resuming ovulation (spontaneously or with medications) can eliminate hyperplasia. If this doesn't work, a D&C is the next logical step. A hysterectomy is not necessary unless the hyperplasia persists after the lining is removed. If severe hyperplasia persists and keeps redeveloping despite HRT and a repeat D&C, then a hysterectomy may be required.

hyper/hypothyroidism When the body produces either too much or too little thyroid hormone, respectively.

Too little thyroid production (hypo-) may cause two fertility problems: increased prolactin levels and irregular ovulation. Hypothyroidism slows down a woman's metabolism and causes estrogens to build up in the blood. This continual ESTROGEN stimulation tricks the hypothalamus into believing that the OVARY is producing enough estrogen, so it directs the pituitary to reduce LH and FSH stimulation. When this happens, the follicles fail to mature and the ovaries don't produce enough estrogen to trigger the LH SURGE necessary for ovulation.

When the thyroid gland produces too much thyroid hormone (hyperthyroidism), estrogen supply is used up too early and the woman begins to suffer from a lack of estrogen. Since the pituitary never senses that the FOLLICLE has reached maturity (which is signaled by high estrogen levels), it doesn't trigger the LH surge to trigger ovulation.

Treatment

For hypothyroidism, a thyroid hormone supplement will lower prolactin levels and improve estrogen metabolism. Some causes of hyperthyroidism are also treated with thyroid hormone. Taking a thyroid supplement may turn off the overactive thyroid gland and return thyroid hormone levels to normal, so that normal ovulatory cycles resume. However, surgery to remove the overactive thyroid gland is sometimes necessary.

hypogonadotropic hypopituitarism A spectrum of diseases that cause low pituitary gland production of LH and FSH. Men with this disorder have low sperm counts and may lose their virility; women don't ovulate and may lose their secondary sex characteristics.

hypo-osmotic swelling test (HOST) A method to predict whether a SPERM can fertilize an egg. Since normal sperm tails swell in the presence of a special sugar and salt solution, poorly functioning or dead sperm don't seem to have that effect.

The HOST test should not be used to evaluate sperm function but may be used as an optional test of vitality. It is simple to perform and easy to score and gives additional information on the integrity and the compliance of the cell membrane of the sperm tail.

hypospadia A condition in which a male is born with the urethra open near the base or along the underside of the penis, not at the tip. As a result, the penis is usually short and curved, which can lead to problems during sexual intercourse and can contribute to infertility.

If untreated, these males experience normal sperm production but can't ejaculate SPERM directly into the cervix. This can be corrected with plastic surgery, by recreating a new opening at the tip of the penis. See also EPISPADIAS.

hypothalamus A part of the brain that regulates hormones, located next to and above the pituitary gland, both of which are found at the base of the brain. In both men and women, this tissue secretes GONADOTROPIN-RELEASING HORMONE (Gn-RH) every 60 to 90 minutes. Gn-RH enables the pituitary gland to secrete LH and FSH, which stimulate the testicles and ovaries.

The hypothalamus and pituitary gland are essential for normal sexual development. The hypothalamus is an important endocrine gland about the size of a thumbnail; the pea-sized pituitary is linked to the hypothalamus by a tiny structure called the pituitary stalk.

Once the hypothalamus secretes one of its many different hormones, it is delivered to the pituitary gland via the pituitary stalk. The pituitary gland is then encouraged to secrete hormones of its own, which then circulate in the blood. This teamwork is essential for a number of physical and biological processes to be carried out. One of these processes is the regulation of sexual development by the hypothalamus, pituitary gland, and the gonads (testes and ovaries).

Hypothalamic hormones target the pituitary gland and, normally, pituitary hormones are released in response, which then target the gonads. These pituitary hormones have two main functions: to encourage and maintain the body's secondary sexual characteristics and to promote fertility. The feedback mechanisms linking the gonads to the hypothalamus and pituitary gland normally ensure that these hormones are always available in the correct amounts.

hypothyroidism   See HYPER/HYPOTHYROIDISM.

hysterectomy   A surgical procedure involving the removal of the uterus, usually including the cervix but not necessarily the ovaries and fallopian tubes. One in four women in the United States has a hysterectomy by the age of 60.

Each year U.S. doctors perform about 500,000 hysterectomies, making it one of the most commonly performed major operations in the country. Some of these operations are necessary to stop the growth of cancers of the UTERUS, ovaries, or cervix, but most are performed to treat noncancerous conditions such as uterine fibroids, excessive menstrual bleeding, and other reproductive problems.

In the past, medical experts often thought of the uterus as something a woman didn't need once she was past childbearing years, and the uterus was sometimes removed during fibroid surgery to eliminate the chance of uterine cancer. Nowadays, a hysterectomy is not recommended unless it's absolutely necessary.

For many women, the biggest problem with a hysterectomy is the loss of fertility. Some experience a loss of sexual desire, although this problem is usually associated with removal of the ovaries and is treatable with hormone therapy.

Hysterectomy is required for women with ovarian or uterine cancer, very large uterine fibroids or ovarian cysts, advanced PELVIC INFLAMMATORY DISEASE, or severe complications during pregnancy. Cesarean hysterectomy may be performed after delivery to stop life-threatening bleeding from the uterus. Conditions that don't usually require hysterectomy include abnormal menstrual bleeding, uterine fibroids not associated with symptoms, ENDOMETRIOSIS, uterine prolapse, precancerous cervical lesions, or chronic pelvic pain. A second opinion is often advisable before considering a hysterectomy.

A hysterectomy requires a hospital stay of a few days, followed by at least a month of rest at home. Women who have abdominal hysterectomies usually need to stay in the hospital a day or two longer than women who have vaginal hysterectomies. (Vaginal hysterectomies don't require an incision of the abdomen.)

Some studies suggest that up to 40% of women experience a decrease in sexual response after the operation. This may be related to a TESTOSTERONE deficiency that can develop if the ovaries are removed, which in turn reduces the production of male hormones. This imbalance can be treated with hormones, including the use of natural testosterone creams applied vaginally. (Most hysterectomies spare the ovaries, however, thus sparing ovarian hormonal function.) Since contractions of the uterus can contribute to orgasm, some women report that they have more difficulty reaching a satisfying orgasm.

Other studies have found that women don't have a problem with sex after hysterectomy—and still others say they find sex more enjoyable than before.

hysterosalpingogram (HSG)   An X ray of the pelvic organs as a radio-opaque dye is injected through the cervix into the uterus and fallopian tubes. This test is used to check for malformations of the uterus or blocked fallopian tubes in suspected infertility. It is performed after a menstrual period is over but before OVULATION.

In this procedure, the doctor inserts a small tube into the woman's cervical canal and injects dye into the uterus, which then flows out along the fallopian tubes. The progression of the dye can be watched on an X-ray screen as it fills the uterus and moves through the tubes. If either or both tubes are blocked or scarred, this test will help to make that diagnosis. In addition to determining whether the tubes are open or blocked, the test can reveal the presence of polyps, fibroid tumors, or scar tissue.

Medications such as ibuprofen (Motrin or Advil) can prevent the cramping that sometimes occurs during the procedure.

Several studies have found that pregnancy rates slightly increased in the first months following a hysterosalpingogram. This may be because the flushing of the tubes with the contrast could open a minor blockage or clean out some debris that may be a factor preventing the couple from conceiving. Some of these studies suggest that using oil-based contrast dye triggers a higher increase in pregnancy rates than does the use of water-based contrast.

Complications

Rarely, a woman may have an allergic reaction to the dye, which usually manifests as a rash, although it can be more serious. Pelvic infection or uterine perforation are also possible, yet rare, complications.

If a woman has multiple sexual partners or is at risk for sexually transmitted diseases, she should be screened with cervical cultures before doing an HSG. Some doctors prescribe several days of antibiotics before the test to reduce the risk of infection after the procedure.

hysteroscopy A surgical procedure to check for abnormalities within the uterus. It is performed by placing a small, thin telescope-like instrument through the cervical canal to inspect the inside of the uterus. The procedure can be used both to diagnose and treat problems, since minor surgical repairs also can be done during operative hysteroscopy.

This procedure usually takes place in an operating room, usually under general anesthesia, or in a doctor's office with or without sedation. There is usually minimal discomfort during hysteroscopy with local anesthesia. Most women are able to resume normal activities immediately. If required, a short-acting narcotic may be given.

Because the inside of the uterus is not naturally inflated but is more like a collapsed dome, it is necessary to distend it with either a liquid or a gas in order to see. For this reason, gas or liquid is introduced into the uterus through the hysteroscope to separate the walls and allow inspection of possible fibroids, polyps, scarring, abnormal shape, and malignancy. Hysteroscopy is usually performed during the first half of the cycle to avoid interrupting a pregnancy.

Hysteroscopy may be used not just to diagnose but to treat. Instruments can be inserted through the hysteroscope to remove polyps, to cut adhesions, and do other procedures. In many situations, operative hysteroscopy may offer an alternative to hysterectomy.

Risks

Risks include bleeding, infection, and effects from the anesthetics.

ICSI   See INTRACYTOPLASMIC SPERM INJECTION.

idiopathic infertility   The medical term for unexplained INFERTILITY.

immune system and fertility   The immune system plays an important role in human reproduction. Inflammatory cells and their secretory products are involved in the processes of OVULATION and preparation of the uterine lining for implantation of a fertilized egg.

On the other hand, a malfunctioning immune system can interfere with the normal reproductive processes and cause INFERTILITY. Experts estimate that an immune factor may be involved in up to 20% of couples with otherwise unexplained infertility. Although many of these links to infertility remain unproved, there is solid scientific evidence to implicate the formation of antibodies against sperm as an important infertility factor.

There are a number of ways in which the immune system of either the mother or the father can affect the reproductive system, causing fertility problems.

For example, the woman's body may produce antibodies that attack the cells responsible for the placenta and the placenta's blood supply, or that attack the nuclei of the uterine or placenta cells. Or the woman's system might fail to produce antibodies that prevent her immune system from attacking her own fetus. Sometimes her system may just have too many natural killer cells.

The father's immune system can also cause problems, such as producing antibodies that attack his own sperm. Any one of these problems can be significant enough to prevent conception or cause a miscarriage. Some women undergoing assisted reproduction may experience failed IVF cycles, implantation failure, clinical miscarriages, or other difficulties due to immune problems.

immunobead tests   Tests that detect the presence of ANTISPERM ANTIBODIES attached to cells (such as SPERM cells), which may lessen the fertilizing potential of sperm. Antibodies are substances that interact with foreign substances such as proteins, toxins, or bacteria that the body perceives as harmful. Antisperm antibodies mistakenly attack a person's own sperm and can interfere with the physical changes that the sperm must undergo to successfully swim through the cervical mucus and penetrate the egg for fertilization.

The immunobead test uses tiny polyacrylamide "beads" coated with specific antibodies that bind to antisperm antibodies. They identify many classes of immunoglobulins (a protein with antibody activity; classes are abbreviated as "IgG," "IgA," etc.).

The immunobead test can distinguish the location on the sperm where the antibody is located (head, midpiece, or tail). There are two types of immunobead testing:

- Direct method measures the binding of beads to the target sperm.
- Indirect (passive) includes an additional procedure in which antibody is transferred to the donor sperm from the body fluid in question

(cervical mucus, follicular fluid, blood or semen).

Antisperm antibodies have been found in some men who have undergone VASOVASOSTOMY (reversal of a VASECTOMY) and who have experienced repeated sexually transmitted diseases or other types of testicle injury or twisting. The antibodies also may appear after improper descent of the testes, inflammation of the testes, and long-term increased numbers of white blood cells in the sperm.

implantation   The embedding of the embryo into tissue so it can establish contact with the mother's blood supply for nourishment. Implantation usually occurs in the lining of the UTERUS; however, in an ECTOPIC PREGNANCY it may occur elsewhere in the body.

implantation bleeding   Bleeding that occurs when an EMBRYO attaches itself to the mother's uterine wall. This bleeding can be confused with a menstrual period.

implantation rate   In IN VITRO FERTILIZATION, the proportion of transferred embryos that produce a gestational sac that can be seen on ULTRASOUND examination—that is, the chance that an embryo will result in an early pregnancy sac.

impotence   See ERECTILE DYSFUNCTION.

incompetent cervix   See CERVICAL INCOMPETENCE.

infertility   The inability to conceive after a year of unprotected, well-timed intercourse, or the inability to carry a pregnancy to term. Infertility affects 6.1 million American couples—or about 10% of the reproductive age population. That means that one out of every six couples will at one point have a problem with infertility. Of course, that number may be misleading: Many couples give up on the idea of children rather than seek treatment for their infertility. Other couples suffer recurrent pregnancy losses that are, in a way, a form of infertility, but these couples aren't technically considered "infertile" because they are able to conceive.

Most doctors advise couples who are having problems getting pregnant not to worry until they have been trying to conceive for at least a year. However, if the woman is over age 35 or has a history of pelvic inflammatory disease, painful periods, miscarriage, irregular cycles—or if her partner has a known low sperm count—the couple should seek help before a year passes. This is important because the peak rate of conception occurs in both men and women at age 24 and begins to decline significantly after age 35, so that for every 5 years, the length of time required for conception doubles.

Willingness to seek help may be complicated by the fact that many couples are reluctant to admit that they may be infertile, hoping after each menstrual period that pregnancy will occur.

Causes

Infertility may be the temporary or permanent result of many different problems, many of which can be corrected. In any case, it's neither exclusively a "man's" nor a "woman's" problem: 35% of the time, the problem is a MALE FACTOR INFERTILITY; 35% is due to FEMALE FACTOR INFERTILITY. In addition, 25% of infertile couples have more than one factor that contributes to their infertility. The rest of the cases either are caused by problems in both partners or the reason for the infertility is unknown.

A man may be infertile because he doesn't have enough SPERM, because the sperm don't move or function properly, or because he has blocked passageways. Disease, fevers or infections, and abnormalities present since birth can contribute to these problems in men. Between 30% to 40% are caused by oligospermia, increased semen viscosity, decreased sperm motility (ability to move), or decreased semen volume. Less than 5% of cases are caused by abnormal sperm or abnormal cervical mucus penetration or ANTISPERM ANTIBODIES.

A woman may be infertile because some parts of her reproductive system are not functioning properly because of disease, infections, problems with hormone production, or abnormalities present since birth. In women, 15% to 20% of cases of infertility are due to ovulatory dysfunction, 30% to 40% to pelvic factors such as ENDOMETRIOSIS, adhesions, or tubal disease. Commonly, a woman may simply not have enough eggs, or she may suffer from blocked fallopian tubes, endometriosis, or POLYCYSTIC OVARY SYNDROME. These factors may interfere with reproduction in a number of ways: ovulation may not occur; the uterus may not be properly prepared to receive the developing embryo; the tubes may be blocked, diseased, or bound by scar tissue; or there may not be adequate CERVICAL MUCUS for the sperm's survival.

In about 10% to 15% of couples, no direct cause of infertility can be found. However, with further evaluation and treatment, occasionally factors such as poor sperm penetration or abnormal-appearing eggs are discovered. This group is referred to as having unexplained infertility.

While most cases of infertility are caused by physical problems, there are a host of other factors that can influence fertility success:

- Substance abuse: In women, alcohol boosts prolactin levels, which can interfere with ovulation and impair fertility.
- Coffee: Caffeine may interfere with fertility, although the data aren't conclusive; to be safe, couples should limit caffeinated coffee to two cups per day.
- Marijuana: Some studies suggest that men who smoke marijuana have lower sperm counts.
- Bacterial vaginal infection: A bacterial infection in your vagina can kill sperm; a woman may need a cervical culture before trying to conceive.

- Smoking: Toxins in smoke can lower sperm count or slow down the sperm's ability to swim.
- Douches, lubricants, soap: These products introduced into the cervical canal during or immediately following sex are potential sperm killers.
- Weight: Women who weigh 30% more or less than their ideal body weight may have irregular periods and, thus, more problems conceiving (very thin women may stop ovulating altogether).
- Stress: Severe life stress can interfere with ovulation, which can make it harder to get pregnant.
- Overheating: For healthy sperm, the testes should be cooler than a man's body temperature, so men with low or borderline sperm counts should avoid hot tubs, saunas, and steam rooms if they're trying to conceive.
- Herbs: Taking large doses of echinacea, ginkgo biloba, or St. John's wort over a long period of time damages hamster sperm, according to a recent report in *Fertility and Sterility*. More studies need to be done with humans to see if the risk is real.
- Environmental toxins: Pesticides, chemicals, and lead may be to blame for some cases of infertility.

Infertility can lead to stress and tension in a relationship. Couples may find it hard not to get discouraged. It is a time when a couple needs to be especially supportive of each other and may need to turn to professional counseling.

Diagnosis

Patients interested in seeking advice from an infertility specialist should get a referral and then schedule a meeting to discuss the issues, because it's important to find a specialist who meets a couple's needs. Most specialists prefer to see a couple together at the first appointment.

It is very important to regard infertility as a "two-patient" disorder, which means that both man and woman must be thoroughly evaluated, counseled, and included in the decision-making process. Often, couples will be asked to complete a questionnaire before the first visit exploring prior conceptions, BIRTH CONTROL METHODS, and sexual frequency and techniques.

Both partners will be screened for drug and alcohol use, since these substances may affect fertility. Research suggests that men who are heavy marijuana users show reduced TESTOS-TERONE levels, decreased sperm counts, and impotency. Alcohol is well known to affect sexual interest and potency. Moreover, lower levels of GONADOTROPIN and ovulation problems have been found among women who abuse drugs or alcohol. Cigarette smoking has also been linked to early menopause, reduced sperm production, and decreased steroid production. Other research suggests that smokers typically take longer to conceive than do nonsmokers.

The initial evaluation of the infertile couple requires a detailed history and physical examination. After the history and physical examination of both partners, an initial diagnosis should be made. The history and physical examination may clearly point to one or more causes of infertility. During the first evaluation, initial laboratory and diagnostic tests should be ordered. The assessments include a SEMEN ANALYSIS, assessment of ovulatory function, and evaluation of fallopian tube health by using HYSTEROSALPINGOGRAPHY (HSG). Further evaluation of pelvic anatomy (either by LAPAROSCOPY or HYSTEROSCOPY) is considered part of the initial workup if the HSG finds an abnormality, or later if no cause for infertility can be found. Other procedures such as POST-COITAL TESTING, ANTISPERM ANTIBODIES, SPERM PENETRATION assay, or other tests of sperm function may be employed in certain cases. In addition, FOLLICLE-STIMULATING HORMONE (FSH) and ESTRADIOL levels obtained on the third day of the menstrual cycle may be useful in women over age 35.

In the first month of evaluation, the couple should use condoms or barrier contraceptives. The following tests would then be scheduled:

Day 1: The woman should begin the BASAL BODY TEMPERATURE CHARTING.

Day 7–11: An HSG is scheduled between these days of the cycle to avoid menstruation and the possibility of radiation exposure of an embryo.

Day 10–18: Home urine LH tests.

Day 21: A progesterone blood level is obtained (or, more accurately, obtained 7 days after the LH surge).

Day 25–28: An endometrial biopsy (again most accurately dated to the LH surge) is done. During this time a semen analysis is also obtained.

In the second month, a follow-up visit is scheduled. This may be done between days 12 and 14 or after the LH surge, at which time a postcoital test is performed if indicated. At this time, test results, HSG films, and other data are reviewed with the couple.

Male Exam

The doctor will first perform a complete physical exam and then focus on the genitals, with careful inspection of the penis. A semen analysis is the next step. The man is asked to bring a sample of his semen into the lab for examination. SEMEN ANALYSIS includes

- check of the sperm's shape and appearance (SPERM MORPHOLOGY)
- measurement of sperm volume and pH
- sperm count, expressed as millions of sperm per milliliter of semen
- sperm movement (motility), expressed as the percentage of moving sperm
- cultures that may be requested to detect bacterial and mycoplasma infections

If there is any question about the findings, additional tests may be conducted, or the husband may be referred to a UROLOGIST (a doctor who specializes in matters involving the urinary tract, testes, and related reproductive organs).

Female Exam

A detailed physical exam will be performed, together with tests to identify any vaginal or cervical infections. The cervix should be carefully examined for abnormalities due to intrauterine exposure to DIETHYLSTILBESTROL or prior cervical surgery, including cryotherapy, cautery, or laser. A thorough pelvic examination will reveal any cervical and uterine tenderness and pelvic masses. A sterile plastic catheter can be used to check for cervical stenosis and to measure the depth and direction of the uterine cavity; this information may aid in future intrauterine insemination or embryo transfer.

The doctor will find out if the woman is producing an egg each month, since ovulatory factors account for up to 25% of cases of infertility. The results determine whether additional tests are needed. This can be done in several ways:

- BASAL BODY TEMPERATURE (BBT) charting
- ultrasound to monitor follicle development
- urinary LH tests
- PROGESTERONE TEST
- ENDOMETRIAL BIOPSY

To find out whether the fallopian tubes are open, a doctor can perform an X-ray examination of the tubes, called a HYSTEROSALPINGOGRAM; a contrast dye can reveal the shape of the uterus. The test should be performed as soon as menstrual bleeding has stopped. This eliminates the risk of performing the procedure during early conception. There has been some evidence that an HSG itself is therapeutic, and pregnancies have been reported after the procedure. While HSG rarely causes an allergic reaction or infection, women who are allergic to iodine or are suspected of having an infection should not undergo this procedure.

The tubes also can be examined using laparoscopy, a technique that allows the doctor to check the organs for disease by looking into the abdomen with a miniature light-transmitting telescope called a LAPAROSCOPE. Experts suggest that laparoscopy should not be performed until 3 months after a normal HSG because of the potential therapeutic effect of HSG. However, laparoscopy should be performed after a normal HSG if pregnancy has not occurred by 6 months to 1 year because of the high incidence of pelvic problems.

Although routine screening of infertile women isn't required, it is extremely helpful to screen for anemia and to identify blood type, including Rh or antibody status. If a woman has never been exposed to rubella, she should be immunized before infertility treatment. Testing for AIDS is essential among women at high risk, women undergoing ASSISTED REPRODUCTIVE TECHNOLOGY (ART), or women who are receiving frozen gametes.

Treatment

Recent improvements in medication, microsurgery, and IN VITRO FERTILIZATION (IVF) techniques make pregnancy possible for the vast majority of couples pursuing treatments. Some obstetrician-gynecologists and urologists are trained to deal with patients having difficulty getting pregnant. Doctors with specific training who specialize in infertility are often board-certified in REPRODUCTIVE ENDOCRINOLOGY, which means that the doctor has also passed a rigorous examination. Experience is the most important characteristic in infertility treatment. At least one of the physicians in the practice should be available 7 days a week, 24 hours a day, if a protocol requires monitoring (and most of them do).

If an infertile couple wants to conceive a child, the first step is to have a complete infertility evaluation, beginning with the medical history of the couple followed by a brief physical exam. The couple is also asked about their sexual relations to find out if their infertility may be related to such factors as the timing or frequency of intercourse.

In some cases, FERTILITY DRUGS may be prescribed to treat an underlying disease or hormone deficiency. For more difficult infertility problems, recent advances over the past 15 years have improved the chances of treating infertility.

Effectiveness

How effective any one particular treatment is depends on its appropriateness. Age, in addition to other factors, affects the likelihood of success.

Cost

The cost of treatment varies tremendously depending on the diagnosis and resulting treatment protocol. Clomid alone can cost about $100 a month, plus another $150 for an ultrasound and $75 for a progesterone level blood test. IVF with INTRACYTOPLASMIC SPERM INJECTION (ICSI) can cost from $12,000 to $15,000.

Prevention

Sexually transmitted diseases can be a major cause of infertility, so couples should always have protected sex. See also ALCOHOL AND INFERTILITY; ANTISPERM ANTIBODIES; ASSISTED REPRODUCTION TECHNIQUES; CAFFEINE AND INFERTILITY; MARIJUANA AND INFERTILITY; SMOKING AND INFERTILITY; STRESS AND INFERTILITY.

infertility around the world   Between 8% and 12% of couples around the world have problems conceiving a child at some point in their lives. In some parts of the world, more than one-third of couples are infertile. In a few developing countries (such as Nigeria), infertility is the leading reason for gynecological consultations.

Although infertility affects both men and women, especially in developing countries it is women who often bear the sole blame for barren marriages; in many places infertility is a socially acceptable reason for a husband to divorce his wife.

Most infertile couples around the world suffer from primary infertility, which means that the woman has never conceived. However, sub-Saharan Africa is a striking exception: In this region most couples (52%) were infertile after having previously conceived. (This is called secondary infertility.) While Latin America also has a relatively high rate of secondary infertility (40%), only 23% of infertile couples in Asia and 16% in North Africa experience secondary infertility.

Causes

While it is hard to accurately compare infertility rates from different countries, it is clear that the level and causes of infertility vary widely. For example, the Demographic Health Survey and World Fertility Survey have found that infertility in sub-Saharan Africa ranges from 11% to 20% in the 27 countries surveyed, yet these national rates conceal wide ethnic and geographic variations. For example, Namibia's national infertility rate of 19% is an average of rates ranging from 14% to 32% among the country's major ethnic groups.

Throughout the world, about 5% of couples suffer from anatomical, genetic, endocrinological, and immunological problems that cause infertility. The rest are infertile largely because of preventable conditions, including sexually transmitted, infectious, and parasitic diseases; poor health care practices; and exposure to potentially toxic substances. The factors that contribute to these conditions vary from region to region. Varying degrees of the availability of medical care make comparisons between countries difficult.

Reproductive tract infections (especially sexually transmitted diseases—STDs) are the leading preventable cause of infertility. The WHO multinational study found that 64% of infertile women in sub–Saharan Africa had STD-related infertility, about double the rate of other regions. Tubal problems and other infection-related diagnoses also are associated with postpartum and postabortion complications.

infertility, absolute   See STERILITY.

infertility, complete   Absolute infertility in which there is no chance of a pregnancy occurring without help, usually because there is either no SPERM, no OVULATION, or a complete blockage so that egg and sperm can't meet.

infertility, secondary The inability of a couple to achieve a second pregnancy. This strict medical definition includes couples for whom the pregnancy did not last the full 9 months.

In popular terms, "secondary infertility" refers to a couple who has one biological child but is unable to conceive another. Secondary infertility is even more common than primary infertility: About 3.3 million American couples have secondary infertility; 2.8 million couples have primary infertility.

The same factors responsible for primary infertility are the cause, such as pelvic scarring, blocked FALLOPIAN TUBES, ENDOMETRIOSIS, defective OVULATION, or poor SPERM quality or quantity. Whatever the cause, the condition was either present initially but the couple was "lucky" or the condition developed or worsened since the first birth. Complications during labor and delivery could have triggered a problem, or the infertility may be age related.

Treatments for primary and secondary infertility are the same.

infertility, unexplained In some cases of infertility, doctors can't pinpoint any reason why a couple can't conceive. "Unexplained infertility" doesn't mean that there is no reason for the infertility, just that the doctor can't identify the reason. Although between 10% and 30% of all infertile couples will have unexplained infertility, about 20% of these couples will become pregnant each year for 3 years. FERTILITY DRUGS and a number of ASSISTED REPRODUCTIVE TECHNOLOGIES are effective treatments for unexplained infertility.

Critical factors to be considered in evaluating and managing unexplained infertility include the age of the woman and how long the infertility has lasted. Couples with unexplained infertility who are infertile for more than 3 years have spontaneous conception rates of only 1% to 2%

a month, compared to normal fertility of 20% per month.

It's clear that aging lessens the ability to conceive and raises the chances of miscarriage, particularly after a woman reaches age 35. Tests of reproductive capacity (ovarian reserve), which may include levels of FOLLICLE-STIMULATING HORMONE (FSH) and ESTRADIOL and/or the CLOMIPHENE CITRATE CHALLENGE TEST, may help evaluate how well the ovaries are functioning.

Infertile couples in which the woman is older than age 35 should be encouraged to actively pursue treatment after only 6 months of trying to conceive or if a known infertility-related problem exists.

Treatment

Both simple and more complex treatments for unexplained infertility exist. A doctor will often begin treating the woman with OVULATION INDUCTION drugs (such as CLOMIPHENE CITRATE) for three to six cycles combined with INTRAUTERINE INSEMINATION (IUI) (inserting prepared semen directly into the uterus) followed by IN VITRO FERTILIZATION or GAMETE INTRAFALLOPIAN FERTILIZATION (GIFT). GIFT is an assisted reproductive technique that involves injecting a mixture of eggs and sperm directly into the fallopian tube.

Recent research indicates that pregnancy rates with these therapies are equal to or higher than pregnancy rates of couples with other infertility diagnoses. As experts better understand human reproductive physiology, more effective therapies for patients with unexplained infertility will be developed.

infertility specialists See FERTILITY SPECIALIST.

inhibin A hormone produced in the testicles and ovaries that regulates the hormone FOLLICLE-STIMULATING HORMONE (FSH).

Insler score A score on a scale of 1 to 12 that rates the quality of CERVICAL MUCUS. Named after the infertility specialist who invented it, the total score is reached by grading each of the following from 0 to 3:

- open cervix
- volume of mucus
- clear, watery, and stretchy mucus
- mucus producing a FERNING pattern when dried on a microscope slide

The first two criteria will vary on OVULATION from one woman to the next, but they should be consistent in the same woman from one ovulation to another.

insurance coverage for infertility treatment

Traditionally, infertility treatment has not been a covered benefit of insurance policies. Some insurers don't recognize infertility as a "disease," and others classify medically accepted treatments as "experimental." Some even regard infertility treatments as "medically unnecessary." Since many insurance policies are open to interpretation, patients should review their policies and request information in writing about coverage options and limitations.

Although no federal law requires insurance coverage for infertility treatment, 13 states have enacted some type of infertility insurance coverage law. Each law is different, but most can be generally described as either a "mandate to cover" or a "mandate to offer" coverage. These 13 states that address infertility coverage include Arkansas, California, Connecticut, Hawaii, Illinois, Maryland, Massachusetts, Montana, New York, Ohio, Rhode Island, Texas, and West Virginia. However, the laws in these states differ quite a bit, one from another. For example, Massachusetts mandates that infertility treatments be covered. California only requires the insurance company to offer the coverage to employers—it doesn't require that coverage be provided or mandate the employer to provide coverage.

Many insurance plans specifically exclude coverage for IN VITRO FERTILIZATION. HMOs are required by federal law to provide certain benefits, but that law says IVF isn't one of them. The high costs of IVF in nonmandated states encourages patients who can only afford one cycle of IVF to request that more embryos be transferred at one time, so as to increase the overall pregnancy rate with a high-risk multiple birth.

In 1997, about 20% of all employers with 500 or more workers provide coverage of in vitro fertilization, up from 16% in 1996. Only about half of all large employers provide any coverage for any type of infertility treatment. At the same time, some insurance companies and employers are cutting back coverage. For example, Aetna/U.S. Healthcare, the nation's largest health insurer, now offers IVF coverage to new customers only as an option employers can buy separately. The insurance companies say it's because the cost of these programs is astronomical. This is not substantiated by the observation that the incremental cost per family for infertility benefits is only a few dollars per year. Companies that include IVF in their benefits say they have seen little change in their health care costs.

A couple planning on undergoing infertility treatment should get a copy of their insurance plan's contract. The couple should get a written predetermination of coverage before any procedures are finished.

Mandate to Cover

Arkansas. Mandates insurance carriers (excluding HMOs) to cover IVF, and allows insurers to impose a lifetime benefit cap of $15,000.

Hawaii. Insurance carriers must cover one cycle of IVF, only after several conditions have been met.

Illinois. Insurance carriers must cover comprehensive diagnosis and treatment of infertility, including assisted reproductive technology procedures, but limits first time attempts to four complete oocyte retrievals, and to two complete oocyte retrievals for a second birth. Insurance carriers are not required to provide this benefit to businesses (group policies) of 25 or fewer employees.

Maryland. Insurance carriers (excluding HMOs) must cover IVF, only after several conditions have been met. Insurance carriers are not required to provide this benefit to businesses (group policies) of 50 or fewer employees.

Massachusetts. Insurance carriers must cover comprehensive infertility diagnosis and treatment, including assisted reproductive technology procedures.

Montana. HMOs must cover infertility treatment as a "preventative health care service" benefit.

New York. Insurance carriers must cover the "diagnosis and treatment of correctable medical conditions." Insurers may not deny coverage for treatment of a correctable medical condition solely because the condition results in infertility.

Ohio. HMOs must cover infertility treatment as a "preventive service" benefit.

Rhode Island. Insurance carriers must cover comprehensive infertility diagnosis and treatment, including assisted reproductive technology procedures, and permits insurers to impose up to a 20% copayment requirement for this benefit.

West Virginia. HMOs must cover infertility treatment as a "preventive service" benefit.

Mandates to Offer

California. Insurance carriers must offer group policy holders coverage of infertility diagnosis and treatment (excluding IVF but including GIFT).

Connecticut. Insurance carriers must offer coverage of comprehensive infertility diagnosis and treatment, including assisted reproductive technology procedures, to group policy holders.

Texas: Insurance carriers must offer coverage of infertility diagnosis and treatment (including IVF) to group policy holders.

intermenstrual bleeding   Bleeding between menstrual periods. The timing of this bleeding is important in determining its cause: Bleeding after sex is called postcoital bleeding; bleeding a few days before the start of a menstrual period is PREMENSTRUAL SPOTTING; and bleeding (or spotting) while on oral contraceptives is called BREAKTHROUGH BLEEDING.

International Council on Infertility Information Dissemination (INCIID), The   A nonprofit organization dedicated to educating infertile couples about the latest methods to diagnose, treat, and prevent infertility and pregnancy loss. INCIID operates primarily on the Internet and, since its inception in April 1995, has become the largest infertility advocacy site on the web. This popular site offers fact sheets written by experts and hosts dozens of subject-specific bulletin boards and chats.

INCIID's goal is to help people find appropriate care. The staff includes six doctors, two psychologists, a social worker who specializes in alternative family planning, an attorney specializing in insurance and donor gamete issues, an insurance expert, and others who volunteer to answer consumer questions. For more information, contact The International Council on Infertility Information Dissemination, Inc., PO Box 6836, Arlington, VA 22206; phone: (703) 379-9178. Website address: http://www.inciid.org.

intracytoplasmic sperm injection (ICSI)   A lab procedure in which a single SPERM is injected through the outer shell of the egg (ZONA PELLUCIDA) to enable FERTILIZATION in couples where the male partner has a very low sperm count. In this type of microinsemination technique, a single sperm is inserted directly into the cytoplasm of a mature egg using a glass needle. This procedure replaces two earlier micromanipulation techniques: PARTIAL ZONA DISSECTION (PZD) and SUBZONAL SPERM INSERTION (SUZI), because it results in higher overall fertilization rates.

In the past, the only way to get a sperm to fertilize an egg outside the womb was to incubate the egg with millions of sperm, which was successful in fertilizing about 75% of eggs. Microinsemination techniques were developed to improve these odds.

This procedure is designed to help couples who have male factor infertility. In these cases, either there isn't enough sperm, the sperm don't swim properly or at all, or their abnormal shape interferes with the ability to penetrate the egg. This technique is not usually successful when used to treat fertilization failures that are primarily due to poor egg quality. It can also be used to treat

- problems with sperm binding to and penetrating the egg

- ANTISPERM ANTIBODIES (immune or protective proteins that attack and destroy sperm)

- prior fertilization failure with standard IN VITRO FERTILIZATION culture and fertilization methods

- frozen sperm collected before cancer treatment that may be limited in number and quality

- absence of sperm due to blockage or abnormality of the ejaculatory ducts, or an irreparable VASECTOMY

Using a microscope, the embryologist gently draws one sperm into a pipette, which is then guided into an egg. As the egg is held in place with another pipette, the sharpened tip of the pipette with the sperm is inserted into the egg. At this moment, the embryologist injects the sperm into the egg and removes the tip of the pipette. The entire technique takes less than 10 minutes.

The technique, which was developed by Belgian reproductive specialists to help couples overcome the inability of sperm to fertilize an egg, represents one of the most important recent advances in ASSISTED REPRODUCTIVE TECHNOLOGY.

Success Rate

Rarely, some eggs can be difficult to pierce. In other cases, the egg may be fertilized but then fail to divide, or the embryo may stop developing early on. Fertilization rates are 50% or better, with cleavage rates of 80% or more. Pregnancy rates vary with age and other factors. Poor egg quality and the age of the woman may cause these percentages to drop.

Risks

As with regular IVF, multiple pregnancies are common with ICSI, and research published in the 2000 issue of the journal *Human Reproduction* reports that babies born through ICSI had slightly more birth defects than children conceived naturally; these abnormalities were associated with multiple births. Other reports have showed a slightly higher frequency of chromosome abnormalities (X chromosome) in ICSI babies. An amniocentesis (test to diagnose birth defects) during the pregnancy is therefore a good idea.

intrauterine adhesions   Scar tissue found inside the endometrial cavity. It is caused by an inflammatory process that occurs during curettage in the presence of a uterine infection, or treatment for hemorrhage after the birth of a baby.

The most common cause of intrauterine adhesions is trauma to the uterine cavity after dilation and curettage (D&C), an outpatient surgical procedure during which the cervix is dilated and the tissue contents of the uterus are emptied. In addition, adhesions may occur as the result of prolonged use of an intrauterine device (IUD), infections of the endometrium (ENDOMETRITIS), or following surgical procedures involving the UTERUS (such as removal of fibroids).

Symptoms

There may be no symptoms, but many women experience light or infrequent MENSTRUATION—or no periods at all. INFERTILITY or recurrent MISCARRIAGES are also possible. Less often, there may be pelvic pain or painful menstrual periods.

Diagnosis

An X-ray procedure called HYSTEROSALPINGOGRAPHY (HSG) can diagnose intrauterine adhesions. During an HSG, a solution is injected into the uterus to allow a doctor to determine if the uterus is normal and the FALLOPIAN TUBES are open. Alternatively, a doctor may perform HYSTEROSCOPY, inserting a thin, telescopelike device through the cervix to visualize the uterine cavity. Although HSG is a useful screening test, hysteroscopy is a more accurate way to evaluate adhesions. Both HSG and hysteroscopy can be performed in an office setting without general anesthesia.

Treatment

Surgical removal of intrauterine adhesions is recommended, followed by temporarily placing a plastic catheter inside the uterus to keep the uterine walls apart and prevent adhesions from reforming. Hormonal treatment with estrogens, progestins, and nonsteroidal anti-inflammatory drugs are often prescribed after surgery to lessen the chance of adhesion reformation.

Prognosis

Whether a woman can become pregnant after this procedure depends on the type and extent of the adhesions. After treatment, about 70% to 80% of women with mild to moderate adhesions achieve a full-term pregnancy, and menstrual problems are often alleviated. Alternatively, patients with severe adhesions or extensive destruction of the endometrial lining may only have full-term pregnancy rates in the 20% to 40% range after treatment.

intrauterine device (IUD) A plastic device that contains either copper or a natural hormone, inserted into the uterus to block implantation of an embryo. The IUD is one of the most popular birth control devices in the world, although in the past it has received some negative publicity in the United States.

Today there are only two types of IUDs legally available in the United States: the Paragard Copper T-380A and the Progestasert Progesterone T. The Paragard IUD can remain in place for 10 years; the Progestasert IUD must be replaced every year.

It isn't entirely clear how IUDs prevent pregnancy. Until about 1980, doctors thought that the IUD worked mainly by causing an inflammatory response in the uterus, interfering with implantation of a fertilized egg. More recent studies support the conclusion that copper IUDs prevent fertilization by reducing the number and viability of sperm reaching the egg, and by impeding the number and movement of eggs into the uterus. Experts believe that the continuous release of copper from the coils and sleeves of the Copper T-380A into the uterine cavity enhances the contraceptive effect of the IUD.

Contraindications

Many of the contraindications to IUD use are linked to infections. An IUD is not an appropriate method for a woman who has

- a sexually transmitted disease (STD)
- a high risk of STDs because she or her partner has multiple sexual partners
- acute PELVIC INFLAMMATORY DISEASE or a history of PID
- untreated acute cervicitis or vaginitis, including bacterial vaginosis (until infection is treated)
- leukemia, AIDS, or intravenous drug abuse

Failure Rate

IUDs have one of the lowest failure rates of any contraceptive method. In the population for which the IUD is appropriate (those in mutually monogamous, stable relationships who aren't at a high risk of infection), the IUD is a very safe and very effective method of contraception. It has an expected failure rate of between 1% and 2% depending on the type, and a typical failure rate of about 3%.

Complications

During the 1970s, an IUD known as the DALKON SHIELD was taken off the market in the United States because it was associated with a high incidence of pelvic infections and infertility, and some deaths. Today, serious complications from IUDs are rare, although IUD users may be at increased risk of developing a serious infection called pelvic inflammatory disease. Other problems can include perforation of the uterus at insertion, abnormal bleeding, and uterine cramping. In fact, menstrual cramps and excessive bleeding are the most common reason why some women have their IUDs removed during the first year:

The initial insertion can be associated with cramping. Complications occur most often during and immediately after insertion; antibiotics can be taken to prevent potential infection.

Because women who haven't yet had children experience a higher risk of developing pelvic inflammatory disease with the IUD that can impair fertility most clinicians won't recommend an IUD for a woman who still wants to have children at some later date.

In the Future

Several types of IUDs are currently under development or are now being used in other countries. The Levonorgestrel IUD (LNg-20) is shaped like a "T" and contains a progestin called levonorgestrel that is released steadily into the uterus for up to 7 years. The LNg-20 is made and sold in Finland. In other new developments, two "frameless" IUDs are being used in European clinical trials. It is hoped that they will cause less cramping because there is no rigid frame to press against the uterus.

Insertion

The clinician first performs a pelvic examination to determine the size, shape, depth, and position of the uterus. Next, the IUD is guided through the vagina and the cervix to the top of the uterus. As the IUD is inserted, the woman may feel some pain or cramping.

Many clinicians prefer to insert an IUD within 7 days of the onset of menstruation when pregnancy is unlikely and the cervical opening is slightly dilated, making insertion easier. Insertion of the IUD early in the cycle is likely to result in less discomfort, cramping, and spotting for the patient.

Removal

The IUD should be removed only by a trained health care provider in the clinic and takes only a few minutes. It can be removed whenever the woman wishes or at the end of 10 years, whichever comes first. In addition, some conditions require removal:

- unexpected pregnancy
- unexplained, severe, or prolonged vaginal bleeding or discharge
- severe pelvic or lower abdominal pain or cramps
- unexplained fever with pelvic tenderness
- disappearance of the IUD's strings
- continued pain during sexual intercourse

intrauterine insemination (IUI)   A relatively simple ASSISTED REPRODUCTION TECHNIQUE (ART), which deposits washed SPERM directly into the UTERUS, bypassing the cervix and allowing the sperm to enter the FALLOPIAN TUBES where FERTILIZATION normally occurs. The procedure is used to treat hostile cervical mucus, unexplained infertility, and MALE FACTOR INFERTILITY. It can be performed either during a natural cycle or following ovarian stimulation with CLOMIPHENE CITRATE or FOLLICLE-STIMULATING HORMONE (FSH) to encourage multiple eggs to mature.

TRANSVAGINAL ULTRASOUND (two or three times per treatment cycle) is used to monitor the cycle.

Alternatively, timing with the urine ovulation detection kit may be used.

Unlike IN VITRO FERTILIZATION or GAMETE INTRAFALLOPIAN TRANSFER (GIFT), IUI does not require an egg retrieval or general anesthetic.

The success rate lies between 10% and 20% per cycle, although rates vary with age and other factors. A doctor might recommend four cycles of IUI, and if these fail, he might recommend other methods, such as in vitro fertilization or GIFT.

Risks

Complications are rare but can include infection, brief uterine cramps, transmission of venereal disease, multiple pregnancy, or OVARIAN HYPER-STIMULATION SYNDROME if medications are used.

in vitro fertilization (IVF)   Literally meaning "in glass," the term refers to fertilization that takes place outside the body in a small glass dish. After other treatments have failed to result in a pregnancy, more and more infertile couples turn to in vitro fertilization.

This procedure involves stimulating the ovaries, retrieving released eggs, fertilizing the eggs, growing the embryos in a laboratory, and then implanting the embryos in the woman's UTERUS to develop naturally. It is one of many types of assisted reproduction, in which a man's SPERM and the woman's egg are combined in a laboratory dish so that fertilization can occur. Usually, two to four embryos are transferred with each cycle.

The first successful IVF offspring were rabbits born in 1959; the next success came with laboratory mice in 1968. Animal research in this procedure was crucial for the development and use of IVF in humans. In 1978, the first IVF baby, Louise Brown, was born in London. Since that time, this procedure has been used with increased success rates to produce offspring from patients with various infertility problems.

Assisted Reproductive Technology

IVF is only one of a number of innovative techniques available worldwide that can enable infertile couples to achieve a family. As couples exhaust all clinical and surgical treatments for their infertility problems, they turn to the rapidly growing group of new technologies to bring children into the world, called ASSISTED REPRODUCTIVE TECHNOLOGIES (ART). Artificial insemination (AI) is one of the most frequently used ART techniques. Artificial insemination involves the transfer of male sperm directly into the reproductive tract of the female. This technology works best when the infertility problem is identified as the male's inability to produce or deliver viable sperm into the female's reproductive tract. A choice may be made to use IVF in cases when the woman has blocked fallopian tubes or other problems that could prevent the successful release or fertilization of an oocyte.

In vitro fertilization was the first of the ART techniques to be developed. Next came GIFT (GAMETE INTRAFALLOPIAN TRANSFER): The eggs are stimulated to develop by the same medications, but instead of removing the eggs for fertilization, the doctor performs a minor surgical procedure (LAPAROSCOPY) to remove the eggs from the ovaries and immediately replace them into the far end of the fallopian tubes along with prepared sperm. (Alternatively, the procedure can be performed through the vagina guided by ultrasound.) Once the egg is fertilized, it moves into the uterus for implantation and normal fetal development.

GIFT is indicated if a woman has unexplained infertility or ENDOMETRIOSIS but normal fallopian tube function. At most infertility centers, the success rate for each transfer is about 20% to 30%. IVF and GIFT have similar success rates, but since IVF doesn't require surgery it's more popular than GIFT.

ZIFT (ZYGOTE INTRAFALLOPIAN TRANSFER) combines IVF with a laparoscopic surgical procedure to transfer the embryos not into the uterus but directly into the fallopian tube. Since transferring embryos through the cervix with IVF gives the same pregnancy rate as ZIFT—and it avoids surgery—IVF is also more popular than ZIFT.

Only about 8% of couples with infertility problems choose in vitro fertilization; more than 90% use easier and less expensive treatments ranging from FERTILITY DRUGS to INTRAUTERINE INSEMINATIONS (IUIs). The average cost of IVF varies from one center to another, but the average is about $5,000 per cycle, including hospital, lab, surgical, and medication costs. Some insurance companies provide partial or full coverage for IVF procedures. Basically, IVF has four steps:

1. maturation of the egg
2. retrieving the eggs
3. fertilizing the egg and allowing the embryo to grow
4. replacing the embryo back into the uterus

Egg Ripening

A woman begins step 1 by taking drugs to trigger the formation of eggs in her ovaries. Various hormone products can be used alone or in combination to induce several ovarian follicles to develop.

These drugs trigger multiple follicles to develop so that several eggs can be retrieved, which improves the chances of fertilization. Typically, a combination of CLOMIPHENE CITRATE, HUMAN MENOPAUSAL GONADOTROPINS, and a Gn-RH AGONIST (a drug that stimulates the release of gonadotropins from the pituitary gland) is used to stimulate the ovaries so that many eggs will mature.

These hormones, which have been used for more than 20 years, do not seem to cause birth defects or miscarriage. After the stimulating drugs are given and the eggs develop, a second hormone is injected to allow the eggs to be prepared for ovulation or egg retrieval. Without using this medication, it would be hard to time the ripening of the eggs correctly.

Egg Retrieval

Eggs are collected from the follicles either during a laparoscopic procedure or needle aspiration guided by ultrasound scan.

Fertilization

Once the eggs have been retrieved, they are placed in a special solution for 2 to 3 hours. A semen sample is obtained and brought to the lab, where it is washed, incubated, and placed in the medium with the egg. They are examined after about 18 hours and allowed to remain in the medium for about 40 hours. If the egg develops normally, it will be replaced into the uterus from 1 to 3 days later.

Embryo Replacement

This procedure is simple and does not require anesthesia. Three or four embryos are transferred from the culture dish into the mother's uterus with a thin tube, where they continue normal fetal development. The woman may need to remain in a head-down position for between 2 to 4 hours and rest for between 24 and 48 hours after that.

Additional embryos can be frozen in liquid nitrogen to be used later if pregnancy doesn't occur. Despite the transfer of several embryos, the chances of producing one full-term baby are only about 18% to 25% each time eggs are placed in the uterus.

Variations

Other possibilities include the use of donor eggs or transfer of frozen embryos to a surrogate mother. However, these techniques raise moral and ethical issues, including questions about the disposal of stored embryos (especially in cases of death or divorce), legal parentage if a surrogate mother is involved, and SELECTIVE REDUCTION of the number of implanted embryos (similar to abortion) when more than three develop.

in vitro maturation The laboratory maturation of an egg that was retrieved from an immature follicle. This is a different procedure from standard IN VITRO FERTILIZATION (IVF), in which the eggs are removed from the mother in a more mature state.

The procedure was developed by a team of Canadian doctors, who believe it is safer and cheaper than more traditional IVF because it does not require the use of expensive drugs to stimulate the ovaries and avoids potential drug side effects. The technique has not been perfected and is not widely available.

in vitro mucus penetration test (IVMP) One of several ways to test the ability of SPERM to penetrate CERVICAL MUCUS. The mucus is obtained around OVULATION time and placed in a test tube. One end of the tube is dipped in SEMEN so that penetration and movement of sperm in the mucus can be measured. In addition, the test can be used to determine if the partner's cervical mucus is hostile to sperm. See also POSTCOITAL TEST.

IUD See INTRAUTERINE DEVICE.

IUI See INTRAUTERINE INSEMINATION.

IVF See IN VITRO FERTILIZATION.

IVM See IN VITRO MATURATION.

Kallmann's syndrome   A HYPOTHALAMUS dysfunction present at birth that leads to impaired release of GONADOTROPIN-RELEASING HORMONE (Gn-RH). The syndrome can either be inherited or develop spontaneously, but almost all sufferers who have inherited Kallmann's syndrome are male. According to recent estimates, it affects around 1 in 10,000 men and 1 in 70,000 women.

Kallmann's syndrome is named after New York geneticist and psychiatrist Franz J. Kallmann, who in 1944 was the first to offer a genetic explanation for a medical condition he observed in some of his patients who were both sexually immature and unable to smell.

Symptoms
Symptoms include delayed puberty, small-sized penis (microphallus), infertility, and/or undescended testes (CRYPTORCHIDISM). Other symptoms of Kallmann's syndrome include a lack of the sense of smell.

Teenagers may have normal growth, with a height-age greater than bone-age and testes smaller than 2 cm in diameter. Although prepubertal LH and FSH levels may be within the low-normal range, blood TESTOSTERONE levels are low. The Gn-RH stimulation test will produce an increase in both LH and FSH.

Women experience a lack of a menstrual period and no egg production (ANOVULATION). A woman with the condition will not be able to produce LUTENIZING HORMONE (LH) and FOLLI-CLE-STIMULATING HORMONE (FSH). A man with Kallmann's syndrome has no sperm in his ejaculate. Besides infertility, men with this syn-drome tend to be tall and thin, and have soft, small testicles. Both men and women with the syndrome have no sense of smell.

Diagnosis
Kallmann's syndrome is extremely rare, and it is very difficult to diagnose in a young child. However, alert pediatricians can sometimes detect early signs, especially if the child can't smell. The disease is more easily diagnosed in a teenager or adult who has failed to go through puberty and in whom an abnormal sense of smell is observed, but many are too embarrassed about their lack of sexual development to see a doctor.

A teenager failing to go through puberty and who is not seen by a specialist may be told that he or she is a "late developer." The main difference between delayed puberty and Kallmann's syndrome is that in the former case puberty eventually occurs. In Kallmann's, puberty can only occur with the help of hormonal therapy.

If a hormonal disorder or delayed puberty is suspected, an ENDOCRINOLOGIST can establish exactly why puberty has failed to occur. If delayed puberty is eliminated as a possible cause, the next step is to look at hormonal causes. It is relatively easy to establish an initial diagnosis of Kallmann's syndrome by performing a smell test to assess the extent of anosmia (lack of smell). There are two main types of smell tests: The first involves smelling and identifying the contents of small bottles; the second type of test uses "scratch & sniff" cards. If there is an absent or exceptionally weak sense of smell, then this is a strong indication that the problem is indeed Kallmann's syndrome. If it turns out the patient has a normal sense of smell, the problem could be a different form of hypogonadism.

Once these initial tests have been carried out, more tests may be required to confirm a diagnosis of Kallmann's syndrome. One of the most common is a blood test to measure the levels of LH and FSH, as well as testosterone or estrogen. Very low levels of these hormones mean that there is a problem with either the hypothalamus or pituitary gland.

Treatment

Fertility drugs are used to treat this disorder. Providing hMG (a combination of FSH and LH) can stimulate the testicles to produce testosterone so that male sexual characteristics develop. HCG and LH-RH are other hormones that can stimulate the testicles into normal sperm production. A woman with this condition must take hormone supplements to achieve puberty, to maintain secondary sex characteristics, and to become fertile.

Klinefelter's syndrome A male genetic abnormality characterized by having one Y (male) and two X (female) chromosomes. This results in a male with an extra X chromosome. Men with this syndrome have no SPERM. Klinefelter's syndrome is probably the best known of the genetic disorders that cause infertility in men, occurring in about 1 of every 500 live births. Often, it is not diagnosed until puberty.

Normal women have two X chromosomes (XX), whereas normal men have an X chromosome and a Y chromosome (XY). In Klinefelter's the affected male has a genetic signature of "XXY" with a total of 47 chromosomes within each bodily cell (the usual number is 46).

Symptoms

Testicular failure is due to hardening of the seminiferous tubules within the testes. In some individuals, more complicated genetic patterns (called mosaicism) such as "XXYY," "XXXY," or "XXXXY" have been found. Skeletal abnormalities are more common among men with multiple X chromosomes. Patients with chromosomal

"mosaics" (XXY/XY) have a less severe form of Klinefelter's syndrome and may be fertile, since a normal ("XY") group of sperm-producing seminiferous tubules may exist within the testes.

Men with Klinefelter's syndrome are typically sterile. Although sexual function may be normal, sperm are not produced. In adolescent boys, Klinefelter's syndrome may produce small, firm testes, overdevelopment of the male breasts, slowed growth of facial hair, and incomplete masculine bodybuild. Most young men with Klinefelter's syndrome are tall (the average height is about 6 feet), but they may not be coordinated or athletic. Psychological, social, and learning problems are common in this group, as is mental retardation. Other associated conditions include glucose intolerance (the inability to metabolize sugar) and varicose veins in the legs.

High levels of GONADOTROPINS are usually found in the blood, and SEMEN samples show lack of sperm. There is an imbalance in blood levels of ESTRADIOL (a form of the female sex hormone ESTROGEN) vs. ANDROGEN (male sex hormone). Although most adult men with Klinefelter's syndrome have normal sexual function with adequate erection and ejaculation, some may be impotent or have a low sex drive, and they may exhibit incomplete development of the scrotum or penis.

Treatment

Sex hormone therapy may help boys with Klinefelter's syndrome, especially if their blood testosterone levels are low. Specialists generally recommend hormone therapy to ensure sexual development, including growth of pubic and facial hair, increased size of the penis and scrotum, deepening of the voice, and increased muscular size and strength. This includes use of synthetic testosterone. This treatment, however, does not repair the sperm production problems.

Kremer test One type of IN VITRO MUCUS PENETRATION test involving assessments of the interaction between sperm and mucus. The test assesses

- male partner's sperm and female partner's mucus
- male partner's sperm and known good mucus
- known good sperm and female partner's mucus
- known good sperm and known good mucus

laparoscope A small telescope that can be inserted into an incision in the abdominal wall to allow a doctor to inspect the internal organs. The device is used to diagnose and treat a number of fertility problems, including ENDOMETRIOSIS and abdominal adhesions. Examination of the pelvic region by using a laparoscope is called a LAPAROSCOPY. See also MINILAPAROSCOPE.

laparoscopy A minimally invasive surgical procedure in which a telescope-like instrument called a LAPAROSCOPE is inserted through a small incision in the abdominal wall to view the inner organs in order to diagnose suspected reproductive problems.

Before placing the laparoscope through the abdominal wall, carbon dioxide gas is introduced into the abdomen to elevate the abdominal wall so that the doctor can better visualize the pelvic organs. Small incisions in the lower abdomen allow for the introduction of special surgical instruments.

Using a camera attached to the laparoscope, the doctor can perform the procedure while visualizing it on a TV monitor. Laparoscopy is performed in an operating room under general anesthesia.

Laparoscopy can be used to diagnose and treat ENDOMETRIOSIS, tubal pregnancy, uterine FIBROIDS, and ovarian tumors, and to investigate potential causes of INFERTILITY. A dye may be injected through the cervical canal and into the cavity of the uterus and the FALLOPIAN TUBES to determine if the tubes are open. If the tubes are open and normal, the dye can be seen running

out through the ends of the fallopian tubes. Laparoscopy is also used to access the fallopian tubes for some assisted conception procedures, such as GAMETE INTRAFALLOPIAN TRANSFER or ZYGOTE INTRAFALLOPIAN TRANSFER.

The examination also can help identify the cause of pelvic pain. It may detect endometriosis, an ECTOPIC PREGNANCY, PELVIC INFLAMMATORY DISEASE, ovarian tumors, or infertility. When used as a diagnostic aid, laparoscopy takes about 30–60 minutes.

Risks

Laparoscopy carries the same risk as does any surgical operation: bleeding, general anesthesia problems, or damage to internal organs such as the bladder, bowel and blood vessels. The risk of these complications is low (about less than 1 in 1,000). Very rarely, death has resulted from these complications. The potential risk of infection is decreased if antibiotics are given as a precaution. See also MINILAPAROSCOPY.

laparotomy for fertility Major abdominal surgery in which an incision is made through the abdominal wall, so that more extensive repairs to the reproductive organs can be corrected and fertility restored. A laparotomy must be performed for microsurgical operations on the FALLOPIAN TUBES or to remove extensive scars that can't be removed with LAPAROSCOPY. There are several options to repair a blocked fallopian tube with a laparotomy:

• fimbrostomy: a procedure that corrects damage to the fimbria

- SALPINGOSTOMY: a procedure in which the fimbrial end of the fallopian tube is opened, and damaged tissue is removed
- tubal reimplantation: a procedure in which the damaged portion of a tube is removed and the fallopian tube is reconnected to the uterus.

The operation requires a hospital stay of several days. The incision is usually a low horizontal incision just above the pubic bone; some numbness along the scar is common for several months.

Latin American Parents Association   A non-profit volunteer organization of adoptive parents committed to helping people seeking to adopt children (as well as those who already have) by researching new sources of ADOPTION in Latin America, supplying materials to orphanages, and providing educational and social activities. To work more effectively, the group has created files of all members who have completed a Latin American adoption by country and adoption source. LAPA has approved sources in Brazil, Chile, Colombia, and Guatemala, based on excellent reports in feedback questionnaires and interviews with adoptive parents and source personnel. Contact: PO Box 339, Brooklyn, NY 11234; phone: (718) 236-8689; website http://www.lapa.com.

leukocyte immunization therapy (LIT)   Injecting a woman with her husband's or a donor's white blood cells (leukocytes) to increase her fetal-blocking antibodies and lower her natural killer cells. Women who have high levels of white blood cell antibodies have a history of carrying pregnancies longer than women who have low levels. This treatment is highly controversial and its effectiveness unproven.

leuprolide acetate (Lupron)   A fertility drug containing a Gn-RH (GONADOTROPIN-RELEASING HORMONE) ANALOG that following an initial stim-ulation, suppresses FSH (FOLLICLE-STIMULATING HORMONE) and LH (LUTEINIZING HORMONE) secretion. Leuprolide is similar to a hormone normally released from the hypothalamus gland called Gn-RH. By suppressing LH and FSH stimulation of the ovary, ovulation is suppressed, as is the production of the ovarian hormone estrogen. Since fibroids and ENDOMETRIOSIS grow in response to estrogen, Gn-RH analogues are used to treat these conditions.

Side Effects
Blurred vision; burning, itching, redness, or swelling at place of injection; decreased interest in sexual intercourse; dizziness; headache; nausea or vomiting; swelling of feet or lower legs; swelling or increased tenderness of breasts; trouble in sleeping; weight gain.

levonorgestrel   A type of progestin used in BIRTH CONTROL PILLS and implantable birth control (such as NORPLANT SYSTEM) that when combined with natural or synthetic estrogens can prevent ovulation and pregnancy. In general, a combination of ESTROGEN and progestin works better than a single-ingredient product to prevent ovulation and pregnancy.

BIRTH CONTROL PILLS such as the combination ethinyl estradiol/levonorgestrel tablets can be used under specific circumstances for emergency contraception after unprotected sex. They also can help regulate menstrual flow, treat acne, or may be used for other hormone-related problems in women.

Leydig cell   The testicular cell that produces the male hormone TESTOSTERONE and perhaps other hormones. The Leydig cell is stimulated by LH (LUTEINIZING HORMONE) from the pituitary gland. It is also called the cell of Leydig or the interstitial cell of Leydig.

The cell gets its name from German anatomist Franz von Leydig (1821–1908), who in 1850 discovered and described the interstitial cell in a detailed account of the male sex organs. In 1857 he published a major text on the histology of humans and animals that was a major account of histology's development up to that time. The Wolffian duct was discovered and described by him in 1892.

LH   See LUTEINIZING HORMONE.

LH kit   A kit a woman can use at home to predict OVULATION by detecting LH hormone in the urine. Before ovulation, the pituitary gland produces a sudden increase in LUTEINIZING HORMONE (LH). This sudden boost is called the LH SURGE; ovulation usually follows about 24–36 hours later. The LH surge occurs about 14 days before the next menstrual period.

Urine testing should begin on cycle day 10. A woman's fertile time usually occurs the day after the LH surge. Intercourse is recommended at this time. See OVULATION TEST KIT.

LH surge   A sudden large release of LUTEINIZING HORMONE (LH) from the pituitary gland that culminates in the release of a mature egg from the follicle (OVULATION) about 36 hours after the surge begins. This occurs by day 14 of a typical 28-day cycle. Once released, the egg is taken up by the fimbria at the end of the FALLOPIAN TUBE and then travels down the tube on its way to possible FERTILIZATION. After the egg has been released from the FOLLICLE, LH signals the remains of the follicle to transform itself into the CORPUS LUTEUM, which will then produce the major female sex hormone progesterone.

During IN VITRO FERTILIZATION (IVF), medications such as Lupron are used to suppress the LH surge. This surge must be suppressed before HUMAN CHORIONIC GONADOTROPIN (which is biologically similar to LH) is given to cause the eggs to mature. The egg retrieval is timed before ovulation is possible (36 hours after hCG).

live birth rate per egg retrieval   A figure offered by a FERTILITY CLINIC that tells how many births occurred in relation to the number of egg-retrieval procedures performed.

live birth rate per egg stimulation   The number of live births per IN VITRO FERTILIZATION (IVF) cycle in which medications are started. This number is meaningful because it includes all patients who started a cycle, including those who were canceled or had no FERTILIZATION or embryo transfer, as well as those who ultimately had a pregnancy test performed.

loop electrocautery excision procedure (LEEP) A procedure used to remove abnormal cells from the cervix using an electric cutting wire. It is similar to CONIZATION.

LPD   See LUTEAL PHASE DEFECT.

lubricants and infertility   Most lubricants used during sexual intercourse, such as petroleum jelly and vaginal creams, have a toxic effect on sperm. This can be a problem if the woman lubricates poorly during sexual arousal and finds sex without use of lubricants to be irritating and uncomfortable. Only water-soluble lubricants should be used if fertility is a concern.

Lunelle   A new type of monthly injectable contraception that was approved in October 2000 by the FDA. Lunelle contains both ESTROGEN and progestin, rather than just progestin alone like DEPO-PROVERA, which only has to be injected every 3 months. Lunelle causes fewer menstrual irregularities than Depo-Provera, with fewer reports of amenorrhea (absence of a menstrual period), infrequent bleeding, irregular bleeding, and extra-long menstrual bleeding.

This new type of BIRTH CONTROL METHOD is 99% effective in preventing pregnancy if women get Lunelle injections at the right time every month. This means that if 100 women get the injections correctly, one woman will get pregnant in a year.

Many proponents see the shot as an alternative to the BIRTH CONTROL PILL, which is taken daily as a means of birth control, considering it a type of "monthly injectable pill" that will need to be taken only 13 times a year rather than daily.

Lunelle is made by Pharmacia, which also produces Depo-Provera, (MEDROXYPROGES-TERONE). Lunelle may interfere with a woman's fertility for up to 4 months, whereas Depo-Provera can block conception for a year or more after the last injection—longer than some women might wish.

Side Effects

Lunelle is an injectable method of contraception, containing two hormones like the pill, so it has the same side effects as the pill, like a much more regular cycle of (menstrual) bleeding, and it is highly effective. Other side effects include breast tenderness, weight gain, acne, and mood swings. The estrogen in Lunelle can cause different complications, including cardiovascular events such as heart attack and stroke. But the likelihood of those occurrences are exceedingly low. For women who can't remember to take a pill every day, Lunelle might fill that niche and provides another option that meets birth control needs in a slightly different way.

Lunelle costs about the same as a month of birth control pills: between $30 to $37. The shots are given in a doctor's office or clinic, much the way patients get allergy or flu shots.

Lupron See LEUPROLIDE ACETATE.

luteal phase The second half of the menstrual cycle that occurs between the release of an egg (OVULATION) and the menstrual period. In turn, it causes the uterine lining to secrete substances to support the implantation and growth of the early embryo. It lasts about 14 days, unless FER-TILIZATION occurs, and ends just before a menstrual period.

In the luteal phase, the ruptured FOLLICLE closes after releasing the egg and forms a CORPUS LUTEUM, which secretes increasing quantities of PROGESTERONE and ESTROGEN. This causes the uterine lining the thicken so it can support the

implantation and growth of the embryo. The progesterone triggers a slight rise in body temperature during the luteal phase, which remains higher until a menstrual period begins. This rise in temperature can be used to estimate whether ovulation has occurred.

The corpus luteum breaks down after 14 days, and a new menstrual cycle begins unless the egg is fertilized. If the egg is fertilized, the corpus luteum begins to produce HUMAN CHORIONIC GONADOTROPIN. This hormone maintains the corpus luteum, which produces progesterone, until the growing fetus can produce its own hormones. Pregnancy tests are based on detecting increased levels of human chorionic gonadotropin.

luteal phase defect (LPD) A condition that occurs when the uterine lining does not develop adequately, either because of inadequate PROGES-TERONE release or because the uterine lining can't respond to progesterone stimulation. LPD may prevent implantation of the EMBRYO or cause an early miscarriage. It is also known as inadequate luteal phase or luteal phase insufficiency. This luteal phase is often shorter than the normal 11–14 days. The diagnosis should be confirmed by two properly timed endometrial biopsies.

Symptoms

Normally, after OVULATION the OVARY produces progesterone so that the uterine lining can develop enough to support implantation of a fertilized egg. In the case of an LPD, a woman's ovarian function becomes disrupted so that there isn't enough progesterone produced after ovulation (the luteal phase).

Luteal phase defect can interfere with early embryo implantation; if a fertilized egg has already implanted, it can cause a woman to menstruate too early, which would end a pregnancy within a few days after implantation.

Treatment

Treatment involves supplemental progesterone or medications that improve progesterone production from the ovary (for example, CLO-MIPHENE CITRATE).

The concept of LPD has been recognized for 30 years. However, experts recently have questioned whether the condition actually causes INFERTILITY. Given the discomfort associated with two endometrial biopsies and the fact that clomiphene is often recommended no matter what the biopsy result, many clinicians don't believe making an LPD diagnosis is important.

luteinizing hormone (LH) A pituitary hormone (also known as a GONADOTROPIN) that stimulates the ovaries or TESTICLES. In a man, LH is necessary for the production of SPERM and TESTOSTERONE. In a woman, LH is necessary for the production of ESTROGEN and to stimulate the release of an egg.

When estrogen reaches a critical peak, the pituitary releases a surge of LH near the middle of the menstrual cycle, which causes the egg to mature. Ovulation occurs about 24 to 36 hours after the LH surge.

LH is suppressed by GN-RH AGONISTS and GN-RH ANTAGONISTS.

luteinizing hormone-releasing hormone (LH-RH) Another name for GONADOTROPIN-RELEASING HORMONE (Gn-RH).

male birth control pill   A BIRTH CONTROL PILL for men has long eluded scientists, although many have tried to come up with a viable product. Recently, Chinese scientists report a male birth control pill that is 90% effective in stopping sperm production with "hardly any" of the side effects associated with the pill taken by women. The pill contains the hormone progestin, a key ingredient in oral contraceptives for women; TESTOSTERONE implants were also given to maintain sex drive.

Combining these two hormones reduces the negative effects of using testosterone alone: weight gain, aggression, increased sex drive, and more body hair. As with any steroid, muscle mass tends to increase and the testes shrink. Extra testosterone also seems to interfere with cholesterol levels, raising concerns about the possibility of heart problems.

After men stopped taking the pill, researchers at the Shanghai Institute of Family Planning report that SPERM counts return to normal in 2 to 3 months. The men in the study who took the pills were in their 30s and reported little weight gain and no mood swings. They did not experience loss of sex drive because of the testosterone implants, which slowly released the male hormone into their bloodstream. But success rates are much lower in Caucasians than in Asians: typically 90% to 95% effective in Asians but only 40% to 60% effective in Caucasians. Experts believe that the pills are more effective in some races because of the difference in height and fat ratios between Asians and Caucasians.

In the past, male birth control pills using testosterone alone were more effective in Asians than in Caucasians. But again, success rates are much lower in Caucasian men, and among those men whose sperm counts did not drop all the way to zero, 8% of their partners still got pregnant—an unacceptable failure rate.

A third approach is to use the French abortion pill RU-486 (MIFEPRISTONE), which has been shown to immobilize sperm in hamsters and other lower species. A study by the World Health Organization last year showed that injections of RU-486 markedly reduced sperm production in fertile men. However, the drug is very expensive, and injections must be given so often that they aren't practical.

male factor infertility   Infertility caused by a problem with the male partner. While many people tend to believe that infertility is mostly a woman's problem, in fact infertility occurs about equally in both men and women. In approximately 40% of infertile couples, the male partner is either the sole cause or a contributing cause of the inability to conceive a child.

Causes
The most common cause of male infertility is a problem in sperm production. In addition, male infertility may be caused by abnormalities in the testes or other areas of the male reproductive tract, as well as immune system defects.

A man may be infertile because of

- a lack of normal sperm production from the testicles
- sperm that don't move or function properly

- blocked passageways through which the sperm must travel
- antibodies against sperm
- injury to the testicle
- undescended testicles (CRYPTORCHIDISM)
- TESTICULAR TUMORS
- retrograde ejaculation
- sexually transmitted diseases
- problems with hormone production
- varicose vein around the testicle (VARICOCELE)

Childhood disease, fevers or infections, and medications or congenital abnormalities can contribute to these problems in men.

Diagnosis

The evaluation of the male begins with a medical history. The doctor will pay special attention to details about previous surgeries, infections, chronic illnesses, or hospitalizations, including any recent pelvic injuries, illnesses, high fever or viral infections, venereal diseases, or tuberculosis. Also helpful will be complete information on smoking and recreational drug and alcohol use. The physician also will ask about exposure to harmful environmental and occupational toxins, chemicals, drugs (for example, chemotherapeutic medications and steroids), excessive heat, or radiation. If possible, the physician should be given a list of all medications, including nonprescription products, plus the dates of any exposure to environmental toxins, occupational toxins, chemicals, drugs, heat, or radiation. In addition, the doctor will ask about specific childhood illnesses and developments such as mumps, orchitis (inflammation of the testes), any injury or twisting to the testicles, undescended testes, and onset of puberty. Also important is the patient's family history: relatives with cystic fibrosis, androgen receptor deficiency, diabetes, and so on. Any history of previous pregnancies will be discussed.

The history interview will be followed by a complete physical exam. The doctor will carefully feel the scrotum while the patient is in a variety of positions to detect abnormalities of the testes, abnormalities of the vas deferens, and seminiferous vesicles, as well as whether varicose veins (VARICOCELES) are present. The doctor will also check for abnormalities of the testes, penis, prostate, or secondary sex traits. Next, the doctor will look for indications of delayed sexual maturity, as shown by lack of normal secondary sex characteristics, including

- abnormal male hair distribution: thin hair on the face, pubic area
- underarms, and body; lack of hair recession at the temples
- small penis, testes, and prostate; underdeveloped scrotum
- underdeveloped muscle growth and low muscle mass
- lack of sense of smell

The physician also will want to identify any irregularities of the penis, such as abnormal curvature, underside opening of the urethra, or too-tight foreskin over the glans.

The doctor will look for evidence of overdevelopment of the male breasts, which could indicate a hormonal imbalance that can affect fertility. This may be normal at certain stages (birth, adolescence, and old age). However, male breast enlargement also can be caused by low levels of the male sex hormone testosterone, high levels of the female sex hormone estrogen, or the use of certain drugs.

Finally, the doctor will want to check for other physical signs of hormonal malfunction. Thyroid disease may be suggested by enlarged thyroid gland or knots of tissue. Likewise, an enlarged liver may suggest other hormonal problems. A large percentage of men with cirrhosis of the liver will have enlarged breasts, impotence, and wasting away of the testes.

A SEMEN ANALYSIS checks for the number of sperm in the ejaculate and their shape and size. The semen analysis isn't a perfect test for fertility, because it does not test certain aspects of sperm function, such as whether the sperm can actually penetrate an egg. Several other optional tests can provide even more information about the fertilizing ability of sperm, which can help define specific sperm problems or diseases of the male reproductive system. However, the clinical usefulness of these tests is questionable.

No semen test can fully predict the fertilizing ability of sperm because of the variability of other factors, including those in the female partner. Therefore, a complete infertility evaluation of the woman is also necessary.

Optional semen tests may include

- vital staining: determines numbers of living and dead sperm
- urinalysis: sperm in the urine suggests retrograde ejaculation; white blood cells suggest infection
- ANTISPERM ANTIBODIES: tests for antibodies that bind to sperm and may affect fertility
- strict morphology: detailed examination of sperm shapes
- peroxidase staining: checks for infection by differentiating white blood cells from immature sperm
- hypo-osmotic swelling: assesses the sperm membrane for structural integrity
- biochemical analysis: measures various chemicals in semen, such as fructose (which is absent when there are no seminal vesicles or when the ejaculatory ducts are obstructed)
- hormone evaluation: measures blood levels of hormones (such as FOLLICLE-STIMULATING HORMONE and TESTOSTERONE) involved in sperm production
- post-coital/cervical mucus test: checks the compatibility of a sperm with the partner's cervical mucus
- sperm penetration assay (hamster test): measures the sperm's ability to penetrate the egg of a hamster

- human ZONA PELLUCIDA binding tests: measures the ability of sperm to bind to the outer covering of the egg, including the HEMIZONA ASSAY
- computer-assisted semen analysis (CASA): measures precise characteristics of sperm motion

There are several additional tests that may be recommended in special cases. A TESTICULAR BIOPSY can determine the ability of the sperm-producing cells to produce normal sperm. A VASOGRAPHY provides an X-ray of the vas deferens, which can reveal a blockage. High-resolution scrotal ultrasounds help identify varicoceles that are too small to be felt. Ultrasound also allows study of sex glands like the prostate and seminal vesicles for blockages.

marijuana and infertility The effects of marijuana on reproduction have been well established; men who have smoked marijuana for a long time produce less sperm and tend to have lower TESTOSTERONE levels, less SPERM MOTILITY, and more abnormally shaped sperm than nonsmokers. Some findings suggest that marijuana may lower blood testosterone levels. Marijuana use, like alcohol use, has been associated with the development of abnormally large male breasts. See also MALE FACTOR INFERTILITY.

maturation arrest A testicular condition in which at one stage of sperm production all sperm development stops throughout all testicular tubules.

Mayer-Rokitansky-Kustur-Hauser Syndrome See ROKITANSKY SYNDROME.

medications and fertility There are a number of medications that can affect fertility in both men and women.

Women

Prescription drugs that affect the female fertility cycle include antibiotics, tranquilizers, and cortisone. Among the medications that can potentially reduce fertility are many used to treat chronic disorders, as well as antidepressants, hormones, painkillers, and even over-the-counter medications such as aspirin and ibuprofen (if taken midcycle).

Antibiotics

Occasionally, women who take antibiotics have noticed a change in the normal cervical mucus pattern. However, it's hard to tell whether the antibiotics themselves or the stress caused by the illness for which the drugs were prescribed are responsible for the change in the mucus secretions.

Tranquilizers

Drugs used to treat migraine, nausea and vomiting, and some drugs used for motion sickness may boost levels of prolactin in the bloodstream and so can delay or suppress ovulation.

Cortisone

These preparations are often prescribed for allergies such as hay fever, asthma, and rheumatic problems. There is a close link between adrenal hormones (cortisone) and ovarian hormones, and the use of cortisone over long periods of time may cause irregular menstrual cycles.

Cold/flu Remedies

These medicines are designed to dry up mucous membrane secretions, and since the cervix is a mucous membrane, there is always the risk that this drying effect will also disrupt secretions of cervical mucus. Taking acetaminophen (Tylenol) regularly may reduce estrogen and luteinizing hormone levels, although its effects on fertility are unproven. In most cases, however, once the illness is treated or medication stopped, fertility is often restored.

Men

Many medicines are commonly prescribed without knowing whether they impair fertility. Studies have shown that a number of drugs can affect male fertility, including corticosteriods, narcotics, alcohol, tranquilizers, some antidepressants, and high blood pressure medicine. These drugs may interfere with potency and the ability to ejaculate, and cause retrograde ejaculation.

Specifically, drugs known to affect male fertility include cimetidine (Tagamet), sulfasalazine (Azulfidine), colchicine, methadone, methotrexate (Folex), phenytoin (Dilantin), spironolactone (Aldactone), and thioridazine (Mellaril). Cancer drugs such as busulfan (Myleran), chlorambucil (Leukeran), and cyclophosphamide (Cytoxan, Neosar) can destroy developing sperm as well as cancer cells. Anabolic steroids (which are those abused by weight lifters and other athletes) are known to severely impair sperm production.

Other drugs (such as methotrexate, salazopyrine, and antimalarials) may be associated with defects of sperm cell production. Narcotics can affect the hypothalamis and pituitary and prevent normal production of FSH and LH, lowering sperm production.

Reducing the dose or changing the medication will usually reverse the effects but may take many weeks to show an improvement.

medroxyprogesterone acetate (MPA)   A type of birth control marketed as a tablet (Provera) or injection (DEPO-PROVERA) that contains a synthetic hormone called progestin. This chemical is similar to the natural hormone PROGESTERONE that is produced by the ovaries during the second half of the menstrual cycle.

An injection can prevent pregnancy for 12 weeks by stopping the ovaries from releasing eggs and thickening cervical mucus to keep sperm from meeting an egg. The injection also prevents pregnancy by changing the lining of the uterus to make it less likely that the egg could implant.

Intramuscular MPA is one of the most effective reversible methods of birth control. Of every 100 women who use it, fewer than one will become pregnant during the first year. It works as well as STERILIZATION or NORPLANT. It is more effective than the BIRTH CONTROL PILL because it is not dependent upon correct daily usage. (Some women get pregnant taking birth control pills if they take pills incorrectly or miss pills.)

Protection is immediate if Depo-Provera is given during the first 5 days of a woman's period. Otherwise, an additional method of contraception should be used for the first 2 weeks. However, it does not protect against sexually transmitted diseases.

Women who use this type of birth control like its convenience, since it doesn't need to be taken daily or used before having sex, and it doesn't require surgery; they also like the fact that it doesn't use estrogen. It also lessens menstrual cramps and protects against both endometrial and ovarian cancers.

However, the method doesn't protect against sexually transmitted diseases, so latex condoms should be used for increased protection. Depo-Provera may reduce the risk of PELVIC INFLAMMATORY DISEASE if CHLAMYDIA or GONORRHEA is contracted.

Depo-Provera is not for everyone. A woman needs to get an injection every 3 months, and the effects can't be reversed immediately. A woman may not be able to get pregnant for a full year after stopping.

Side Effects

Irregular bleeding or light spotting is the most common side effect. Periods become fewer and lighter for most women—most will have no periods after 5 years. It may take a year for periods to begin again after a woman stops using the shot.

Less common side effects include increased appetite and weight gain, headache, sore breasts, nausea, nervousness, dizziness, depression, rashes, or spotty darkening of skin, hair loss, increased facial or body hair, and increased or decreased sex drive.

Side effects may continue for up to 8 months until the medication is cleared from the body.

Candidates

This medication is especially helpful for women who want very effective long-lasting contraception, who want long-term birth spacing, and who can't take estrogen.

It's not a good choice for those women who worry about gaining weight, or those who have diabetes, major depression, a recent history of liver disease (such as hepatitis), or blood clots in the eyes, legs, or lungs.

Women should absolutely not use Depo-Provera if they are pregnant, want to get pregnant within 18 months, or have unexplained vaginal bleeding, a serious liver disease or growths of the liver, a known or suspected breast cancer, CUSHING'S SYNDROME, or if they are being treated with Cytadren.

menopause A natural state a woman experiences after her ovaries have stopped producing eggs and when menstruation ends. The typical age for menopause is between 40 and 55 years, averaging about age 51.

The period of time when a woman's hormones begin to fluctuate as menopause approaches is called perimenopause, and may take from a year or two to more than 10 years, culminating in the arrival of menopause. During perimenopause, women experience a range of symptoms, including hot flashes, memory problems, and mood swings.

menotropins HUMAN MENOPAUSAL GONADOTROPINS (hMG) are extracted from the urine of postmenopausal women, and contain high concentrations of FSH or LH—either in combination or as pure FSH. HMG such as Pergonal, Repron, Repronex contain FSH and LH and are produced by purifying the urine of postmenopausal women. Although they are not as pure as the newer preparations of FSH produced by recombinant DNA technology they are of comparable effectiveness.

FSH therapy is usually prescribed after other simpler therapies have failed. FSH medications such as hMg are used to treat OVULATION problems, unexplained infertility and IVF. The drugs are administered by injection.

Estrogen levels must be frequently monitored, together with frequent ultrasounds, because FSH medications can overstimulate the ovaries, causing estrogen levels to rise to dangerously high levels. If hyperstimulation is severe (which is rare), hospitalization may be required.

menstrual cycle The monthly series of reproductive changes in the UTERUS and other organs that averages about 28 days, measured from the onset of menstrual flow to the next. Menstruation (the shedding of the uterine lining and some blood) occurs each month unless a woman is pregnant or there are other changes that interfere with menstruation. The menstrual cycle marks the reproductive years of a woman's life, extending from the start of MENSTRUATION (menarche) during puberty until menopause.

The first day of normal bleeding is counted as the beginning of each menstrual cycle (day 1), which ends just before the next menstrual period. Typically, menstrual cycles range from about 21 to 40 days; only 10% to 15% of cycles are exactly 28 days. The intervals between periods are generally longest in the years right after menstruation begins and right before it ends (menopause).

The menstrual cycle can be divided into three phases: follicular, ovulatory, and luteal.

Proliferative (Follicular) Stage

After blood loss from the uterine lining, the lining again becomes thicker. During this time, the FOLLICLE is maturing and secreting estrogens. This phase varies in length but averages 14 days and extends from the first day of bleeding to immediately before a surge in the level of luteinizing hormone, which triggers ovulation.

During the first half of the phase, the pituitary gland slightly increases its secretion of FOLLICLE-STIMULATING hormone (FSH), stimulating the growth of 3 to 30 follicles, each containing an egg. Only one of these follicles continues to grow to become the "dominant follicle"; the rest degenerate. The phase ends when the dominant follicle ruptures and releases the egg. After about 14 days, the next period begins.

Ovulatory Phase

This is the phase during which the egg is released, starting with a surge in the level of LUTEINIZING HORMONE (LH). The follicle releases the egg, usually 36 hours after the LH surge begins. Around the time of OVULATION, some women feel a dull pain on one side of the lower abdomen (MITTELSCHMERZ), which may last for a few minutes to a few hours. Although the pain is felt on the same side as the OVARY that released the egg, the precise cause of the pain isn't known. The pain may precede or follow the rupture of the follicle and may not occur in all cycles.

Egg release doesn't alternate between the two ovaries and appears to be random. If one ovary is removed, the remaining ovary releases an egg every month.

Luteal Stage

The LUTEAL PHASE follows ovulation and is the part of a woman's cycle between the release of an egg (OVULATION) and the next menstrual period. The uterine lining gets thicker and swells during this period. The ruptured follicle now becomes CORPUS LUTEUM and produces PROGESTERONE. This phase lasts for 10 to 14 days unless fertilization occurs, and ends just before a menstrual period. Progesterone causes the uterine lining to thicken so it can support the implantation and growth of the embryo. The progesterone triggers a slight rise in body temperature during the luteal phase, which remains higher until a menstrual period begins. This rise in temperature can be used to estimate whether ovulation has occurred.

The corpus luteum breaks down after 14 days and a new menstrual cycle begins unless the egg is fertilized. If the egg is fertilized, the pregnancy begins to produce HUMAN CHORIONIC GONADOTROPIN. This hormone is biologically similar to LH and maintains the corpus luteum, which continues to produce progesterone to maintain the pregnancy. Pregnancy tests are based on detecting increased levels of human chorionic gonadotropin. If pregnancy has not occurred, the lining of the uterus begins to shrink a day or two before menstruation begins. This phase lasts for 2 days and ends when constricted arteries open and patches of the uterine lining break off, signaling the beginning of the menstrual period.

menstruation   The periodic discharge of blood and tissue from the UTERUS occurring at an average of every 28 days. It is triggered by a drop in ovarian hormones (especially PROGESTERONE) when a released egg does not become fertilized. Menstruation begins at puberty (age 9 to 17) and continues more or less regularly throughout a woman's life until MENOPAUSE.

The endometrium consists of three layers. The top and most of the middle layer are shed, leaving the bottom layer to produce new cells to rebuild the other two layers. The flow lasts on average from 3 to 7 days and recurs about every 28 to 31 days. It stops during pregnancy and may not return until after breast-feeding is completed. It ends permanently with the onset of menopause. At other times, it may cease as a result of severe weight loss, excessive exercise, physical disorders, hormonal disorders, pregnancy, and some psychological states.

The amount of monthly blood loss ranges from 1/2 to 10 ounces, averaging 4.5 ounces, and it's the single most common cause of iron deficiency in women. Blood loss is increased with the use of some types of contraceptive devices (such as IUDs) and drops or disappears with the use of oral contraceptives. Excessive blood flow may be characterized by the need to change a tampon or sanitary pad every hour, by the appearance of blood clots larger than a half inch, by clots that appear on any day but the first, or by flow that lasts longer than a week.

A sanitary pad or tampon, depending on the type, can hold up to an ounce of blood. Menstrual blood usually doesn't clot unless the bleeding is very heavy.

The absence of periods is called AMENORRHEA; slight flow is OLIGOMENORRHEA; painful periods is dysmenorrhea; excessive flow is menorrhagia; and bleeding between expected periods is called metrorrhagia.

menstruation, retrograde   Menstrual fluid that flows backward through the FALLOPIAN TUBES into the peritoneal cavity.

menstruation, suppressed   Failure of MENSTRUATION to occur when expected.

methotrexate   A chemotherapy drug that destroys the cells of the placenta, commonly used to treat early ECTOPIC PREGNANCY.

Metrodin   An injectable form of HUMAN MENOPAUSAL GONADOTROPIN (hMG) from which LUTEINIZING HORMONE (LH) has been removed, leaving pure FOLLICLE-STIMULATING HORMONE (FSH) as the primary active substance. Metrodin HP (Fertinex) is even more pure and has no LH activity at all.

Metrodin is used to stimulate follicle growth and release of the egg (OVULATION). Metrodin is usually given when CLOMIPHENE CITRATE hasn't worked, for IVF, or to supplement INTRAUTERINE INSEMINATION treatments. Women with POLYCYSTIC OVARY SYNDROME typically have high levels of LH and low to normal levels of FSH, and are often treated with Metrodin.

Metrodin is usually given daily early in the cycle for about a week; ovulation usually occurs about a week or two after treatment.

Women taking this drug are usually monitored with ultrasound and estrogen level tests. They also usually are given an injection of HUMAN CHORIONIC GONADOTROPIN to stimulate follicle release.

metroplasty   A surgical procedure designed to change the shape of the uterine cavity, usually in the case of a BICORNUATE UTERUS.

microepididymal sperm aspiration Selecting suitable SPERM cells using microsurgery to dissect the EPIDIDYMIS or testis. Once located, the sperm are aspirated, isolated, and prepared for an assisted conception procedure (usually INTRACYTOPLASMIC SPERM INJECTION).

microfertilization See INTRACYTOPLASMIC SPERM INJECTION.

micromanipulation The use of high magnification and special instruments to manipulate SPERM, eggs, and embryos during IN VITRO FERTILIZATION. These newer methods include INTRACYTOPLASMIC SPERM INJECTION (ICSI) and ASSISTED HATCHING. ICSI is the newest micromanipulation method, in which a single sperm is injected into the egg itself. This procedure is recommended for couples with very low sperm count.

Assisted hatching is a similar micromanipulation technique, in which an opening is made in the outer covering of the embryo to help a normal growing EMBRYO emerge from the covering and implant itself into the uterus.

micromanipulation of eggs Techniques to introduce material into a human egg. The most common example of micromanipulation is INTRACYTOPLASMIC SPERM INJECTION (ICSI), in which a single SPERM is injected into an egg. ICSI is commonly used to treat sperm problems and IVF with failed FERTILIZATION. The two other types of experimental egg micromanipulation are oocyte nuclear transfer and CYTOPLASMIC TRANSFER.

In oocyte nuclear transfer, researchers remove the nucleus of an infertile woman's egg using very delicate instruments. This nucleus is then placed into a donor's egg that has had its nucleus removed. This highly experimental technique may one day be used to help older women who need donor eggs get pregnant. Scientists suspect that it could be possible that the donor's cytoplasm (the part of the egg surrounding the nucleus) may be all that is required to boost the infertile older woman's eggs into fertilizing and developing normally. While some early success with this technique has been reported, it is still highly experimental.

In cytoplasmic transfer, on the other hand, a small amount of normal cytoplasm is removed from a donor egg and injected into an egg of an infertile older woman. Doctors hope that this donor cytoplasm will give the infertile woman's egg a boost so that a pregnancy will result. However, so far this technique has produced only a few pregnancies and births, and is considered experimental.

microscopic surgery Laser techniques can be used to treat some types of INFERTILITY. These procedures are especially useful in correcting conditions that block, scar, or displace the FALLOPIAN TUBES. The use of a surgical microscope to magnify the small tubes and tissues with a highly focused beam of light called a laser to make delicate repairs has improved this type of reconstructive procedure. In appropriate cases, this can be done through laparoscopic surgery, which does not require an overnight hospital stay.

mifepristone (Mifeprex) Popularly known as RU-486 or the "French abortion pill," this early-abortion drug was approved by the Food and Drug Administration (FDA) on Sep. 28, 2000 after a 12-year struggle to bring the medication to the United States. Studies show mifepristone is 92% to 95% effective in causing early ABORTION by blocking action of a hormone essential for maintaining pregnancy. Without that hormone (PROGESTERONE), the uterine lining thins so that an EMBRYO cannot remain implanted and grow.

Referred to as a medical (as opposed to surgical) abortion, the pills are dispensed in a doctor's office. The regimen requires three doctor's visits. At home, the woman experiences the equivalent of a planned miscarriage. Side effects include bleeding, cramping, and, possibly, nausea, headaches, and diarrhea.

The vast majority of today's 1.3 million annual U.S. abortions are surgical, although doctors in 1995 began publicizing the fact that a drug already sold to treat cancer (methotrexate) also could be used to induce abortion.

Mifepristone is used in combination with a prostaglandin such as misoprostol to induce abortion when administered in early pregnancy, providing women with a medical alternative to suction abortion. Unlike suction abortion, which is not often performed before the seventh or eighth week of gestation, mifepristone can be used as soon as pregnancy is discovered. It is most effective when used in the first weeks after fertilization and implantation, when progesterone is being produced mostly by the ovaries. As pregnancy proceeds, the placenta takes over progesterone's role, and the antiprogestins are less effective.

Proponents say the pill, which has been used by millions of women in 13 countries, could transform abortion in the United States by making it more accessible and more private. The pill-caused abortion should cost the same as surgical abortion, but it can be used only in the earliest days of pregnancy. Worried about antiabortion violence that has sprung up in recent years, the FDA kept secret the names of the medical officers who reviewed the drug.

Regimen

To ensure the pill is used accurately and safely, the FDA mandated that women be given special brochures called "MedGuides" explaining who is eligible for a pill-caused abortion and what side effects to expect. The drug can be used only within 49 days of the beginning of a woman's last menstrual period. To begin the process, the woman takes three mifepristone pills, and 2 days later she returns to the doctor for a second drug (misoprostol) that causes uterine contractions to expel the embryo. She returns for a follow-up visit within 2 weeks to make sure the abortion is complete.

The FDA will allow mifepristone to be distributed only to doctors trained to accurately diagnose pregnancy and to detect ectopic pregnancies, because those women can't take mifepristone. The FDA also restricted mifepristone's use to doctors who can operate in case a surgical abortion is needed to finish the job or in cases of severe bleeding. Doctors who have made advance arrangements for a surgeon to provide such care to their patients may also prescribe the drug. Some state regulations require abortion providers to increase their office space, provide beds, and even hire additional staff.

At Planned Parenthood, a woman seeking a medical abortion will first undergo ultrasound to verify the pregnancy and determine whether she is within the 49 days since her last period, as required by the FDA. The woman then reviews the procedure with a doctor or nurse practitioner, including potential side effects and the necessity of having a surgical abortion if the regimen fails. After signing a consent form, she can take the medication in the office.

History

The abortion pill was approved in France more than 10 years ago and is widely available throughout Europe, where it is considered to be a safe, effective, acceptable option for women seeking abortion during the first several weeks of pregnancy. Approximately 500,000 women in Europe have had medical abortions using the mifepristone regimen. More than 2,000 American women have used the drug during clinical trials.

During the long fight to legalize its use, abortion rights organizations said that the drug reduced the need for riskier surgical abortions; opponents argue that the drug is dangerous to a woman's health. Even while the use of mifepristone expanded from France to the United Kingdom and Sweden, manufacturer Roussel-Uclaf announced that it had no intention of marketing the drug in the United States or in any other country where political and social conditions were not receptive.

However, following public hearings on the subject, the FDA Advisory Committee for Reproductive Health Drugs recommended approval of mifepristone in the summer of 1996. The FDA issued an approvable letter for mifepristone in September of that year, indicating that the drug was safe and effective but that the manufacturer needed to provide additional manufacturing, labeling, and other information in order to obtain final approval.

Health experts say that mifepristone won't increase abortions—that didn't happen in Europe. But the FDA's formal approval may encourage more doctors who don't offer surgical abortions to offer the pill, thus making it easier for women, particularly in rural areas, to get an abortion without traveling hundreds of miles or entering surgical clinics often staked out by protesters.

The National Abortion Federation, which accredits abortion providers, said 240 of its member clinics were already prepared to offer Mifeprex, and it is training other physicians in how to use the pill.

Side Effects

The pill-induced abortion can be painful, and symptoms are similar to those of a spontaneous miscarriage, causing bleeding and nausea. Heavy bleeding is a potentially serious side effect, but an effect that the FDA determined is rare. In safety testing of the first 2,100 American women who took mifepristone, 4 bled enough to need a transfusion.

minilaparoscope   An extremely small instrument (just a few millimeters in diameter) used to perform minilaparoscopy. This minute device makes it possible to perform outpatient surgery without general anesthesia. However, some conditions (such as for ENDOMETRIOSIS) are more difficult to treat using this device.

minipill   Another type of oral contraceptive that contains only one hormone (progestin) instead of two (progestin and estrogen). These pills work by reducing and thickening cervical mucus to prevent sperm from reaching the egg.

They also keep the uterine lining from thickening, which prevents a fertilized egg from implanting in the uterus. They prevent a woman's body from releasing an egg during her monthly menstrual cycle, although they don't have this effect in every menstrual cycle.

Some doctors advise that the best time of day to take minipills is late afternoon or early evening, since it takes about 4 hours for the cervical mucus to thicken and create the most effective barrier against sperm. Since bedtime is typically when sex occurs, taking a minipill several hours earlier may be the best time to protect against pregnancy.

Benefits

Because they lack estrogen, these pills are slightly less effective than combined oral contraceptives. Women who take the minipill late (even by as little as 3 hours) have a higher chance of pregnancy.

Some women prefer minipills because they can decrease menstrual bleeding and cramps, as well as the risk of endometrial and ovarian cancer and PELVIC INFLAMMATORY DISEASE. Because they contain no ESTROGEN, minipills don't present the risk of blood clots associated with estrogen in combined pills.

Minipills also are a good option for women who can't take estrogen because they are breastfeeding or because estrogen-containing products cause them to have severe headaches or high blood pressure.

Side Effects

Menstrual cycle changes, weight gain, and breast tenderness are typical side effects. See also BIRTH CONTROL METHODS.

miscarriage   Spontaneous loss of an EMBRYO or fetus before the 20th week of pregnancy. Most miscarriages occur during the first 14 weeks of pregnancy. The medical term for miscarriage is spontaneous abortion. Approximately 20% of all pregnancies (one in five) end in miscarriage. A miscarriage is often a traumatic event for both partners and can cause feelings similar to those for the loss of a child or other member of the family.

Risk of Miscarriage

There is an overall risk to pregnancy loss that increases with age. Between the ages of 15 to 24, the risk of miscarriage is about 9.5%. This continues to rise steadily with age. By age 30 the risk of pregnancy loss has increased to 11%, and by age 40 it is 33%. Women over age 44 have a whopping miscarriage risk of 53%. Since there is a parallel increased risk of chromosome abnormalities in live births in women over 35, the same mechanisms are probably responsible for increased risk of miscarriage.

There are other risk factors besides age. Women who smoke raise their risk by 50%. Other risks include infection, exposure to toxins such as arsenic or lead, multiple pregnancy, or poorly controlled diabetes.

However, 90% of women who have had one miscarriage go on to have a normal pregnancy and a healthy baby; 60% are able to have a healthy baby after two miscarriages. Even a woman who has had three miscarriages in a row still has more than a 50% chance of having a successful pregnancy the fourth time.

Causes

There are many reasons for a miscarriage, including an abnormal UTERUS, exposure to DIETHYLSTILBESTROL (DES), incompetent cervix, bacterial infection, immune problems, or lack of PROGESTERONE.

Chromosomal Abnormality

The most common cause of any pregnancy loss is a chromosome abnormality, which is often a problem in the egg. In fact, only about half the eggs a woman produces in her lifetime are capable of a successful pregnancy, and most of these fertilized eggs are never identified as pregnancies. Either they don't divide to produce an embryo or fetus, or the conception is lost very soon after implantation of the early embryo.

Sometimes in the formation of a sperm or egg some genetic material gets lost, either because of the loss of a part of a chromosome or because the missing genetic material is attached to another chromosome. Large errors of genetic material are lethal to the developing fetus, and a miscarriage will occur. These errors are different from inherited genetic diseases. They probably occur during development of the specific egg or sperm, and therefore are not likely to occur again.

Uterine Abnormalities

In about 10% of cases, a problem with the structure of the cervix or uterus results in pregnancy loss. The biggest problem is an incomplete formation of the uterus, sometimes resulting in a SEPTATE or BICORNUATE (or "two-horned") uterus. A uterine septum increases the miscarriage risk considerably. A bicornuate uterus carries only a slight increased risk of miscarriage. Today, a relatively simple surgical procedure can remove a uterine septum.

Uterine abnormalities such as a small malformed uterus are especially common in women whose mothers used diethylstilbestrol (DES) when pregnant with them. DES was used many years ago to prevent miscarriages. Unfortunately, now experts know that its use not only increases the risk of a very rare vaginal cancer in exposed women, but it also can lead to decreased fertility and increased risk of pregnancy loss. It is easy to diagnose the uterine abnormality associated with DES with an X ray of the uterus and fallopian tubes, called a HYSTEROSALPINGOGRAM.

Incompetent Cervix

A common cause of second trimester loss is an "incompetent cervix." The incompetent cervix painlessly dilates in early– to mid–second trimester, and the pregnancy is painlessly expelled. Placing special sutures in a purse string fashion around the cervix is sometimes helpful to treat the condition, especially for future pregnancies.

Bacteria

Some infectious agents have been incriminated in pregnancy loss, but the evidence is not clear-cut. The focus has primarily been on several types of bacteria called *Mycoplasma hominis, Ureaplasma urealyticum,* and *Chlamydia,* although the data supporting *Chlamydia's* role as a cause for pregnancy loss is even less strong than for the other two.

Immune Problems

About 10% of couples with recurrent pregnancy loss have immune problems that may contribute to their loss. The immunology problem is called lupus anticoagulant, but it's not related to the disease called lupus and it isn't an anticoagulant. Instead, the immunology problem actually may cause clotting in the small blood vessels of the placenta.

Luteal Phase Defect

Many ob-gyns have suspected that some women don't produce enough progesterone to support an early pregnancy. Although this may be uncommon, on some occasions it may be responsible for pregnancy loss.

Symptoms

The most common symptom of miscarriage is bleeding from the vagina, which may be light or heavy. However, bleeding during early pregnancy is common and is not always serious. Many women have slight vaginal bleeding after the egg implants in the uterus (about 7 to 10 days after conception), which can be mistaken for a threatened miscarriage. A few women bleed at the time of their monthly periods through the pregnancy. However, any bleeding in the first 3 months of pregnancy is considered a threat of miscarriage and should not be ignored. In addition to signaling a threatened miscarriage, it could also indicate ECTOPIC PREGNANCY, a potentially life-threatening condition. In an ectopic pregnancy, the fetus implants outside the uterus, most often in the fallopian tube.

Cramps are another common sign of a miscarriage as the uterus tries to push out the pregnancy tissue. If a pregnant woman experiences both bleeding and cramping, the possibility of miscarriage is more likely than if only one of these symptoms is present.

Diagnosis

If a woman experiences any sign of impending miscarriage she should see a doctor or nurse for a pelvic examination to check if the cervix is closed, as it should be. If the cervix is open, miscarriage is inevitable. An ultrasound examination can confirm a missed abortion if the uterus has shrunk and the patient has had continual spotting with no other symptoms.

Treatment

Women who experience bleeding and cramping should rest until symptoms disappear, and they should avoid sexual intercourse until the outcome of the threatened miscarriage is determined.

It is not usually helpful to examine the product of miscarriage for chromosome abnormalities, since usually it is abnormal. It is done to evaluate the chromosomes of couples with repeated losses to determine if one of them is at increased risk of making an egg or sperm with the improper number of chromosomes. If there is such a problem, it is necessary to consider donor sperm or donor egg in order to carry a pregnancy to term.

An incomplete miscarriage or missed abortion may require the removal of the fetus and placenta by a dilatation and curettage (D&C), a procedure that empties the contents of the uterus.

After a miscarriage, a doctor may prescribe rest or antibiotics. There will be some bleeding from the vagina for several days to 2 weeks after miscarriage. To give the cervix time to close and avoid possible infection, women should not use tampons or have sex for at least 2 weeks. Couples should wait for one to three normal menstrual cycles before trying to get pregnant again.

Prognosis

A miscarriage that is properly treated is not life threatening and usually does not affect a woman's ability to deliver a healthy baby in the future. Feelings of grief and loss after a miscarriage are common. In fact, some women who experience a miscarriage suffer from major depression during the 6 months after the loss. This is especially true for women who don't have any children or who have had depression in the past. The emotional crisis can be similar to that of a woman whose baby has died after birth.

Prevention

Most miscarriages can't be prevented because they are caused by genetic problems present at conception. Some doctors advise women who have a threatened miscarriage to rest in bed for a day and avoid sex for a few weeks after the bleeding stops. Other experts believe that a healthy woman (especially early in the pregnancy) should continue normal activities instead of protecting a pregnancy that may end in miscarriage later on, causing even more profound distress.

If her miscarriage was caused by a hormonal imbalance (LUTEAL PHASE DEFECT), a woman can be treated with progesterone to help prevent subsequent miscarriages. It's also important to treat genital infections, eat a well-balanced diet, and refrain from smoking and using recreational drugs.

miscarriage, incomplete   A miscarriage that does not result in all of the tissue being expelled. Doctors can establish whether a miscarriage is incomplete (which leaves some immature pregnancy tissue behind) by performing a TRANSVAGINAL ULTRASOUND. Any tissue that remains must be removed.

miscarriage, inevitable   In the past, an inevitable miscarriage was any vaginal bleeding during early pregnancy combined with an opening of the cervix. Today doctors can diagnose an inevitable miscarriage much sooner through the use of TRANSVAGINAL ULTRASOUND, which can

reveal an abnormal EMBRYO, even before the clinical symptoms develop.

miscarriage, menstrual   Loss of an early EMBRYO during the time when menstruation is expected. A woman usually will not know she has been pregnant and is having a miscarriage without testing the level of HUMAN CHORIONIC GONADOTROPIN in her blood.

mittelschmerz   The discomfort felt on one side of the lower abdomen at the time of OVULATION.

monoamniotic twins   Identical twins in which the split has occurred after the BLASTOCYST has formed, so that they share the same amniotic cavity. There is a higher risk of complications when twins share the same amniotic sac. Such twins are also called monozygotic twins.

monozygotic twins   See MONOAMNIOTIC TWINS.

monthly fecundity   Medical term for the monthly chance of getting pregnant, also called monthly fertility.

monthly fertility   Medical term for the monthly chance of getting pregnant, also called monthly fecundity.

"morning after" pill   An imprecise term for the EMERGENCY CONTRACEPTIVE PILL, which is a type of EMERGENCY CONTRACEPTION that can prevent pregnancy after unprotected sex in cases of unanticipated sexual activity, contraceptive failure, or rape. ECPs actually involve more than one pill; they don't need to be taken on the "morning after"; and they should not be confused with the so-called abortion pill (RU-486), because ECPs can't terminate an established pregnancy. See also BIRTH CONTROL METHODS.

motility   See SPERM MOTILITY.

Mothers of Supertwins (MOST)   An international nonprofit support network of families with triplets and more founded in 1987 by several mothers of triplets. MOST provides information, resources, empathy, and good humor during pregnancy, infancy, toddlerhood, and school age. The group also conducts medical and psycho/social research projects annually. Contact Mothers of Supertwins (MOST), P.O. Box 951, Brentwood, NY 11717-0627; phone: (631) 859-1110; website http://www.mostonline.org. See also MULTIPLE BIRTHS AND FERTILITY DRUGS.

mucus, hostile   Cervical mucus that slows down the natural progress of sperm through the cervical canal.

Mullerian ducts   The fetal structures that fuse to form the uterus.

multifetal reduction   A process used to reduce the number of developing fetuses in the case of a multiple pregnancy in order to improve the chances for survival of the remaining babies. Although multifetal reduction has been performed on women with naturally occurring multiple pregnancies, most are used to reduce the number of fetuses resulting from fertility drugs, IN VITRO FERTILIZATION, and other reproductive techniques.

More than 20% of pregnancies resulting from the use of FERTILITY DRUGS involve more than one fetus, in contrast to a rate of 1% to 2% in the general population. While most of these pregnancies are twins, a significant percentage are triplets or more.

In the general population, about 1 birth in 100 will be twins (1.2%), and 1 in 8,000 will be triplets. In 1996, CDC statistics show about 43 twins and triplets per 100 births for women under age 35 years. Twin and triplet pregnancies increase the likelihood of premature birth and its significant related problems.

Multiple births are risky for mothers and babies. The more fetuses, the greater the risk of pregnancy loss, premature delivery, birth defects, pregnancy-induced high blood pressure, hemorrhage, and other significant complications. Twins are seven times more likely to be born smaller than single infants. More than half of all twins weigh less than 5.5 pounds, compared to 6% of single babies, and 4 of every 100 twins die. The risk of low birth weight and death only increases with multiple births. For example, more than 90% of triplets born each year weigh less than 5.5 pounds and 10 of every 100 die. There are also risks to the mother of multiples, including premature labor and delivery, pregnancy-induced high blood pressure or pre-eclampsia, diabetes, and hemorrhage.

Despite these risks, the rate of multiple births increased 24% between 1983 and 1993, with 2.5% of all 1993 babies born as twins, triplets, quadruplets, or quintuplets. In 1993, the most recent year tabulated, babies born weighing 5.5 pounds or less accounted for 7.2% of all births—the highest low-birthweight rate since 1976. Just as the number of multiple births rises, so does the number of low-birthweight babies.

While neonatal intensive care continues to save many of these tiny babies, some public health specialists worry that if the trend continues, their numbers could drive up pre- and postnatal medical costs and perhaps the infant mortality rate.

Because of these risks, nearly 300 clinics in the United States perform multifetal reductions. While there are many advantages to performing these reductions, there are also risks, including

- the accidental loss of pregnancy
- the performance of the procedure on the wrong "healthy" fetuses
- inflammation of the tissues surrounding the fetus
- premature delivery
- permanent damage of the surviving fetuses
- severe depression in the mother after the procedure

Technique

There are many techniques used in multifetal reduction, but the most common technique involves the injection of potassium chloride into the heart of each fetus to be eliminated. Other techniques include transcervical suction, transabdominal and vaginal needling of the heart, and air injection. Except for transcervical suction, these techniques target the developing heart, because once the heart is destroyed the fetus immediately dies.

Multifetal reduction is usually performed as soon as possible, because the longer the mother carries the multiple fetuses, the greater the potential harm for those remaining. Most reductions are done between the 9th and 13th weeks of pregnancy, when the doctor usually eliminates the fetuses that are most easily accessible rather than those that are weakest. However, reductions done during the 18th to 24th week are based more on eliminating weak or abnormal fetuses.

Controversy

Multifetal reduction is not without critics and controversy, especially among those who feel it is a form of abortion, and that the termination of life is unjustifiable even if the process will increase the chances of survival of the remaining fetuses.

Multiple pregnancy of an order higher than twins involves great danger for the woman's health and also for her fetuses, which are likely to be spontaneously aborted or to be delivered prematurely with a high risk of either dying or being damaged. In such circumstances, proponents consider reduction justifiable and indicated.

Where interruption of pregnancy for severe fetal abnormality is considered ethically justified, the same ethical principles apply to the reduction of a multiple pregnancy in which one (or more) fetus is abnormal, provided that every effort is taken to ensure the health of the woman and the normal survival of the remaining fetus or fetuses.

Guidelines

While there is no legal limit to the number of embryos a clinic can transfer into a woman's uterus, the American Society for Reproductive Medicine issues general guidelines on how many embryos should be transferred in an ART cycle. However, this final decision is up to the couple and their doctor. The ASRM recommends that

- for young women with healthy embryos, no more than three embryos are usually transferred
- for women aged 35 to 40, no more than four embryos are usually transferred

In women over age 40 (or those who have had unsuccessful treatment cycles) up to five embryos are usually transferred

History

Over the years, clinics have tended to implant more and more embryos at a time; the chance for successful implantation by transferring two embryos is 20%, but with three it rises to 25%, and so on; the transfer of six embryos gives a successful implantation rate of nearly 40%. As clinics compete to boost success rates, some have been transferring more and more embryos in a cycle—not two or three but as many as eight—to increase the odds of pregnancy. This is not in the best interest for everyone. With IVF the pregnancy rate is not often the most important way to judge a program.

FERTILITY DRUGS have had a significant effect on the frequency of births. According to the Centers for Disease Control and Prevention, rates for births of triplets or greater have risen from 29 per 100,000 births in 1971 to 174 per 100,000 in 1997, largely because of infertility treatments. New guidelines for treating patients with fertility medications advise doctors to limit multiple births and provide strategies for doing so, but not everyone agrees that high-order multiple births should be limited. Some are opposed because they consider reducing the number of viable fetuses as abortions. Some patients are reluctant to reduce the number of fetuses because they're paying for fertility treatments themselves or because their insurance companies place strict limits on coverage. See also FETAL REDUCTION.

multiple births and fertility drugs Known medically as "multiple gestation," up to 20% of pregnancies resulting from FERTILITY DRUGS are multiple, in contrast to a rate of 1% to 2% in the general population. While most of these pregnancies are twins, a significant percentage are triplets or more. This is a concern because the more fetuses, the greater the risk of pregnancy loss, premature delivery, birth defects, pregnancy-induced high blood pressure, hemorrhage, and other significant complications.

The average length of pregnancy is 39 weeks for a single gestation, 35 weeks for twins, 33 weeks for triplets, and 29 weeks for quadruplets. In general, the risk of complications due to premature delivery is significantly less once the pregnancy reaches 32 to 34 weeks gestation. The more babies, the higher the risks of MISCARRIAGE, birth defects, premature birth, and the mental or physical problems that can result from a premature delivery. There are also risks to the mother of multiples, including premature labor and delivery, pregnancy-induced high blood pressure, or pre-eclampsia, DIABETES, and hemorrhage.

FERTILITY DRUGS have had a significant effect on the frequency of births. According to the Centers for Disease Control and Prevention, rates for births of triplets or greater have risen from 29 per 100,000 births in 1971 to 174 per 100,000 in 1997, largely because of infertility treatments.

New guidelines for treating patients with fertility medications advise doctors to limit multiple births and provide strategies for doing so, but not everyone agrees that high-order multiple births should be limited. Some are opposed because they consider reducing the number of viable fetuses as ABORTIONS. Some patients are reluctant to reduce the number of fetuses because they're paying for fertility treatments themselves or because their insurance companies place strict limits on coverage.

The American Society for Reproductive Medicine issues general guidelines on how many embryos should be transferred in an ART cycle. However, this final decision is up to the couple and their doctor. The ASRM recommends that

- for young women with healthy embryos, no more than three embryos are usually transferred
- for women aged 35 to 40, no more than four embryos are usually transferred
- in women over age 40 (or those who have had unsuccessful treatment cycles) up to five embryos are usually transferred

Women undergoing GIFT may have one additional embryo added to each category above.

In the general population, about 1 birth in 100 will be twins (1.2%) and 1 in 8,000 will be triplets. In 1996, CDC statistics show about 43 twins and triplets per 100 births for women under age 35 years. Twin and triplet pregnancies increase the likelihood of premature birth and its significant related problems. See also SELECTIVE REDUCTION.

mumps An acute, contagious viral disease that causes painful enlargement of the salivary or parotid glands. Mumps virus affects glandular tissue, and the second most common gland it affects (after the salivary glands) are the TESTICLES. This is why a common complication in boys who get mumps after puberty is inflammation of the testicles (ORCHITIS); however, it is rare to become infertile from mumps orchitis. In addition, mumps may also affect the ovaries, leading to an inflammation (oophoritis).

Mumps is caused by the paramyxovirus, which is spread from person to person by saliva droplets or direct contact with articles that have been contaminated with infected saliva. The parotid glands (the salivary glands between the ear and the jaw) are usually involved. Children between the ages of 2 and 12 are most commonly infected, but the infection can occur in other age groups. The incubation period is usu-

ally 12 to 24 days. Because of widespread vaccination, only 4,000 cases were reported in United States in 1991.

myoma   See FIBROIDS AND INFERTILITY.

nafarelin (Synarel) A Gn-RH AGONIST similar to Lupron (LEUPROLIDE ACETATE) and Zoladex (GOSERELIN). Nafarelin is given as a nasal spray to trigger the release of LH (LUTEINIZING HORMONE) and FSH (FOLLICLE-STIMULATING HORMONE) from the pituitary. This allows the doctor to induce OVULATION with great precision by suppressing normal ovarian function. By eliminating the natural Gn-RH production, the doctor can then begin to prescribe the exact amounts of FSH and LH needed to induce ovulation without having to worry about natural FSH and LH released by the woman's body.

These drugs have been especially helpful for women who are intending to use ASSISTED REPRODUCTIVE TECHNOLOGY. Long-acting forms of these drugs are sometimes given to women with POLYCYSTIC OVARY SYNDROME, ENDOMETRIOSIS, or polycystic ovaries.

Side Effects

Side effects are typical of those seen during MENOPAUSE, including hot flashes, headaches, mood swings, vaginal dryness, painful intercourse, reduced breast size, and bone loss.

National Adoption Center A national organization that promotes the ADOPTION of children throughout the country (especially those with special needs) and maintains a significant Internet presence offering photos of hard-to-place children for adoption. Since 1972, the center has found families for more than 13,000 children. The National Adoption Center is a member organization of Children's Charities of America and a participant in the Combined Fed-

eral Campaign. Contact 1500 Walnut Street, Suite 701, Philadelphia PA 19102; phone: 800-TOADOPT or (215) 735-9988; website http://www.adopt.org.

National Adoption Information Clearinghouse A comprehensive resource on all aspects of ADOPTION, provide as a service of the Children's Bureau, Administration on Children, Youth and Families in the Department of Health and Human Services. The clearinghouse is a national resource for information on all aspects of adoption for professionals, policy makers, and the general public. Clearinghouse services include technical assistance to professionals and policy makers, a library collection, publications, databases on adoption resources, and information on federal and state legislation. Services are generally provided free of charge; however some directory publications have a nominal charge to cover printing and shipping/handling charges.

Contact: National Adoption Information Clearinghouse, 330 C Street, SW, Washington, DC 20447; phone: (703) 352-3488 or (888) 251-0075; e-mail: naic@calib.com; website: http://www.calib.com/naic/.

natural family planning A method of natural birth control that basically involves avoiding sex on the days when a woman is most fertile.

During each menstrual cycle, a woman's ovaries release an egg (OVULATION) that moves toward the uterus through the FALLOPIAN TUBES, where FERTILIZATION may take place. Because SPERM may live in a woman's reproductive tract for up to 7 days and the egg remains fertile for about 24 hours, it's possible to get pregnant from 7 days before ovulation to 3 days afterward. To practice natural family planning, a couple needs to figure out the woman's fertile time by using a method based on her menstrual cycle, changes in cervical mucus, or changes in body temperature.

There are two basic ways to do this: the ovulation method and the symptothermal method. In the ovulation method, a woman determines the days just before and just after ovulation by checking her cervical mucus. When a woman is most likely to get pregnant, the cervical mucus is stretchy, clear, and slick, rather like an uncooked egg white.

In the symptothermal method, a woman takes her temperature each day with a special thermometer and tracks it on a chart. At ovulation, a woman's temperature will rise slightly. The woman also checks the consistency of her cervical mucus. She may also notice other changes, such as pain in the area of the ovaries, bloating, low backache, and breast tenderness.

In both methods, couples use a special chart to keep track of the changes in the woman's body.

These methods can help a couple avoid pregnancy if the couple is trained and carefully follows all instructions. When used correctly, both methods can be 90% to 98% effective (2 to 10 pregnancies per 100 couples). However, if a couple doesn't follow the instructions completely, these methods will be much less effective. In practice, these methods may not be as reliable as other forms of birth control.

As many as two of three couples who don't have fertility problems become pregnant if they have sex on the days that the cervical mucus is clearest and most stretchable.

While not especially reliable or effective, for religious or health reasons some women choose this type of birth control to limit family size or space out pregnancies. See also BIRTH CONTROL METHODS; RHYTHM METHOD.

necrospermia   See NECROZOOSPERMIA.

necrozoospermia   A total absence of moving SPERM. If sperm are seen but aren't moving, it is important to find out if the visible sperm are alive. It's possible to have sperm with normal reproductive genetics that are deficient in one or several of the factors necessary for movement. It is possible to inject healthy, nonmoving sperm directly into the egg using INTRACYTOPLASMIC SPERM INJECTION.

nonoxynol-9   A type of SPERMICIDE that effectively kills sperm but will not prevent the spread of HIV, the virus that causes AIDS.

Norplant   A method of implantable birth control that is one of the newest types of birth control options. Contraceptive implants are small, matchstick-sized tubes containing a progestin or LEVONORGESTREL inserted just under the skin of a woman's arm. Once in place, the implants release a small amount of hormone each day for 5 years, blocking OVULATION and thickening cervical mucus. Other than a VASECTOMY, the implants are probably the most effective method of contraception available.

The implants begin to work within 8 to 24 hours of the procedure, and they don't require maintenance of any kind, nor do they affect the use of the arm once the site has healed. They can be felt if the insertion site is touched, and their outline may be visible in thin arms. Women should plan on returning for a checkup within 3 months of insertion followed by yearly checkups to monitor the recipient's progress. Once the implants are removed, a woman can become pregnant again.

Implants are a good choice for women who want to delay pregnancy for several years but hope to bear children later on. Although failure is rare, pregnancies do occur (especially among heavier and younger women).

Insertion

The implants can be inserted during an office visit. First, the skin is numbed with local anesthetic, and then the tubes are embedded under the skin of the upper arm. They must be surgically removed (which may be difficult).

The six-rod Norplant implant provides protection for up to 5 years (or until it's removed), while the two-rod Norplant 2 protects for up to 3 years. Norplant failures are rare but occur more often with increased body weight.

Removal

When the time comes to remove the implants, the insertion site is again anesthetized, and a small incision is made in the arm. Removal can be uncomfortable and is more difficult than the original procedure if scar tissue has formed over the implants. It usually takes 15 to 20 minutes, although it may require more than one visit. The implants' contraceptive action wears off a few hours after removal, and fertility is restored within a couple of weeks. If the user wishes, new implants can be inserted as soon as the old ones are removed.

Side Effects

While implants are very effective, they can cause all of the side effects typically related to hormonal types of birth control. Like other progestins, levonorgestrel thins the lining of the uterine and prevents it from shedding. Menstrual disorders—spotting between periods, longer or heavier periods, or no periods at all—are, therefore, the most common side effects and the main reasons why women discontinue the Norplant system. More serious symptoms include arm pain, pus or bleeding at the insertion site, expulsion of the implant, and delayed menstrual periods after a long time of regular periods.

Other potential problems include weight gain, headaches, breast tenderness, mood changes, and acne. In many cases these problems subside as time passes, or they can be substantially reduced by other therapies.

Some studies have reported an association between depression and Norplant use. In one study, however, after 2 years, many Norplant users who had severe depression at the beginning showed improvement.

About 3% of users suffer a reaction to the local anesthetic or experience tissue or nerve damage due to poorly placed implants or problems in removal.

Certain medications, including antiseizure drugs and rifampin (rifampicin), an antibiotic used to treat tuberculosis, interfere with Norplant. For this reason, a doctor must always be informed of any medications the patient is taking, even if they are unrelated to gynecologic problems.

There have been some reports of strokes, unexpected pressure in the brain, and clotting abnormalities in women using implants, but there is no evidence that Norplant was the cause of these rare events.

Who Should Not Use Implants

Women should not use implants if they have

- breast cancer
- acute liver disease or tumors
- blood clots
- undiagnosed vaginal bleeding
- blood clots in the veins or lungs
- take antiseizure drugs
- take rifampin

Women who are breast-feeding must wait until 6 weeks after delivery to receive the implants. Women at risk for breast cancer, osteoporosis, heart disease, DIABETES, high blood pressure, blood clots, liver disease, or stroke should consider a nonhormonal birth control method. Because of a link between bone calcium loss and progestin contraceptives, women at risk for osteoporosis should consider nonhormonal methods. The implants don't protect against sexually transmitted diseases, so women at risk for infection should use a barrier contraceptive in addition to the implants or as an alternative.

obstetrician-gynecologist A specialist in the evaluation and treatment of women's reproductive health problems, including prenatal care and delivery of babies. Following a residency training program, the obstetrician passes a written examination and becomes "board eligible," with board certification only following both the written and oral examinations.

Although physicians who are board-certified in general obstetrics and gynecology receive some training in the diagnosis and treatment of infertility, they may lack the additional training and experience of physicians who specialize in reproductive medicine.

Ob-gyns who are most experienced in infertility are those who devote most or all of their practice time providing treatment to infertile couples. Ready access to laboratories and qualified and experienced staff who can assist with semen analysis, inseminations, and other ASSISTED REPRODUCTIVE TECHNOLOGIES may be important.

OHSS See OVARIAN HYPERSTIMULATION SYNDROME.

oligomenorrhea An irregular menstrual cycle that is usually longer than 35 days. This condition is usually caused by irregular hormone levels produced by the ovaries. An irregular menstrual cycle can make it more difficult to conceive.

oligospermia The term for a low number of sperm cells in the ejaculate. About one-third of all cases of infertility are caused by oligospermia.

In many cases of low sperm count, there may be a minor surgical problem, such as a VARICOCELE, that can be corrected. But if severe structural problems within the sperm ducts caused by previous infection, trauma, or even surgery (such as a VASECTOMY), occur, major surgery may be needed.

In blocked sperm ducts, surgery can sometimes restore function, but this does not necessarily mean that a pregnancy will be possible. In fact, in many cases of previous vasectomy or injury, the men may have produced antibodies to his own sperm that may interfere with future attempts to have a baby.

In a relatively small number of cases of male infertility, the failure to produce an adequate quality of sperm is linked to reduced secretion by the pituitary gland of those hormones necessary to stimulate sperm production. In men, the pituitary gland produces two important hormones that affect testicular function: FOLLICLE-STIMULATING HORMONE (FSH) and LUTEINIZING HORMONE (LH). LH's main function is to act on LEYDIG CELLS in the testicles that produce the male hormone TESTOSTERONE. Therefore, a drop in FSH production can cause male infertility. Usually, a drop in either LH or FSH means the other will also be low.

Women produce eggs in a cyclic manner. In men, sperm are produced continually and each sperm takes 3 months to be produced. Therefore, any treatment to improve sperm production can be properly tested only after waiting for about 100 days.

To assess the potential of a male to respond to FERTILITY DRUGS aimed at stimulating the testicles to produce more sperm and male hormone, it's necessary first to measure both FSH and LH, which are produced by the pituitary gland, as well as the male hormones TESTOSTERONE, androstenedione, dehydroepiandrosterone, and prolactin. Measurement of these hormones gives an indication as to whether the man is likely to respond to treatment with FSH or FSH/LH.

The most common drug used to boost sperm production is CLOMIPHENE CITRATE, a hormone that acts on the brain to stimulate the pituitary gland to produce large amounts of FSH. The FSH, in turn, stimulates sperm production. Measures of semen, FSH, LH, and male hormones are taken right before beginning clomiphene citrate treatment and then repeated afterwards. The final assessment of a man's response to the drug can only be made 100 days after starting treatment. Clomiphene citrate is basically harmless to men, although a few side effects may include spots in front of the eyes, dry mouth, headaches, slight mood changes, and, rarely, hot flashes. These side effects all stop when treatment ends.

If clomiphene citrate therapy doesn't work, it's possible to administer FSH alone or in combination with LH to try to stimulate testicles directly. In certain cases of male infertility, this regimen might be combined with the administration of the hormone HUMAN CHORIONIC GONADOTROPIN (hCG), which is also a natural hormone with a similar function to LH. These drugs are usually given three times a week for 100 days; the same hormonal and sperm tests are given. This treatment is safe; minor side effects stop when treatment ends.

oligozoospermia   See OLIGOSPERMIA.

oocyte   The biological term for an egg.

oocyte maturation inhibitor (OMI)   A protein found in the follicular fluid that keeps the egg from maturing.

oogenesis   The production of eggs in the ovaries of a fetus.

oogonium   The earliest recognizable form of an egg in the ovaries of a fetus. After multiplication, it develops into OOCYTES.

oophorectomy   See OVARIECTOMY.

opiates and infertility   Heroin, morphine, and other opiates, in addition to related drugs like methadone, have been linked to the inhibition of gonad-stimulating hormones (GONADOTROPINS) secretion and with reduced levels of TESTOSTERONE in the blood.

oral contraception   See BIRTH CONTROL PILL.

orchidopexy   A surgical procedure to move an undescended testicle (CRYPTORCHIDISM) down into the scrotum so it can develop normally and produce SPERM cells. Undescended TESTICLES that remain in the abdomen for many years can cause infertility or a malignant tumor in later years.

In normal fetal development, the testicles develop in the abdomen and descend into the scrotum during the last months before birth. In a small percentage (0.04%) of newborns (more often among the premature), one or both testicles fail to descend into the scrotum. In these cases, orchidopexy is recommended for infants over 1 year of age whose testicles haven't descended into the scrotum. Most often, only one side is affected.

After general anesthesia, the procedure begins with an incision in the groin, where most undescended testicles are lodged. The spermatic cord is freed from surrounding tissues, and a small incision is made in the scrotum. After a pouch is created, the testicle is located and carefully pulled down into the scrotum. The testicle is stitched in place in the scrotum, and the incisions are stitched closed. Orchidopexy is successful in most cases, and the long-term prognosis for hormone production and fertility is excellent.

The surgery may be done on an outpatient basis and should be followed by bedrest for the first 2 to 3 days. Strenuous activity should be avoided for at least a month.

orchitis   An inflammation of one or both of the TESTICLES. Orchitis may be caused by numerous bacterial and viral organisms; the most common viral cause is mumps (see MUMPS AND INFERTILITY). Between 15% to 25% of men who have mumps after puberty will develop orchitis during the course of the illness. BRUCELLOSIS is a rare disease in which orchitis develops in 2% to 20% of men with the disease. Sometimes, orchitis leads to permanent infertility in men.

Symptoms
Symptoms may include scrotal swelling; a tender, swollen, "heavy feeling" in the testicle or groin on the affected side; fever; blood in the semen; pain in the groin or testicle or during urination, intercourse, or ejaculation.

Diagnosis
The condition is diagnosed with a urinalysis and culture, tests to screen for chlamydia and gonorrhea, a complete blood count, and a blood chemistry.

Treatment
When inflammation is caused by a virus, only pain relievers are prescribed, together with bedrest, elevation of the scrotum, and ice packs applied to the area. Normal function of the testicle is usually preserved, but the outcome of mumps orchitis is unpredictable; sterility has followed mumps orchitis. The inflammation may cause infertility and atrophy (diminished size) of one or both testicles.

Organization of Parents Through Surrogacy, The   A national surrogacy support organization for both couples through surrogacy as well as surrogate mothers. The country's oldest and only

nonprofit support group for surrogacy, the organization offers information, networking, support, and advocacy. Membership offers person-to-person contact with experienced parents and surrogates together with online support through the group's listserv, a packet of newsletters, resource guides, book lists, regional meetings, legislative information, and advocacy. OPTS is not affiliated with any surrogacy practitioner, agency, or lawyer. The organization offers support services to all regardless of where they might be in the process or how they have chosen to proceed. See also SURROGATE MOTHER. Contact: OPTS, P.O. Box 611, Gurnee, IL 60031; phone: (847) 782-0224; website http://www. opts.com.

ovarian cancer and fertility drugs   While a few controversial data associate ovulation stimulation drugs like GONADOTROPINS to a higher risk of future ovarian cancer, most studies have found no connection between fertility drugs and cancer.

The risk of ovarian cancer seems in part related to the number of times a woman ovulates. Infertility increases this risk; BIRTH CONTROL PILL use decreases it. While research is underway to help clarify this issue, the careful use of gonadotropins is still reasonable, especially considering that pregnancy and breast-feeding reduce cancer risk. Most doctors will not advise taking any fertility drug for more than several months at a time, and certainly not for more than a total of 6 months to a year.

ovarian cyst   A fluid-filled sac inside the OVARY. Typically, ovarian cysts are not related to any disease and disappear on their own. Such a cyst might form during ovulation, when a follicle grows but fails to rupture and release an egg. Instead of being reabsorbed, the fluid within the follicle remains and forms a cyst. Cysts usually disappear within 2 months without treatment. These ovarian cysts are relatively common, and they occur most often during childbearing years. No known risk factors have been identified.

An ovarian cyst may be found together with ovulation disorders, tumors of the ovary, and ENDOMETRIOSIS. Functional ovarian cysts should not be confused with other conditions involving cystic ovaries, such as POLYCYSTIC OVARY SYNDROME or ovarian cancer.

Symptoms

Cysts may not cause any symptoms at all. If symptoms do appear, they may include abnormal uterine bleeding, menstrual cycle changes, pelvic pain, pain during sex, pelvic pain, nausea/vomiting, or breast tenderness. Prolonged symptoms may be associated with polycystic ovary syndrome and include abnormally light or lack of menstrual periods, infertility, obesity, swollen abdomen, and increased growth of body hair.

Treatment

Functional ovarian cysts typically disappear within 60 days without any treatment. Oral contraceptives may be prescribed to help establish normal cycles. See also CHOCOLATE CYST.

ovarian dysgenesis   A condition that leads to female sterility present at birth, caused by an abnormality in the second X chromosome. The disease is inherited in the autosomal recessive pattern, which means that an abnormal gene from each parent is required to cause the disease. People with only one abnormal gene in the gene pair are called carriers, but since the gene is recessive they don't exhibit the disease.

In Finland, where the only studies have been conducted, the incidence is 1 in 8,300 newborn girls, with almost three times more cases in the north central part of Finland. How common this disease might be in other countries is not yet known. The possible effects of this mutation in males are also not known.

Cause

The mutation disturbs the action of the FOLLICLE-STIMULATING HORMONE (FSH) that controls ovarian function, thus preventing the production of eggs and causing lack of menstruation with infertility.

Treatment

Although ovarian dysgenesis itself cannot be corrected, hormonal replacement therapy can improve ovarian function.

ovarian factors and infertility   There are a number of ovarian disorders and problems that can affect the development and release of eggs. OVULATION is the primary function of the ovaries, and problems with ovulation cause as many as 33% of female infertility problems.

Because ovulation is controlled by hormones, anything affecting the HYPOTHALAMUS, pituitary, or ovaries can cause a problem with egg release (ANOVULATION). Other endocrine systems may not directly affect ovulation, but they may also influence ovulation, such as thyroid disease, DIABETES, or high levels of cortisol. A woman's age also can directly affect her ovarian function.

Other less common problems with a woman's ovaries that may affect fertility include birth defects, POLYCYSTIC OVARY SYNDROME (PCOS), ENDOMETRIOSIS, and some medications.

ovarian failure, premature   A condition involving a loss of ovarian function in women under 40, so that menstrual periods stop, ESTROGEN levels drop, and FOLLICLE-STIMULATING HORMONE (FSH) levels rise. The cause of this rare disorder is often undetectable, but possible explanations can include genetics, surgery, radiation, chemotherapy, or immune abnormalities.

POF is sometimes called "early MENOPAUSE," but this term is incorrect—this condition is not menopause. The term "early menopause" was introduced in a few studies when it was thought that, like menopause, the condition was characterized by a total lack of eggs. It was called "premature" to signify that the condition started at an earlier-than-normal age.

However, unlike menopause (which appears to be a permanent loss of ovarian activity), POF may not be permanent. Using pelvic ultrasound to check the ovaries of women with premature ovarian failure indicates that about 40% of the women have structures that appear to be ovarian follicles. In fact, women with POF do intermittently produce estrogen and ovulate. This is why the term "premature ovarian failure" is preferred to "premature menopause"—because menopause refers to a complete cessation of periods. In some cases, premature ovarian failure may be reversible.

POF occurs in 1 in 1,000 women between the ages of 15 and 29, and 1 in 100 women between the ages of 30 and 39, meaning that the condition affects at least 250,000 women in the United States. Most researchers consider that age 39 is the cutoff point; before age 39 ovarian failure is considered POF, but after age 39 it is considered to be an early menopause. The average age of onset is 27.

There is no "typical" menstrual history for women with POF. Some women state that they feel as if they went to bed one night feeling fine and woke up the next morning with POF, but other women notice a more gradual onset. Some have normal periods but develop hot flashes. In some women, the problem becomes apparent after they've had a baby and their periods never return. Others notice a problem when they stop taking BIRTH CONTROL PILLS and their period never returns.

Women with POF have either fewer-than-normal follicles or a dysfunction in their ovaries. The FSH stimulates the development of a follicle, and as the follicles ripen they release estrogen. The estrogen in turn sends a signal back to the brain to turn the FSH off. If a follicle isn't stimulated, there isn't enough estrogen to signal the brain to turn off. So instead of being able to turn off the FSH, the pituitary is driven to send out even more FSH to try and get a follicle to develop. In turn, the FSH level rises.

If there is a dysfunction of the ovaries, experts suspect that a woman produces anti-bodies to her own FSH or to her own ovarian substances.

Women with POF have one of the following:

- a low number of follicles to start with
- eggs that are lost more quickly than normal
- a dysfunction of the follicles

There are several different causes of POF, but most women never find that cause. About 25% to 35% of women with POF have an associated autoimmune disorder. The next most frequent known cause is genetic (a family history of POF occurs in about 4% of women). Finally, there are other reasons, such as a side effect of cancer treatment with radiation or chemotherapy, or hysterectomy with removal of the ovaries. In addition, infections have been associated with POF.

It's possible that POF can develop before a girl even begins to menstruate. About 10% to 15% of women with POF have never had a spontaneous period (primary AMENORRHEA). When primary amenorrhea occurs along with delays in puberty such as breast-budding and hair under the arms, almost 40% of the girls have a chromosomal problem.

Symptoms

Changes begin to occur in a woman's period: the flow may be different or the length of the bleeding may change or periods may stop altogether. Other symptoms include hot flashes, night sweats, irritability, poor concentration, decreased sex drive, painful sex, and thinning and drying of the vagina. Some women discover the problem when they go for fertility testing and discover that they have an elevated FSH. They may not have had any symptoms.

Diagnosis

In addition to a physical and pelvic exam, blood tests should include

- FSH, done at least two times at least 1 month apart. There is debate about the time of the month the FSH is done (such as day 2 or 3 of the menstrual cycle). However, in general the timing during the month isn't that important. It is important that more than one test be performed.

- estradiol
- karyotype; this should be performed as part of the basic laboratory blood work for all women with POF
- autoimmune disorder screening
- serum-free thyroxine
- thyroid-stimulating hormone (TSH)
- antinuclear antibody titer
- fasting glucose
- electrolytes
- antithyroid antibodies, which may be reserved for women with abnormal thyroid function
- corticotrophin stimulation test, for women with signs and symptoms of adrenal insufficiency; a random plasma corticol level is not helpful because blood tests can be in the normal range even with impaired adrenal reserve
- complete blood count
- urinalysis

Treatment

Even if no cause is identified, a woman and her doctor may consider hormone replacement therapy (HRT). This treatment should allow a woman to consider IN VITRO FERTILIZATION with donated eggs. Another benefit of hormone replacement is that it seems to induce remissions of the condition in about 1% to 2% of patients each year. See also PREMATURE OVARIAN FAILURE SUPPORT GROUP.

ovarian hyperstimulation syndrome (OHSS)
A side effect of drug-induced OVULATION in which a woman's ovaries become enlarged and produce too many eggs as a result of being over-stimulated. The medications (usually FSH) cause ovarian enlargement and discomfort; fluid accumulates in the abdomen, which can lead to blood chemistry problems. Usually, ovarian hyperstimulation occurs after the end of treatment with FSH-containing drugs. The problem can begin quickly and peak within 7 to 10 days after FSH treatment.

The condition is more likely to occur when ESTRADIOL levels are high or many follicles exist. It is also more common among women with POLYCYSTIC OVARY SYNDROME. Ovarian hyperstimulation occurs in about 5% of women taking an FSH-containing medication; less than 2% have serious problems.

Symptoms

Early warning signs include pelvic pain, sudden weight gain, abdominal pain, nausea and vomiting, dehydration, and reduced urination. In more severe cases, fluid may build up in the lungs and cause breathing problems.

If an ovary ruptures, blood can build up in the abdomen. Fluid imbalances can occur and very rarely lead to blood-clotting problems, stroke, and lung clots.

Treatment

Mild cases can be treated with bed rest at home and avoiding sex. Moderate to severe cases are treated in the hospital with intravenous fluids. OHSS usually goes away by itself once menstruation begins, but may take longer if pregnancy occurs.

Prevention

Cycles stimulated with these drugs must be carefully monitored with ultrasound scans. OHSS may be prevented by withholding the hCG injection when ultrasound monitoring indicates that too many follicles have matured.

ovarian pregnancy An ECTOPIC PREGNANCY that is found within the OVARY, usually because an egg has been fertilized while still inside the follicle.

ovarian stimulation The use of drugs to stimulate the ovaries to develop FOLLICLES and eggs.

ovarian wedge resection Surgical removal of a portion of a POLYCYSTIC OVARY to produce OVULATION; the OVARY is then sewn back together. This procedure has been effective in decreasing LH (LUTEINIZING HORMONE) and ANDROGEN (male sex hormone) production, and reestablishing regular menstrual periods in more than 75% of patients. Pregnancy rates following ovarian wedge resection vary but have been reported to be as high as 60%. Unfortunately, a major complication of this procedure is the formation of pelvic scar tissue in 30% of patients.

It isn't clear why women with POLYCYSTIC OVARY SYNDROME ovulate after wedge resection. There is no increased risk of multiple pregnancy or OVARIAN HYPERSTIMULATION SYNDROME. If ovulatory cycles fail to restore after the surgery, the doctor may restart ovulation induction.

ovariectomy Surgical removal of an ovary (also called an *oophorectomy*). If only one ovary is removed, the other will still produce eggs, and menstruation will continue as usual. An ovariectomy is performed when there is a cyst or a tumor in the ovary, or if a fertilized egg has become implanted on the ovary. A partial ovariectomy may be performed if there is a benign cyst.

If an ECTOPIC PREGNANCY implants on the ovary, destruction of the ovarian tissue and excessive bleeding may require its removal. The ovary may also have to be removed when it has been entirely replaced with ENDOMETRIOSIS. Sometimes ovarian enlargement caused by a tumor or cyst may cause the ovary to twist and cut off its blood supply.

As long as one ovary is intact, however, fertility should not be compromised. When a woman over 45 years of age has a hysterectomy, both ovaries are often removed in a procedure called a bilateral ovariectomy.

If the ovaries are removed before a woman enters MENOPAUSE, the woman will have an abrupt drop in ESTROGEN and will develop symptoms such as hot flashes. Many gynecologists will start estrogen replacement therapy on young women who have had their ovaries removed before they leave the hospital.

Some premenopausal women whose ovaries have been surgically removed complain of feeling "not themselves" even after their estrogen replacement is adequate, as measured by FSH and estradiol blood tests. Often, small doses of testosterone may be added to the treatment program if the woman still feels uncomfortable within several months after surgery. These are available in many forms, including tablets, pellets, or topical gels.

ovary The female organ that produces eggs, located on each side of the uterus. At birth, the ovaries have thousands of eggs, each surrounded by cells that later develop into a small, fluid-filled blister called a FOLLICLE.

ovary, resistant An ovary that can't respond to FOLLICLE-STIMULATING HORMONE. While primitive germ cells will be present in the ovary, they will not respond to FSH stimulation.

ovulation The release of a mature egg from a FOLLICLE. Typically, a female EMBRYO has about 7 million eggs; by the time the baby is born, that number drops to about 1 million. By the time the girl reaches puberty, the number of eggs has dropped further to about 300,000. This gradual decline continues throughout her reproductive life, until finally she exhausts her supply of eggs, stops having menstrual periods, and enters menopause. Typically, most women ovulate only about 400 times in their lives.

Each egg in the ovary is surrounded by much smaller cells, forming a fluid-filled follicle. On the first day of MENSTRUATION (day 1 of the MENSTRUAL CYCLE), a woman's body releases increasing amounts of FOLLICLE-STIMULATING HORMONE (FSH) produced by the pituitary at the base of the brain. This FSH stimulates a follicle to grow and produce ESTROGEN. The egg also begins to mature at this time.

By about day 14, the pituitary releases a burst of LUTEINIZING HORMONE (LH), a process called the LH SURGE. This sudden burst of hormone triggers ovulation, the release of a mature egg from the follicle. Normally, only one of a woman's two ovaries produces a mature egg each month during her menstrual cycle. Once the egg leaves the ovary, it's swept up into the fallopian tube; as it travels along the tube, another female hormone called PROGESTERONE begins to rise.

If there are no SPERM in the fallopian tube and the egg isn't fertilized, it travels to the UTERUS and is shed, along with the unneeded lining of the uterus, during menstruation.

If there happens to be sperm in the fallopian tubes, the egg will be fertilized, and the resulting embryo continues its trek through the fallopian tube into the uterus, where the higher levels of progesterone have thickened the uterine walls in preparation for a fertilized egg. Here the embryo will implant itself and grow into a baby.

The simple, inexpensive way of finding out the approximate time when a woman ovulates is to take a BASAL BODY TEMPERATURE every morning and record it on a chart. There are other ways to detect ovulation. Nonprescription ovulation predictor urine tests are sold at drug stores. In addition, a woman's body may signal when she is about to ovulate; many women feel twinges in the right and left sides of the lower abdomen. Some women notice clear vaginal discharge at ovulation. In addition, a doctor can request an ultrasound or appropriate blood tests to determine ovulation.

ovulation induction   Drug treatment that triggers the development and release of an egg or eggs from the FOLLICLES in the ovaries. In this procedure, a woman is given a hormone injection that induces an egg to mature. Then the woman is given a second hormone (hCG) that releases the eggs for insemination (or IVF).

Doctors can't know for sure how many eggs will result, but they try to control it by checking a woman's ovaries with ultrasound to search for large numbers of follicles and by measuring a hormone that ovaries produce, called ESTRADIOL. If it looks as if too many eggs are maturing or the estradiol level is too high, the woman is advised to skip the hCG injection that would release the eggs and instead wait for the next cycle. Although skipping the hCG injection may reduce OVARIAN HYPERSTIMULATION SYNDROME and avoid the risk of multiple birth, some women may choose to take on such risks, since the overall pregnancy rate per try is not high.

Several years ago, ovulation induction was more popular than IN VITRO FERTILIZATION. But while ovulation induction is less expensive (about $2,000 to $4,000 per cycle) compared to IVF (about $10,000 per attempt), IVF has a greater chance of success and a lesser chance of multiple births.

Drugs used to trigger ovulation include CLOMIPHENE CITRATE, different formulations of FOLLICLE-STIMULATING HORMONE (FSH), and HUMAN CHORIONIC GONADOTROPIN (hCG). These drugs are used to treat infertility due to lack of OVULATION and to release more than one egg during assisted conception (such as in GAMETE INTRAFALLOPIAN TRANSFER or in vitro fertilization). See also HUMEGON; PERGONAL; OVARIAN HYPERSTIMULATION SYNDROME.

ovulation problems   One of the most common reasons for INFERTILITY in women is related to a problem in the ability of the OVARY to release an egg. Given the intricate interaction of the various hormones necessary for ovulation, it's not surprising that about 33% of infertility cases can be traced to ovulatory and hormonal problems.

A woman who has regular menstrual periods every 26 to 35 days, preceded by breast tenderness, lower abdominal swelling, and mood changes, is ovulating regularly. A woman who has regular menstrual periods without these symptoms also may ovulate.

If a woman is trying to get pregnant but has irregular periods or no periods (AMENORRHEA), the cause is determined before treatment to stimulate ovulation is started.

Ovulation problems may result in the failure of the ovarian FOLLICLE to rupture, an empty follicle, or entrapment of the egg so that it isn't released. Various medical conditions, lifestyle factors such as excessive exercise, eating disorders, or stress can upset normal hormonal rhythm. Even slight irregularities in the hormonal system can result in ovulation disorder.

Ovulation problems can be caused by many factors. Some of the most common causes are medical conditions, excess weight gain or loss, age, too much exercise, or severe emotional stress. These problems can be treated by several different medications that help regulate the cycle and allow ovulation to occur. Some women who don't ovulate have a condition called POLYCYSTIC OVARY SYNDROME or an inherent defect in the way that the pituitary gland releases GONADOTROPINS—the hormones that stimulate the ovaries to work.

Monitoring Ovulation

Determining whether ovulation actually occurs is an important part of an infertility evaluation. Daily measurements of BASAL BODY TEMPERATURE (temperature of the body at rest), usually taken immediately after awakening, may be used to find out if and when ovulation is occurring. A dip in basal body temperature suggests that ovulation is about to occur, whereas a slight, persistent rise of about 0.5°F to 1°F usually indicates that ovulation has occurred. However, basal body temperature is not a reliable or precise indicator of ovulation; at best, it predicts ovulation only within 2 days.

More accurate techniques include ultrasound monitoring and OVULATION TEST KITS that detect an increase in LUTEINIZING HORMONE (a hormone that induces ovulation), which peaks in the urine 24 to 36 hours before ovulation.

It's also possible to measure levels of the hormone PROGESTERONE in the blood, or one of its breakdown products in the urine; a marked increase indicates that ovulation has occurred.

Whether ovulation occurs also can be determined by performing a biopsy: A small sample is removed from the lining of the uterus 10 to 12 days after ovulation is presumed to have occurred; the sample is examined under a microscope. If changes that normally occur in the uterine lining after ovulation are seen, ovulation has occurred.

Treatment

If a woman is unable to ovulate, her doctor may decide to induce ovulation by administering certain drugs selected on the basis of the specific problem. For a woman who hasn't ovulated for a long time (chronic ANOVULATION), CLOMIPHENE CITRATE is usually preferred.

Clomiphene is given for 5 days starting day 3 or 5 of the cycle. A period may need to be induced to get treatment started. Usually, the woman will then ovulate 5 to 10 days after clomiphene citrate is stopped; she will have a period 14 to 16 days after ovulation.

If a woman doesn't have a period after treatment with clomiphene citrate, she takes a pregnancy test. If she isn't pregnant, the treatment cycle is sometimes repeated with higher doses. When the doctor determines the dose that induces ovulation, the woman takes that dose for at least six more treatment cycles.

Most women who get pregnant do so by the sixth cycle in which ovulation occurs. In general, about 75% to 80% of women treated with clomiphene citrate ovulate, but only about 40% to 50% become pregnant.

About 5% of pregnancies in women treated with clomiphene citrate are multiple (mostly twins).

Because there is some concern that prolonged use of clomiphene citrate may increase the risk of ovarian cancer (although this is unproven), doctors will evaluate a woman before treatment, and limit the number of treatment cycles.

If a woman doesn't ovulate or become pregnant during treatment with clomiphene citrate, hormonal therapy with GONADOTROPINS may be effective. Currently, these hormones are extracted from the urine of postmenopausal women, but synthetic and purer versions are now available. Because gonadotropins are expensive and have potentially severe side effects, doctors don't recommend trying this form of therapy until they are sure that intractable ovulation problems, not problems with sperm or fallopian tubes, are the cause of infertility. Even then, treatment cycles are closely supervised by doctors experienced in using these hormones.

Gonadotropins are injected to stimulate the ovarian follicles to mature. To monitor maturation, a doctor measures blood levels of the hormone estradiol and examines ultrasound scans of the pelvis. Doses are adjusted on the basis of the woman's response to the hormones.

After the follicles are mature, the woman is given an injection of a different hormone (HUMAN CHORIONIC GONADOTROPIN) to trigger ovulation. Although more than 95% of the women treated with these hormones ovulate, only 50% to 75% become pregnant. In women treated with HUMAN MENOPAUSAL GONADOTROPINS, 10% to 30% of pregnancies are multiple (primarily twins).

A serious side effect of treatment with human menopausal gonadotropins is OVARIAN HYPERSTIMULATION SYNDROME, which develops in 10% to 20% of the women treated. This syndrome can be severe in less than 5% of cases but usually can be avoided if the doctor closely monitors the treatment and withholds gonadotropins when the woman's response becomes excessive. Human menopausal gonadotropins may increase the risk of ovarian cancer, but current evidence is insubstantial.

Sometimes, ovulation doesn't occur because the HYPOTHALAMUS (the part of the brain that coordinates and controls hormonal activity) doesn't secrete GONADOTROPIN-RELEASING HORMONE, which is necessary for ovulation. In these cases, a synthetic version of gonadotropin-releasing hormone may be used to induce ovulation. The risk of ovarian hyperstimulation is low with this treatment, so intensive monitoring isn't needed.

ovulation test kit   Ovulation predictor test kits are designed to detect LUTEINIZING HORMONE (LH) in the urine, which rises just before OVULATION (ovulation usually takes place within 12 to 24 hours after the rise of LH is detected). The LH kit can be used to time intercourse, insemination, or certain diagnostic procedures.

In general, ovulation occurs 12 to 16 days before the expected start of a woman's next menstrual period. Occasionally, ovulation may not occur in a particular cycle. Persistent failure of a positive test may indicate a problem with ovulation or a problem with the test kit.

To perform the test, urine is collected at the same time each day. If it is impossible to test the urine after it is collected, it may be refrigerated for up to 24 hours. (If refrigerated, the urine should stand at room temperature for 30 minutes before being tested.) To prevent diluting the urine, a woman should avoid drinking for 1 to 4 hours before the sample is collected.

Once the test has registered positive, it isn't necessary to test again until the next menstrual cycle. (Some fertility medications may cause inaccurate results.)

ovulatory failure   See ANOVULATION.

Pap smear A microscopic examination of cells scraped from the cervix to detect cancerous or precancerous conditions of the cervix.

During the procedure, the doctor performs a pelvic exam and inserts a speculum into the vagina. A sample of cells from the outside and the canal of the cervix are removed, placed on a glass slide, and sprayed with a fixative, or put in a bottle containing a preservative and then sent to the lab for examination.

There may be some discomfort and a feeling of pressure during the procedure, and a small amount of bleeding may occur after the test. The test may be affected by colchicines, estrogen, podophyllin, progestins, and silver nitrate.

The test divides the results into three main areas:

- benign: noncancerous
- precancerous: showing some abnormal cell changes
- malignant: possibly cancerous

Test results in either of the two latter groups will usually trigger a follow-up examination, including a repeat Pap smear and possibly other tests. If a woman has never had an abnormal Pap smear before, and the result indicates a mild abnormality, the Pap test is simply repeated in 6 months. If the test result suggests a severe abnormality or cancer, the woman should undergo immediate colposcopic evaluation with biopsies. If a woman has had an abnormal Pap test in the past or has had treatment for a precancerous change, she should have an immediate colposcopy.

Parlodel See BROMOCRIPTINE.

partial zona dissection (PZD) A type of MICROMANIPULATION in which the outer shell of the egg (ZONA PELLUCIDA) is opened to allow the sperm to enter.

pelvic infections See SEXUALLY TRANSMITTED DISEASES AND INFERTILITY.

pelvic inflammatory disease (PID) A general term for infection of the UTERUS, FALLOPIAN TUBES, or ovaries—and the most common preventable cause of INFERTILITY in the United States today. Usually caused by a sexually transmitted disease (STD), 1 million new cases of pelvic inflammatory disease are diagnosed in the United States each year. About one in every seven women is treated for this condition at some point in her life.

The condition can lead to infertility as a result of scars that form inside the fallopian tubes, which can damage or block the tubes completely. The more often a woman gets PID, the greater her risk of becoming infertile. In fact, the risk of infertility doubles with each bout of the disease.

But the risks with PID are not just for infertility; it is also a major cause of illness and death in young women. About 250,000 American women are hospitalized with PID each year, and many of them require surgery because of severe infection. More than 150 women in the United States die from severe PID each year.

Cause

The same organisms responsible for sexually transmitted diseases (such as CHLAMYDIA, GONORRHEA, Mycoplasma) cause 90% to 95% of all cases of pelvic inflammatory disease. After germs infect the cervix, in about 10% of women the bacteria move on to infect the uterus, fallopian tubes, or ovaries. Exactly how these organisms travel from the cervix to these other parts of a woman's body is not known. Occasionally, PID occurs after germs enter the upper portions of the reproductive tract as a result of gynecological procedures such as an induced ABORTION, childbirth, MISCARRIAGE, ENDOMETRIAL BIOPSY, or insertion of an INTRAUTERINE DEVICE (IUD).

PID is most common in young women under age 25 who have more than one sex partner, in those women who have had STDs, and in those who have had a prior case of PID. It is estimated that one in eight sexually active adolescent girls will develop PID before reaching age 20. Since PID is often underdiagnosed, statistics are probably underestimated.

IUD use may increase the risk of developing PID by two to eight times. Some experts suspect that BIRTH CONTROL PILLS may sometimes allow bacteria easier access to tissue, but the pills may in other cases protect against PID because they stimulate the body to produce a thicker cervical mucus, which is harder for bacteria-containing semen to penetrate.

Symptoms

The symptoms of PID range from none to severe, but they are likely to include abnormal uterine bleeding, fever and chills, nausea and vomiting, vaginal discharge with an unpleasant odor or a mild, aching pain in the lower abdomen.

Diagnosis

The diagnosis of PID isn't always easy because the site of infection can't be easily examined. A pelvic exam can reveal if the reproductive organs are tender or swollen. Samples of cervical cells may reveal the organisms that cause gonorrhea and chlamydia infection, and blood tests may also reveal infection. If the diagnosis is not certain, other procedures may be performed, including LAPAROSCOPY and ultrasound of the reproductive organs.

Treatment

In most cases antibiotics alone can cure the infection, but since PID is often caused by more than one type of germ and no single antibiotic kills all of these germs, two or more antibiotics may be necessary. In most cases, antibiotics must be taken for 10 to 14 days to make sure that the infection has been completely cured and to prevent it from returning.

Since most cases of PID are linked to sexually transmitted diseases, it's important to treat the sex partner to prevent repeat infection. All recent sex partners should be examined by a doctor and treated as if they had both gonorrhea and chlamydia infection.

A woman with PID should not have sex again until her sex partners have been treated. Hospitalization may be necessary if the woman's diagnosis is uncertain and appendicitis can't be ruled out. A woman with a very high fever or severe nausea and vomiting may also need to be hospitalized so that intravenous antibiotics can be given. If antibiotics fail or if the doctor suspects a ruptured abscess, surgery may be necessary.

Prevention

Other than completely abstaining from sex, there is no guaranteed method of preventing PID. However, women who are in stable monogamous relationships have very little risk of PID, provided that neither person is already infected with an STD. Some types of birth control, including a CONDOM, DIAPHRAGM, CERVICAL CAP, or SPONGE can protect against STDs, especially when used with spermicides. Women who take oral contraceptives who have more than one sex partner should also use a barrier method with a spermicide to lower their risk of pelvic infection.

Pene Trak This test measures the SPERM's ability to swim through mucus in a test tube. The distance covered in 90 minutes is used to diagnose sperm motility problems.

penis The penis has three distinct anatomic parts: the body, the glans, and the root. The body is the outer portion of the penis; the tip of the penis is called the glans; and at the end of the glans is the opening of the urethra. The root is located within the forward-facing region of the pelvis and is anchored to the pubic bone.

Most sensation within the penis is provided by the penile nerve, which is a branch of the internal pudendal nerves. The pudendal nerves also send signals to the muscles that control ejaculation.

Occasionally, deformity or unusual curvature can interfere with performance, ranging from mild deformity to severe PEYRONIE'S DISEASE, in which the penis can curve so much that penetration is impossible.

Most cases of penile deformity are present from birth. In these cases, the penis seems to be normal when not erect. Most of these patients have no problems in becoming rigid and are capable of good erections. However, occasionally the deformity is severe enough to prevent penetration and can also cause serious psychosexual disturbances. Both of these situations may call for surgical intervention. Surgery is simple, safe, and gives very good results with complete straightening of the penis.

percoll separation A liquid used to filter semen during sperm-washing before IN VITRO FERTILIZATION and INTRAUTERINE INSEMINATION.

percutaneous epididymal sperm aspiration (PESA) A technique that uses a needle to obtain mature SPERM from areas in the upper parts of the EPIDIDYMIS. PESA is useful in men with tubular obstruction and even in those with no vas deferens.

Pergonal The brand name for HUMAN MENOPAUSAL GONADOTROPIN (hMG).

periodic abstinence See RHYTHM METHOD.

peritoneal factors and infertility Women whose history has included appendicitis or abdominal or pelvic surgery may have a scarred abdominal cavity as a result of infection, inflammation, or the surgery itself. These peritoneal factors account for about 25% of female causes of infertility.

PELVIC INFLAMMATORY DISEASE and CHLAMYDIA infection may also form pelvic adhesions, as may the previous use of an intrauterine device (IUD).

The HYSTEROSALPINGOGRAM and LAPAROSCOPY are used as diagnostic tools for suspected peritoneal adhesions.

pesticides and infertility See ENVIRONMENTAL FACTORS AND INFERTILITY; CHEMICALS AND INFERTILITY; WORKPLACE HAZARDS AND INFERTILITY.

Peyronie's disease A condition characterized by the development of nodules or lumps in the penis. The disease, which was named after 18th-century French surgeon Francois Gigot de La Peyronie, affects 1% of the adult male population. It most often appears between ages 40 and 70, although it can occur at any age.

Symptoms
Most patients experience a lump or pain in the penis (especially when erect), bending or deformity of the erect penis, loss of erection, and problems in vaginal penetration. About two-thirds of all patients have pain in addition to a lump, but pain often disappears after the disease has run its full course. The lump is usually about the size of a lima bean, usually located on the upper-middle of the penis. However, the lump can be much larger and may occur in groups. Lumps or deformities that are so extreme they affect performance will require treatment. Not all lumps on the penis indicate Peyronie's disease.

Diagnosis
It is important to examine the penis when erect, after administering a vasodilator drug to allow

objective measurement of the true extent of deformity and the degree of rigidity. A plain soft tissue X ray of the penis can help detect calcific lesions; about a third of all patients with Peyronie's disease will develop calcific changes in the lump. Calcium deposits generally mean the disease has run its full course, and deformity and erection are not going to worsen further.

An ultrasound can help outline the entire extent of the lump in all three dimensions. This is of special help if surgery is being considered. Injections of dye to highlight the arteries of the penis may be done during ultrasound.

Treatment

Several types of treatment have been used to reduce pain and stop the progression of the disease. These include several oral medications, X-ray therapy, topical drugs, electrical therapy, ultrasonic treatment, and local injections. In some cases, Peyronie's disease goes away by itself without treatment, and needless steroid injections into the penis can be damaging. After the disease has run its course, it may even be possible for the patient with minimal penile deformity to rehabilitate himself quite well.

Surgery should be performed as a last resort and only by those especially experienced in dealing with this condition. Surgery is advised for patients with severe deformity (more than 30 degrees) and severe impotence, especially if 12 to 18 months have passed since the first symptom appeared and all other treatments have failed. The type of surgery depends on the location and size of the lump, the degree of deformity, and whether the patient is impotent.

pill, the See BIRTH CONTROL PILL.

pituitary gland The small gland beneath the HYPOTHALAMUS that secretes many hormones, including FOLLICLE-STIMULATING HORMONE (FSH), and LUTEINIZING HORMONE (LH). These are the hormones that stimulate egg maturation and hormone production in the ovary.

pituitary tumor A tumor in the pituitary gland that can cause abnormal hormone levels and infertility. Pituitary adenomas are the most common, causing AMENORRHEA (the loss of menstruation), GALACTORRHEA (the spontaneous flow of milk from the breast), and infertility in women. They cause hypogonadism, decreased libido, and impotence in men.

The pituitary is a pea-sized endocrine gland located at the base of the brain that produces a range of hormones and regulates the secretion of hormones from other endocrine glands.

About 10% of all primary brain tumors begin in the pituitary. Most aren't malignant, but as the tumor grows it can destroy some of the hormone-secreting cells, causing symptoms of underproduction of the pituitary gland (hypopituitarism).

Pituitary tumors may secrete hormones, depending on the cell type of the adenoma. Some tumors produce too much

* growth hormone (causing giantism or acromegaly)
* THYROID-STIMULATING HORMONE (causing HYPERTHYROIDISM)
* adrenocorticotropic hormone (causing Cushing's syndrome)
* prolactin (causing prolactinoma)

The causes of pituitary tumors (adenomas) are unknown but they are not uncommon. They typically appear in early adulthood, equally affecting males and females.

Symptoms

Symptoms are related to hormone deficiencies and pressure on the brain, and can include headache, visual changes, drooping eyelids, personality changes, seizures, nasal drainage, cessation of menstrual periods, decreased sexual drive and impotence in men, skin changes, loss of body hair, weakness, lethargy, intolerance to cold, irritability, constipation, nausea, vomiting, low blood pressure, abnormal milk flow, and breast development in men.

Diagnosis

Tests that help confirm the diagnosis include a cranial CT scan, skull X ray, carotid angiogram, spinal tap, endocrine function tests, MRI scan of the head, and blood and urine tests.

Treatment

Surgery to remove the tumor is possible if the tumor is large and putting pressure on optic nerves. For smaller tumors, the surgeon may wish to remove the tumor through the nose and sinuses. Radiation therapy may be combined with surgery. Certain medications may shrink some types of tumors. While the outcome should be good, spread of the tumor to other brain structures can occur.

Plan B   A brand name for a type of EMERGENCY CONTRACEPTIVE PILLS containing only a synthetic progestin that can prevent pregnancy if taken within 72 hours after unprotected sex (if a contraceptive fails or if no contraception is used). Plan B does not protect against sexually transmitted diseases and should not be used in place of regular contraception.

Plan B is the first progestin-only emergency contraceptive to be approved by the United States Food and Drug Administration (FDA). Although oral contraceptive pills containing progestin have been in use for routine contraception for many years, Plan B contains the first progestin-only tablet specifically developed for postcoital contraception. Plan B is safe for most women and is highly effective.

Each Plan B packet includes a single course of treatment and consists of two tablets, each containing 0.75 mg levonorgestrel, a totally synthetic progestogen. The first tablet should be taken as soon as possible within 72 hours (3 days) of unprotected intercourse. The second tablet must be taken 12 hours later.

According to two randomized, comparative studies conducted by the World Health Organization (WHO), the levonorgestrel-only regimen is highly effective and much better tolerated than the contraception regimen which combines ethinyl estradiol plus norgestrel or levonorgestrel. The incidence of nausea in women taking Plan B was reduced from 50.5% to 23.1%, and the incidence of vomiting was reduced from 18.8% to 5.6%. The studies involved 2,832 women at 22 study centers in 15 countries.

Plan B provides an important safety net for women whose regular contraceptive method may have failed or for women who may have had intercourse without contraception. When unprotected intercourse has occurred, Plan B is second-chance contraception.

Side Effects

Some women experience one or more side effects after taking Plan B. Approximately 23.1% of women taking Plan B experience nausea (compared to 50.5% with the other regimen). Other common side effects include lower abdominal pain, fatigue, headache, dizziness, breast tenderness, and menstrual changes. About 58% of users will have their next menses on time or a few days early or late. See also PREVEN.

Planned Parenthood   Founded in 1916, Planned Parenthood is the world's largest and oldest voluntary family planning organization. The group is dedicated to the principles that every individual has a fundamental right to decide when or whether to have a child and that every child should be wanted and loved. Planned Parenthood believes in the fundamental right of each individual throughout the world to manage his or her fertility, regardless of the individual's income, marital status, race, ethnicity, sexual orientation, age, national origin, or residence.

Planned Parenthood provides comprehensive reproductive and complementary health care services, advocates public policies that guarantee these rights and ensures access to such services, provides educational programs that enhance understanding of human sexuality, and promotes research in reproductive health care. Contact: Planned Parenthood Federation of America, 810 Seventh Avenue, New York, NY 10019; phone: (212) 541-7800; website: http://www.plannedparenthood.org.

polycystic ovaries   A condition of the ovaries in which there are many medium-sized FOLLICLES around the rim of the ovaries that can be seen as part of POLYCYSTIC OVARY SYNDROME.

polycystic ovary syndrome (PCOS)   A metabolic condition associated with irregular (or lack of) OVULATION that may affect about 5 million American women. The syndrome may include obesity, INFERTILITY, and various hormonal problems, such as high TESTOSTERONE and high circulating levels of insulin. Left untreated, PCOS can lead to excessive buildup of the lining of the UTERUS, since MENSTRUATION is irregular. In rare cases, this can lead to cancer of the uterus.

PCOS is a common cause of infertility in the United States. Women with the disorder are also at higher risk for adult-onset DIABETES, high blood pressure, and heart disease. Most experts believe that the syndrome is at least in part genetic. Women with this condition have normal reproductive organs, but the hormonal balance between them is missing.

Symptoms
Although it's possible to have the condition and not have any sign, more typically symptoms may include irregular menstrual cycles, obesity, acne, and facial hair. While there are many symptoms, not all women have all the signs. There is a higher risk of miscarriage and infertility, and a possible higher risk of heart disease because of the excess production of male hormones.

Cause
In a normal cycle, hormones rise and fall in a carefully balanced way until a mature egg is released from a follicle. Women with PCOS often become resistant to their own insulin, which triggers the pancreas to churn out ever-higher amounts of insulin. The resulting high levels of insulin likely stimulate the ovary to produce too much testosterone, which alters the level of other hormones as well, impairing ovulation.

Each month, the body continues to try to ovulate and repeats the attempt month after month, creating more and more immature follicles on the ovary (hence, the term "polycystic ovary syndrome").

Diagnosis
The severity of symptoms varies from one woman to another; the condition is diagnosed by symptoms and blood tests.

Treatment
The treatment of PCOS includes birth control pills to regulate the menstrual cycle and hormone levels, weight loss, and fertility drugs to achieve pregnancy.

Recently, new drugs that help cells use insulin more efficiently are being used to treat PCOS as well. Recent evidence suggests that using medications that lower insulin levels in the blood may be effective in restoring menstruation and reducing some of the health risks associated with PCOS. Lowering insulin levels reduces the production of testosterone, thereby diminishing many of the symptoms associated with excess testosterone, such as hair growth on the body and hair loss on the head, acne, obesity, and heart risk.

There are four drugs currently used to treat PCOS: metformin (Glucophage), pioglitazone (ACTOS), rosiglitazone (Avandia), and troglitazone (Rezulin).

Metformin and troglitazone improve both glucose tolerance and insulin sensitivity, and are approved by the FDA to treat diabetes. Side effects may include temporary symptoms of diarrhea, nausea, vomiting, abdominal bloating, flatulence, and loss of appetite. These symptoms usually disappear after 1 to 4 weeks. Drug dosages should be gradually increased to minimize the chance of side effects.

Pioglitazone works primarily by improving insulin sensitivity and glucose tolerance, and also lowers triglyceride levels. The FDA approved the drug in July 1999 for use in type II diabetes. The medication appears to be well tolerated. Periodic liver function tests are recommended for the first year of therapy. Rosiglitazone works much like Rezulin and pioglitazone, by improving insulin sensitivity.

These drugs can reverse some of the physical and metabolic consequences of PCOS within 2 to 3 months, and can help normalize menstrual cycles. The drugs can help decrease hair loss, lessen facial and body hair growth, regulate menstruation, and lead to weight loss and normal fertility. Some women will actually begin to ovulate on their own, while others may benefit from the combination of one of the newer drugs with CLOMIPHENE CITRATE. In a recent study, almost 90% of women who took metformin for a month ovulated spontaneously or with help from the fertility drug clomiphene; among those taking a placebo, only 12% ovulated even with clomiphene. As the drugs lower insulin levels, testosterone levels also drop.

Complications

All four insulin-sensitizing drugs appear to be relatively safe. However, Rezulin can produce a rare side effect leading to a rise in liver enzymes and possible liver damage, which is why doctors check your liver function by blood analysis for the first 8 months of drug therapy to detect any problems. This drug should not be prescribed to anyone with preexisting liver damage.

Glucophage also has been associated with a rare condition called lactic acidosis. Reported cases have occurred primarily in diabetic patients with severe kidney problems. Although neither ACTOS nor Avandia have been associated with any liver problems, the FDA requires that patients taking any of these drugs be monitored for any signs of liver function abnormalities during the first year of therapy. This is because ACTOS, Avandia, and Rezulin all belong to the same drug class: thiazolidinedione (TZDs).

Polycystic Ovary Syndrome Association, Inc. This organization (also known as PCOSupport) seeks to promote awareness of POLYCYSTIC OVARY SYNDROME, as well as to serve as a support system with accurate information for women with this syndrome. Members are primarily women who have been diagnosed with, or believe they have, polycystic ovary syndrome. The organization promotes research, understanding, and communication of the most up-to-date information concerning PCOS. The organization has 46 chapters in the United States and 11 chapters abroad. In addition to support chapters, the website offers links to a variety of e-mail lists, discussion boards, and online chats. Contact: PCOS Association, PO BOX 80517, Portland, OR 97280; website: http://www.pcosupport.org.

polyspermy Fertilization of an egg by more than one SPERM. The exact cause of polyspermy isn't known, but it may be related to a breakdown in the egg's ability to restrict the entrance of only one sperm.

This type of multiple FERTILIZATION of human eggs is considered a common result of IN VITRO FERTILIZATION (IVF), occurring in approximately 2% to 10% of inseminated eggs.

postcoital contraception See EMERGENCY CONTRACEPTION.

postcoital douche An ineffective attempt at birth control by applying a douche shortly after intercourse. Because SPERM can make their way beyond the cervix within 90 seconds after ejaculation, this method is ineffective and unreliable. In addition, a douche after having sex can wash away spermicidal foam used for contraception, leaving the woman unprotected.

Unless a woman has a medical condition for which a physician has specifically prescribed douches, the practice is considered unnecessary and can even be dangerous. A preliminary study published in the *Journal of Obstetrics and Gynecology* has linked douching to ECTOPIC PREGNANCY, a potentially life-threatening condition, and noted that douching once a week carried twice the risk of ectopic pregnancies compared to women who did not douche at all. Although the exact explanation for this link is still unknown, one likely possibility is that vaginal douching increases the risk of PELVIC INFLAMMATORY DISEASE (PID) by spreading vaginal bacteria or infections past the cervix into the uterus and fallopian tubes.

Because vaginal tissue is self-lubricating and self-cleansing, douching at any time is not necessary, either after a menstrual period or after sexual intercourse. Some vaginal discharge is normal and may vary in color as hormone levels vary. Odors, if any, probably originate from the external genitals.

postcoital test (PCT) This postcoital ("after sex") test is a microscopic examination of the cervical mucus to determine whether SPERM can move through it. The test is also known as the Sims-Huhner or sperm-mucus interaction test.

The test is performed close to the time of OVULATION, when the woman's cervical mucus is thin and watery, so that the sperm are better able to swim through the cervix and fertilize the awaiting egg. The test must be performed just prior to OVULATION so that the mucus will be thin and stretchy.

About 12 hours after sexual intercourse, the woman is examined in the doctor's office, and a small sample of mucus is removed from the cervix. This mucus is evaluated under a microscope; at least six to ten moving sperm indicate a good sperm/mucus interaction. The physician will inspect the female's cervical mucus to see whether enough semen was delivered to the cervix and that sperm are healthy and are swimming energetically through the cervical mucus.

If no sperm are found in the cervical mucus but are present in the vagina, hostile vaginal factor or sperm factor may be suspected, especially if the man's semen analysis is normal. In such cases, the woman may be inseminated with washed sperm to overcome such factors and to help the sperm pass into the cervix.

If many shaking, motionless, clumped, or dead sperm are found in the cervical mucus, the sperm and mucus may be incompatible, or something in the mucus may be attacking the sperm. Reactions can be caused by external factors, such as the use of vaginal lubricants, or by internal factors such as an allergic response to the sperm by the woman or the production of ANTISPERM ANTIBODIES by the man.

The most common explanation for a poor test is improper timing; the test should be done 24 to 36 hours before ovulation, as determined by urinary LH testing.

If a man's semen analysis is normal, INTRAUTERINE INSEMINATION (IUI) may be recommended to treat repeatedly poor results of postcoital tests, PCTs. The presence of significant antisperm antibodies should be treated with IN VITRO FERTILIZATION (IVF).

The exact role of the postcoital test in the modern evaluation of infertility is debatable. Evidence exists to question the predictive value of this quite subjective test. Many physicians no longer perform the test, since most treatments would theoretically treat a mucus problem if it exists or not.

postoral contraceptive syndrome See POST-PILL SYNDROME.

post-pill syndrome Also called post-pill amenorrhea, this is the 3- to 12-month lag time it takes for a woman's cycles to return to normal after stopping the BIRTH CONTROL PILL. About 5% of women who stop taking oral contraceptives won't experience normal cycles for a year. Many of these women had irregular cycles before taking oral contraception in the first place. Birth control pills don't cause INFERTILITY; they may simply cover up an already-existing OVULATION problem.

pre-embryo An embryo from the time it has been fertilized up to implantation.

pre-embryo biopsy The removal of one or two cells from a PRE-EMBRYO for a PREIMPLANTATION GENETIC DIAGNOSIS.

pregnancy A woman becomes pregnant by a complicated series of events that begins on her first day of MENSTRUATION (day 1 of the MENSTRUAL CYCLE), when her body releases increasing amounts of FSH (FOLLICLE-STIMULATING HORMONE) produced by the pituitary at the base of the brain. This FSH stimulates a follicle to grow and produce ESTROGEN. The egg also begins to mature at this time.

By about day 14 of the menstrual cycle, the pituitary releases a burst of another hormone called LH (LUTEINIZING HORMONE). This is called the LH SURGE. This sudden burst of LH triggers the release of a mature egg from the FOLLICLE (OVULATION), where it is swept up into the fallopian tube. As the egg travels along the FALLOPIAN TUBE, levels of another female hormone called PROGESTERONE begins to rise.

If there are no sperm in the fallopian tube and the egg isn't fertilized, it travels to the UTERUS and is shed, along with the unneeded lining of the uterus, during menstruation.

If there happens to be sperm in the fallopian tubes, the egg will be fertilized and the resulting embryo continues its trek through the fallopian tube into the uterus, where the higher levels of progesterone have thickened the uterine walls in preparation for a fertilized egg. Here the embryo will implant itself and grow into a baby.

pregnancy, cervical An ECTOPIC PREGNANCY that is located in the cervix.

pregnancy, cornular A pregnancy in which the fertilized egg implants itself on one side of the uterus very close to where the FALLOPIAN TUBES enter the uterus. This type of pregnancy often ends in MISCARRIAGE.

pregnancy rate The chance of pregnancy per month or treatment cycle, including ECTOPIC PREGNANCY, MISCARRIAGE, STILLBIRTHS, and all live births. Twins and other multiples are not counted more than once.

It takes time for new infertility service providers to establish success rates based on live births. For this reason, some providers cite only national statistics in discussing success rates. Experts say it is fair for new providers to report anticipated births by including those ongoing pregnancies that have progressed beyond 26 weeks—at which point the pregnancy is highly likely to continue to term.

Some providers also favor reporting "cumulative" pregnancy and birth rate claims. Cumulative rates suggest the overall probability of a pregnancy or birth occurring based on women undergoing several successive procedures.

Clinical Pregnancy Rate

The presence of a pregnancy sac on ultrasound examination.

Ongoing Pregnancy Rate

Those clinical pregnancies that have not yet delivered.

Delivery Rate

The percentage of pregnancies that have delivered, also called the TAKE-HOME BABY RATE. (During infertility treatment, a center's pregnancy rate is less important for most people than the take-home baby rate.)

Pregnancy Rate per Attempted Egg Stimulation

This rate refers to the number of clinical pregnancies resulting from all egg-stimulation attempts. This figure does not reveal whether these pregnancies resulted in live births.

Pregnancy Rate per Woman in the Program

This refers to how many clinical pregnancies occurred per woman in the program. Excluded from this figure are the number of births and the number of times an individual woman may have undergone the procedure prior to achieving a pregnancy. This figure is not commonly cited.

Pregnancy Rate per Attempted Egg Retrieval

This rate reflects the number of clinical pregnancies resulting from all egg-retrieval attempts. This statistic does not tell whether these pregnancies resulted in live births and does not include instances where patients began medications but were canceled before egg retrieval.

Pregnancy Rate per Embryo Transfer

This usually refers to how many clinical pregnancies occurred in relation to the number of embryo-transfer procedures performed. This figure does not say how many births occurred or how successful the program was in stimulating egg production, in obtaining egg retrieval, and in fertilizing eggs retrieved.

pregnancy test   A measure of HUMAN CHORIONIC GONADOTROPIN (hCG) in blood or urine. A positive result indicates pregnancy (that implantation has begun).

Pregnyl   The brand name for HUMAN CHORIONIC GONADOTROPIN (hCG) manufactured by Organon.

preimplantation genetic diagnosis (PGD)   The genetic testing of an embryo during IN VITRO FERTILIZATION (IVF) to make sure the genetic makeup of the embryo is normal before transfer to the uterus.

In this procedure, one cell from each embryo (called a blastomere) is removed before implantation so that it can be screened for certain genetic problems. A diagnosis is obtained within a day or so; if some of the embryos do have genetic abnormalities, only the unaffected embryos are replaced.

This enables individuals with serious inherited disorders to lessen the risk of having a child who is affected by the same problem. At present, PGD is only offered in a few centers, but experience with the technique is growing.

PGD was first performed in 1989 and has since been successfully applied to a wide variety of genetic diseases, from single-gene disorders to chromosomal abnormalities. In single-gene disorders where the gene structure is known (such as CYSTIC FIBROSIS or Tay-Sachs), the actual genes of the sampled embryo can be examined for the presence of the condition.

In other genetic conditions, the exact gene defect may not be known, but in those that affect only males (such as Duchenne muscular dystrophy or hemophilia), the DNA of the biopsied cell can be examined to determine the sex of the embryo. If there is concern that the embryo may carry a genetic defect that affects only males, it would be possible to replace only female embryos in the mother's uterus. See also GENDER SELECTION.

Finally, in cases of severe recurrent chromosomal problems such as Down's syndrome, which is characterized by an extra chromosome, the number and character of several chromosomes of the sampled embryo can be determined.

Many, but not all, disorders can be diagnosed with this technique. The most common include

- α-1-antitrypsin deficiency
- CYSTIC FIBROSIS
- fragile X syndrome
- Lesch-Nyhan syndrome
- Charcot-Marie-Tooth disease
- Down's syndrome
- Tay-Sachs disease
- Duchenne muscular dystrophy
- hemophilia A
- retinitis pigmentosa
- Turner's syndrome

Premarin   The brand name for a mixture of ESTROGENS (primarily ESTRONE) in tablet form, obtained from the urine of pregnant mares. Premarin is part of estrogen replacement therapy and may be given to women with hypothalamic pituitary failure and or in cases of premature menopause.

premature menopause See OVARIAN FAILURE, PREMATURE.

Premature Ovarian Failure Support Group A support group for women with premature ovarian failure started by seven Washington, DC, area women patients in 1995. The group offers members a quarterly newsletter, a professional referral list (doctors, adoption lawyers, counselors, and so on), and a confidential "Share List" (names and addresses of women diagnosed with POF who are interested to talk with other women). Contact: POF Support Group, P.O. Box 23643, Alexandria, VA 22304; phone: (703) 913-4787; website: http://www.pofsupport.org/memb.htm. See also OVARIAN FAILURE, PREMATURE.

premenstrual spotting Light bleeding that occurs a few days before the menstrual period really begins. Potential causes include hormonal problems, polyps, or fibroids within the uterus.

PREVEN A kit of EMERGENCY CONTRACEPTIVE PILLS that a woman can take the morning after unprotected sex to prevent pregnancy. Unlike drugs such as RU-486 (the so-called "French abortion pill"), emergency contraception pills can't end a pregnancy that already exists. Instead, the pills in the kit work by preventing OVULATION or by preventing a fertilized egg from implanting in the uterine wall. They are thus acceptable to at least some antiabortion activists.

For decades, European women had been using the emergency contraceptive pills as "morning after" pills. For more than 20 years, U.S. researchers had known that daily contraceptive pills were safe and effective if taken in larger doses as "morning after" pills. But most American doctors did not discuss this method with their patients, and most American women knew nothing about emergency contraception.

In 1996 the FDA convened an expert committee to discuss emergency contraception. The next year, the FDA ruled that six brands of birth control pills were safe and effective as morning-after pills—the first federal acknowledgment of the popular European emergency birth control method. At that time, the agency invited manufacturers to apply for approval to relabel or reformulate birth control pills as emergency contraception, but most companies declined, citing fears of litigation and political disfavor.

Finally, in September 1998, the FDA approved the marketing and sale of the PREVEN kit, which allowed the manufacturer (Gynetics) to package prescription contraceptive pills into kits specifically for emergency use that is about 75% effective in preventing pregnancy.

The PREVEN emergency contraceptive kit includes a step-by-step patient information book with detailed information, a pregnancy test, and two doses of the pills. A pregnancy test is used first to help determine if a pregnancy took place from sex earlier in the month or in previous months. If the test is positive, the pills in the PREVEN kit won't work and should not be taken. However, the test won't be able to tell if a woman is pregnant from sex that took place within the previous 72 hours. Extensive research has found no significant effects on the development of a baby associated with the pills if taken inadvertently during early pregnancy.

The kit contains two doses (each dose contains two pills) of emergency contraceptive pills. The first dose of two pills is to be taken as soon as possible after sex but within 72 hours, and the second dose of two pills is taken 12 hours later.

A woman might need to use emergency contraception if a condom slips or breaks, she miscalculates her "safe" time and has sex without birth control, a diaphragm moves out of position, she is raped, or in any other situation where birth control was not used.

Side Effects

The most commonly reported side effects are nausea and vomiting, but serious as well as minor side effects may occur. Serious risks include blood clots, strokes, and heart attacks. Women over age 35 who smoke have a higher risk of serious side effects. Emergency contraceptive pills do not protect against infection with HIV (the virus that causes AIDS) and other sexually transmitted diseases. See also PLAN B.

Progestasert   An INTRAUTERINE DEVICE (IUD) containing PROGESTERONE that is inserted into a woman's UTERUS as a form of birth control. It works by causing changes in the uterus that help prevent pregnancy.

The FERTILIZATION of the woman's egg with her partner's SPERM is less likely with an IUD in place, but it can occur. Even if an egg is fertilized, however, the IUD makes it harder for the egg to become attached to the uterus walls. The progesterone released from the IUD is believed to improve the effects of the device.

After the IUD is removed, most women trying to become pregnant can become pregnant.

Studies have shown that pregnancy can occur in up to 2 of each 100 women using a progesterone IUD during the first year of use. Other birth control methods such as BIRTH CONTROL PILLS or sterilization are equally or more effective. Methods that don't work as well include CONDOMS, DIAPHRAGMS, vaginal SPONGES, or SPERMICIDES.

IUDs don't protect a woman from sexually transmitted diseases, including the virus that causes AIDS. If an infection is present in the vagina or uterus when the IUD is inserted, the infection may become more serious than it otherwise would have been.

Rarely, a woman can get pregnant while wearing an IUD. If this happens, the IUD should be removed or the pregnancy should be ended within the first 3 months. If the pregnancy continues, removing the IUD decreases the chance of a problem developing, but whether the IUD is removed or not, some problems can occur, including MISCARRIAGE, premature labor and delivery, infection, and, very rarely, death of the mother.

Side Effects

A progesterone IUD may cause some unwanted effects. Although not all of these side effects may occur, if any do occur they may need medical attention. Rare but serious side effects include severe abdominal pain or cramping, faintness, dizziness, or sharp pain at time of IUD insertion, or heavy, unexpected uterine bleeding. More common side effects include pain or cramping on insertion, unusual spotting, or uterine bleeding between periods or on insertion. See also BIRTH CONTROL METHODS.

progesterone   An important ovarian hormone that is normally secreted after OVULATION and during PREGNANCY. Progesterone triggers thickening of the lining of the UTERUS so it can accept implantation of a fertilized egg. Low progesterone levels, also called a LUTEAL PHASE DEFECT, may lead to INFERTILITY or MISCARRIAGE.

Some women don't produce enough progesterone on their own (LUTEAL PHASE DEFECT) which means they may have trouble conceiving. In these cases, supplemental administration of progesterone is required. Supplemental administration of progesterone is also needed when a woman is undergoing certain ASSISTED REPRODUCTIVE TECHNOLOGY (ART) procedures, such as IVF.

Progesterone is administered along with other hormones to mimic a regular menstrual cycle. The combination of hormones allows the uterine lining to mimic the normal cycle and allows implantation to take place. The combination of ESTROGEN and progesterone is used for donor egg recipients and replacement of frozen embryos.

Several forms of progesterone are available commercially such as an intravaginal gel (Crinone) or a capsule (Prometrium). Some must be prepared by a pharmacist, such as vaginal progesterone suppositories. Progesterone may be given by injection, by mouth, or inserted into the vagina. It is often given after ovulation induction for INTRAUTERINE INSEMINATION, GAMETE INTRAFALLOPIAN TRANSFER (GIFT), or IN VITRO FERTILIZATION (IVF). Progesterone can also be compounded into various dosage forms such as an intramuscular injection, vaginal suppositories, or a pill designed to be slowly dissolved in the mouth. The dose of progesterone depends on a woman's need and the specific dosage form of progesterone that is selected. In order to mimic a regular menstrual cycle, therapy with progesterone is usually started a few days after ovulation and is continued until either a woman's period starts or pregnancy is confirmed. If a woman gets pregnant, treatment with progesterone may be continued for up to 3 months. By this time, the placenta is producing enough progesterone for the remainder of the pregnancy.

Side Effects

Adverse effects associated with the use of progesterone include nausea, constipation, breast enlargement and tenderness, headache, drowsiness, vaginal discharge, joint discomfort, and depression. Progesterone may also cause fluid retention; therefore, patients with certain medical conditions such as epilepsy, migraine headaches, asthma, and cardiac or kidney disease require close observation.

progesterone test   A blood test of the hormone PROGESTERONE used to evaluate INFERTILITY. Progesterone is a steroid hormone that is produced and released from the empty follicle after the egg has emerged. In women, the hormone prepares the uterus for pregnancy and the breast for producing milk. After OVULATION, progesterone blocks estrogen-induced buildup of the uterine lining and stimulates the glands of the uterus to begin secretion.

Blood levels of progesterone start to rise in response to a hormone surge from the pituitary (LH SURGE) midway through the menstrual cycle, continue to rise for about 6 to 10 days, and then

fall. Progesterone levels are also very high in early pregnancy. Measurements of progesterone in the blood are obtained at midluteal phase to evaluate the occurrence and adequacy of ovulation and corpus luteum function. Normal values for a woman before ovulation are less than 1.5 ng/ml. After ovulation they rise to 15–20 ng/ml.

Because progesterone is secreted in pulses, a single low level can't diagnose a luteal defect. Therefore, if progesterone is used to determine normal progesterone secretion, it should be measured in multiple cycles, or levels should be drawn every other day during the luteal phase and averaged to yield a single result. However, this is impractical. Although blood levels of progesterone are inadequate to diagnose ovarian production, they may be used to determine if ovulation has occurred. A progesterone level above 2 ng/ml usually indicates that ovulation has occurred. The cost of one test is about $60. Oral contraceptives or progesterone can interfere with the test results.

progesterone withdrawal   A diagnostic procedure used to analyze menstrual irregularity and lack of a menstrual period.

Progesterone induces a menstrual flow only if the uterus has been exposed to estrogen previously. Therefore, a vaginal bleed after progesterone administration means that the woman is producing some estrogen. This is helpful in determining the different causes of menstrual disorder.

progestin   See PROGESTOGEN.

progestogen   A substance similar to, yet more potent than, PROGESTERONE when taken orally. It is combined with ESTROGEN in birth control pills.

prolactin   The pituitary hormone that stimulates the production of milk in breast-feeding women. It also circulates in low levels in the bloodstream of nonpregnant women. During pregnancy, prolactin levels increase approximately 10-fold and stimulate milk formation. Excessive prolactin levels when not breast-feeding may result in INFERTILITY.

Hyperprolactinemia is a condition in which too much prolactin circulates in the bloodstream of nonlactating women. It can produce a variety of reproductive problems, including inadequate PROGESTERONE production during the luteal phase after OVULATION, irregular ovulation and MENSTRUATION, absence of menstruation, and GALACTORRHEA (breast milk production by a woman who is not nursing).

pronuclear stage The stage in embryonic development that occurs after the SPERM penetrates the egg.

pronuclear stage transfer (PROST) Another name for ZYGOTE INTRAFALLOPIAN TRANSFER, or ZIFT. In this procedure, the eggs are retrieved via vaginal ultrasound and then mixed with SPERM in the lab. If FERTILIZATION occurs, the fertilized but undivided eggs (at the PRONUCLEAR STAGE) are introduced into the FALLOPIAN TUBES within 24 hours using LAPAROSCOPY, as in GIFT (GAMETE INTRAFALLOPIAN TRANSFER). This method is rarely used today.

pronucleus A visible structure or two within an egg enclosing the chromosomes from the egg and from the SPERM. The existence of pronuclei indicate FERTILIZATION (three pronuclei suggest that two sperm have penetrated the egg).

prophylactics See CONDOMS.

PROST See PRONUCLEAR STAGE TRANSFER.

prostaglandins A group of hormone-like substances found throughout the body in both men and women that have various effects on reproductive organs.

Drugs that interfere with the production of prostaglandins are used as painkillers and include the nonsteroidal, anti-inflammatory drugs (NSAIDs) such as ibuprofen. These drugs can help lessen uterine contractions during menstrual cramping and premature labor.

Experts suspect that prostaglandins secreted by active, young implants in ENDOMETRIOSIS may interfere with the reproductive organs by causing muscular contractions or spasms. In addition, prostaglandins not washed from sperm can cause severe cramping during intrauterine induction procedures.

They are called prostaglandins because they were first discovered in the PROSTATE GLAND.

prostate gland A walnut-shaped male gland encircling the urethra below the bladder and in front of the rectum in men. It produces a third of the fluid in the ejaculate, including a chemical that liquefies the coagulated semen 20 minutes to 1 hour after entering the vagina. The normal role of the gland is to produce secretions that help to nourish the SPERM. These secretions provide a more hospitable environment for the sperm cells and help to improve their survival in the acidic environment of the vaginal canal.

As part of the male reproductive system, the prostate gland relies on TESTOSTERONE to make it enlarge at puberty and to function properly throughout adult life. In most men, for reasons still unknown, the prostate begins to enlarge again after age 50. Because of the location of the gland, enlargement can sometimes lead to problems in urinating, as the urethra can become blocked.

Provera See MEDROXYPROGESTERONE ACETATE.

puberty The period in human development when sexual maturation occurs.

pyospermia High white blood count in the SPERM. This is caused by an infection somewhere in the body, ranging from sexually transmitted diseases to the flu or colds. To detect infections, cultures of the semen, urine, and, possibly, fluid from the prostate gland will be sent to a laboratory for examination.

In some studies, up to 10% of infertile men have infections but show no symptoms of infection. In women, untreated bacterial infections may reach the FALLOPIAN TUBES, causing most of the structural problems that affect female fertility. In men, untreated bacterial infections tend to affect the prostate gland, causing prostatitis.

A sperm antibody test (of blood and semen) can detect immunological infertility. Sometimes an injury or infection can cause the immune system to attack itself, creating an autoimmune response. Here, the immune system somehow recognizes the sperm as an invader and forms antibodies to it that coat the sperm and ultimately kill them.

radiation Both developing SPERM and eggs are sensitive to radiation, but not all types of radiation are similarly damaging. Diagnostic radiation (for example, a chest X ray) is less of a concern compared to therapeutic irradiation to treat tumors, especially if they are located near reproductive organs.

Sperm and egg cell damage is reversible at low exposures, but permanent INFERTILITY may occur at higher doses. Sometimes irradiation will temporarily destroy sperm or egg formation only to rebound many months later.

If possible, the ovaries and testicles should be protected from radiation when radiotherapy is necessary. See also MALE FACTOR INFERTILITY; OVARIAN FAILURE, PREMATURE.

relaxin A hormone that may be involved in uterine muscle activity and that may be used as part of infertility treatment. The main source of naturally occurring circulating relaxin in the body is the empty FOLLICLE after the egg has emerged (CORPUS LUTEUM). Relaxin is found in a woman's blood throughout pregnancy and also in the blood of nonpregnant women at midcycle. During pregnancy, relaxin is also produced in the tissues of the UTERUS and breast. In men, relaxin is produced in both the prostate gland and cells within the testes. In both men and women, relaxin is also produced in the heart.

Relaxin helps remodel connective tissue during pregnancy to allow the mother's body to accommodate the growing fetus, such as an increase in abdomen size and a loosening of joints and tendons. Relaxin is also believed to have other functions, such as regulating changes in the circulatory system to boost blood flow and oxygenation to the growing fetus, enhancing kidney function, and, perhaps, improving sperm movement and penetration ability.

reproductive endocrinologist An obstetrician-gynecologist who specializes in reproductive endocrinology and who is qualified to manage female fertility. The AMERICAN COLLEGE OF OBSTETRICIANS AND GYNECOLOGISTS certifies this subspecialty for ob-gyns who receive extra training in infertility and endocrinology (the study of hormones). These specialists are trained in the diagnosis and treatment of all types of hormonal problems; disorders involving the pituitary, thyroid, and adrenal glands; the ovaries; and management of the full range of assisted reproductive technologies and fertility medications.

To become board-certified in obstetrics and gynecology, a doctor must graduate from college and medical school and complete a 4-year residency in ob/gyn. In addition, the doctor must pass a written examination, complete a 2-year practice experience, and then pass an oral examination. A doctor who wants to become board-certified in reproductive endocrinology must be board-certified in obstetrics/gynecology, attend a 2- or 3-year fellowship in reproductive endocrinology, pass a written exam, finish a 2-year practice experience in reproductive endocrinology, and then pass a 3-hour oral examination in reproductive endocrinology. Doctors who have completed all but the oral exam and are still in their practice experience in reproductive endocrinology are "board eligible in reproductive endocrinology."

There are about 500 board-certified reproductive endocrinologists in the United States. About another 800 are board-eligible. Lack of board certification in reproductive endocrinology does not prevent a doctor from practicing in infertility.

A couple should consider consulting a reproductive endocrinologist for the following problems:

- microsurgery or treatment for ENDOMETRIOSIS or tubal damage
- history of three or more miscarriages
- irregular menstrual cycle with evidence of irregular ovulation
- low sperm count or motility or poor morphology
- history of pelvic infection
- history of infertility

Reproductive endocrinologists are listed in the Directory of Medical Specialists published by Who's Who and available at most public libraries, listing all ob/gyns and their training. RESOLVE, INC. maintains a physician referral list of more than 700 doctors; a list of specialists in a geographic area is available to RESOLVE members. By calling or writing the RESOLVE national office, a member can also obtain specific data on the physicians regarding their medical training and special expertise and interests.

reproductive endocrinology   A specialized area of medicine that focuses on INFERTILITY, female reproductive hormones, and female reproductive surgery. Specialists are called REPRODUCTIVE ENDOCRINOLOGISTS, who have trained as obstetricians/gynecologists before getting advanced training in reproductive endocrinology and being certified by the American Board of Obstetrics and Gynecology in the subspeciality of reproductive endocrinology and infertility.

Most reproductive endocrinologists limit their practice to infertility and its related procedures, whereas an obstetrician/gynecologist may only treat a few cases of infertility each year and is therefore less experienced in identifying and treating infertility-related problems.

reproductive surgeon   Reproductive surgeons are physicians who are board-certified as obstetricians/gynecologists, UROLOGISTS, or reproductive ENDOCRINOLOGISTS, have received special training, and are experienced in the surgeries common to reproductive medicine. Their training involves microsurgery and reconstructive surgery.

Reproductive surgeons can treat anatomical problems such as blocked FALLOPIAN TUBES, ENDOMETRIOSIS, uterine problems, scarring from PELVIC INFLAMMATORY DISEASE, and other diagnoses that require surgery of the female reproductive organs. Urologists who are also reproductive surgeons treat anatomical problems, obstructions, VARICOCELES, VASECTOMY, and vasectomy reversals. See also REPRODUCTIVE SURGERY; SOCIETY FOR REPRODUCTIVE SURGEONS.

reproductive surgery   A subspecialty that treats anatomical abnormalities that interfere with normal reproductive function. Advanced reproductive surgery requires meticulous surgical technique for best results. Types of reproductive surgery include LAPAROTOMY, LAPAROSCOPY, HYSTEROSCOPY, and FALLOPOSCOPY.

Laparotomy Microsurgery

Microsurgery through an incision allows the most precise cutting and suturing possible and requires magnification. For women, microsurgery can precisely remove scar tissue, destroy active areas of ENDOMETRIOSIS, and repair damaged FALLOPIAN TUBES. It's also possible to reverse a previous TUBAL STERILIZATION. In combination with new anesthetic techniques, microsurgery through a laparotomy can be safely and effectively performed on an outpatient basis.

Laparoscopy

The laparoscope allows a doctor to see the pelvic organs through a very tiny incision. Abnormalities that lead to infertility can be treated surgically through additional small incisions to remove scar tissue or endometriosis, and repair blocked tubes. Many types of female reproductive surgery can be performed on an outpatient basis.

Hysteroscopy

With a hysteroscope, a doctor can directly inspect the uterine cavity through a narrow fiber-optic scope inserted through the cervical canal without having to make an incision. Abnormalities that can be diagnosed and treated through hysteroscopy include endometrial polyps, uterine fibroids, intrauterine adhesions, and a septate uterus. Hysteroscopic surgery is routinely performed in the outpatient setting.

Falloposcopy

This technique allows direct inspection of the inside of the fallopian tube using a tiny flexible fiber-optic scope passed through the cervix and uterus into the tubes. Tubal obstructions can often be corrected through the falloposcope. Falloposcopic examination is also helpful in deciding whether tubal corrective surgery or IVF would be the better treatment for tubal infertility. Falloposcopy is an outpatient procedure, requiring no incision and only minimal anesthesia.

Reproductive surgery can correct physical abnormalities and restore normal reproductive function so that pregnancy can occur naturally. The risks are those of any surgery, such as bleeding, infection, and anesthesia complications. Specific risks during laparoscopy include injuring the intestine or urinary tract. During hysteroscopy or falloposcopy, there is the potential risk of uterine perforation. Tubal pregnancy is a delayed risk of tubal surgery.

reproductive system, female   A woman's reproductive system includes the UTERUS, ovaries, and FALLOPIAN TUBES. The functions of these organs are controlled by hormones produced by the brain and the pituitary gland that regulate the menstrual cycle, pregnancy, and the production of breast milk.

ESTROGEN and PROGESTERONE (the sex hormones) are produced by the ovaries and are responsible for sexual development and for preparing the uterine wall to nourish a fertilized egg every month. These sex hormones also contribute to the basic health of the heart, bones, liver, and many other tissues. Finally, during pregnancy the placenta produces a hormone (HUMAN CHORIONIC GONADOTROPIN, or hCG) that tells the body to support the pregnancy.

A woman is born with all of the eggs that she will ever have, so if her eggs are damaged or destroyed, she won't be able to replace them. Although her ovaries contain about 500,000 immature eggs at birth, only a fraction of these will develop into mature eggs during her lifetime. The rest will be absorbed by her body over the years.

At puberty, a woman begins her menstrual cycles, which enable her to release an egg each month from one of her ovaries. Each cycle begins with a few days of menstrual flow. When each new cycle begins, a new egg starts to grow, and after 2 or 3 weeks, a mature egg is released from the ovary into the fallopian tubes, where it could be fertilized by one of the many sperm that may surround it.

If the microscopic egg is not fertilized, it will be absorbed by the body or lost in the menstrual flow. With the onset of the period (called cycle day 1) a new cycle begins.

If the egg is fertilized, the complex process of reproduction continues. The fertilized egg travels for about a week down the fallopian tube to reach the uterus, where it attaches to the wall. A specialized tissue around the fetus called the placenta forms and the pregnancy grows into the uterine wall. The placenta transfers oxygen and nutrients from the mother to the fetus. During the first 3 months of pregnancy (first trimester), the major fetal organs are formed. During the remainder of the pregnancy, these organs mature and the fetus grows rapidly.

reproductive system, male   A man's reproductive system is found both inside and outside his body. The TESTICLES (or testes) are found inside the scrotum, the fleshy pouch of skin behind the penis. It is inside the testicles that SPERM and the male hormone TESTOSTERONE are produced.

Within each testicle are coiled tubules that contain two different types of cells: immature sperm cells, called GERM CELLS, and SERTOLI CELLS, whose job it is to nourish sperm cells. Between the tubules is another type of cell called a LEYDIG CELL, which is responsible for producing testosterone necessary for sperm production and male sexual characteristics.

Influenced by both Leydig and Sertoli cells, the germ cells begin to develop and mature into sperm. This process continues, taking between 72 and 74 days. As sperm mature, they move from the testicles through the EPIDIDYMIS, an organ that stores and nourishes the sperm as they develop. While sperm have tails when they enter the epididymis, they only begin to move after 18 to 24 hours within the epididymis. It takes sperm about 14 days to move through the epididymis and on into the VAS DEFERENS, a tubal structure connecting the epididymis with the SEMINAL VESCICLES. The seminal vesicles are glands that produce most of the fluid in a man's ejaculate.

As the man ejaculates, sperm combines with fluid from the seminal vesicle and prostate gland, creating semen. This fluid (called ejaculate) is discharged from the erect penis. During sex, it is deposited into the woman's vagina.

During ejaculation, the semen looks like a gel, but it liquefies within a half hour to help the sperm move through the female reproductive tract toward the egg.

The reproductive process in men also depends heavily on reproductive hormones. Pituitary hormones set off the entire sperm production process when they secrete FOLLICLE-STIMULATING HORMONE (FSH) and LUTEINIZING HORMONE (LH). These are the same hormones important in regulating the woman's reproductive system.

In men, FSH stimulates sperm production in the testicles, and LH triggers testosterone production.

resectoscope   A type of hysteroscope with a built-in wire loop that uses high-frequency electrical current to cut or coagulate tissue. It was first developed for surgery of the bladder and the male prostate more than 50 years ago to allow surgery inside an organ without having to make an incision.

Like the standard hysteroscope, the resectoscope is inserted through the cervix. Fluid is used to distend the uterus for a better view. Fibroids, polyps, and adhesions can be corrected with the resectoscope.

Procedures using the resectoscope are almost always done in an operating room such as in an outpatient surgery center. Minor procedures can be done under local anesthesia, but most women prefer general anesthesia.

RESOLVE, Inc.   A nonprofit organization dedicated to providing support and information to people who are experiencing infertility and to increase awareness of infertility issues through public education and advocacy. It is run by a volunteer board of individuals who have experienced medical concerns regarding infertility and who have adopted children, along with members of the professional community.

Founded in 1974 by nurse Barbara Eck Menning, RESOLVE has grown from a small kitchen operation to a national organization with a database of more than 40,000 individuals and providers, more than 50 chapters nationwide, and a national paid staff of 17 that provides services and programs for individuals experiencing infertility. RESOLVE supports family-building through a variety of methods, including appropriate medical treatment, ADOPTION, surrogacy, and the choice of child-free living. The group also advocates on the national and local level for comprehensive insurance coverage for infertility treatment and other family-building issues of concern. The organization offers a helpline and information on local chapters.

Contact: RESOLVE, Inc., 1310 Broadway, Somerville, MA 02144; phone: (617) 623-0744; website: http://www.resolve.org.

rhythm method   A type of natural birth control based on calendar calculations of previous menstrual cycles. This method doesn't allow for normal changes in the menstrual cycle, which are quite common. For this reason, the rhythm method isn't as reliable as either the ovulation method or the symptothermal method of NATURAL FAMILY PLANNING and is generally not recommended. Women who have no variation in the length of their menstrual cycles can use the rhythm method to know when they are ovulating (14 days before the start of their period).

Rokitansky syndrome   A genetic disorder characterized by a malformed vagina and sometimes the absence of the UTERUS. Known medically as Mayer-Rokitansky-Kustur-Hauser syndrome, this condition belongs to a spectrum of genetic defects that cause abnormalities of the reproductive tract. Some of these problems are associated with other defects, such as the absence of a kidney.

The absence of a vagina or uterus would not interfere with the sexual development of the young girl.

Symptoms

Most patients discover that they have no vagina when they don't start having periods during adolescence. Girls with this condition develop breasts and pubic hair like any other woman but never have a period. This is because the ovaries produce normal female hormones that trigger normal development, but the absence of the uterus and vagina means that there is no period. Most girls report this at the ages of 15 or 16 years.

Diagnosis

In addition to a physical exam, the doctor will usually order a blood test to check chromosomes to rule out other genetic problems, and often an ultrasound of the pelvic organs. The ultrasound scan will detect the absence of the uterus but the presence of the ovaries. As some patients with this condition also have kidney problems, a scan or X ray of the kidneys may be recommended.

Treatment

In most patients, a vagina can be created by stretching the short vagina they already have with the use of plastic tubes called vaginal dilators. About 85% of girls are successfully stretched by using this technique alone; the remainder may need an operation to create a vagina known as a vaginoplasty.

During a vaginoplasty, a mold in the shape of the new vagina is sewn into the vaginal space. After the mold is removed, the patient must use dilators or have sex on a regular basis to ensure that the vagina doesn't shorten. Once the vagina has been created, there is no reason why a woman can't enjoy sex normally, since sexual pleasure is obtained from the clitoris rather than from vaginal stimulation.

While it's possible for the vagina to be reconstructed, it's not possible to reconstruct the uterus. If a woman wants to have a child and her ovaries are functioning normally, she should have no problem in producing normal eggs. The retrieved eggs can be fertilized with her partner's sperm in the lab and then transferred into the uterus of a SURROGATE MOTHER.

round spermatic nuclear injection (ROSNI) An experimental technique that uses immature SPERM aspirated from the testes and injected into the egg using INTRACYTOPLASMIC SPERM INJECTION (ICSI). The sperm can either be fresh or frozen. Fresh sperm can be maintained in the laboratory for up to a week; frozen sperm should be thawed and used on the day of the ICSI procedure.

RU-486   See MIFEPRISTONE.

Rubin's test A diagnostic method (also called TUBAL INSUFFLATION) that can be used to determine whether a woman's FALLOPIAN TUBES are blocked.

In this test, the doctor introduces carbon dioxide into the uterus and through the fallopian tubes. The gas escapes into the abdominal cavity if the tubes are not blocked. The abdominal gas may also be revealed on an X ray or fluoroscope. This test is no longer performed and has been replaced by a HYSTEROSALPINGOGRAM.

salpingectomy Surgical removal of a fallopian tube (the tubes through which an egg travels from the ovary to the uterus). There are many reasons why a fallopian tube may need to be removed.

Removal of one tube (unilateral salpingectomy) is usually performed if the tube has become infected (a condition known as SALPINGITIS). Sometimes a tube is in such poor condition that it must be removed so that the remaining, healthy tube will offer a better chance of pregnancy. IN VITRO FERTILIZATION may be more successful if a large, dilated fallopian tube is removed before IVF begins. The tube also may need to be removed due to bleeding from a ruptured ECTOPIC PREGNANCY (a condition in which a fertilized egg has implanted in the tube instead of inside the uterus).

Both tubes are usually removed (bilateral salpingectomy) if the ovaries are going to be removed during a hysterectomy. When the fallopian tubes and the ovaries are both removed at the same time, it is called a salpingo-oophorectomy. For example, this procedure is necessary when treating ovarian and endometrial cancer, because the fallopian tubes and ovaries are the most common sites to which cancer may spread.

The Procedure

The surgery, which is performed under general anesthesia, is performed with the help of a LAPAROSCOPE (a hollow tube with a light on one end). This allows the incision to be much smaller and the recovery time much shorter. The surgeon makes a small incision just beneath the navel and inserts a short hollow tube into the abdomen. Carbon dioxide gas can be used to move intestines out of the way and better view the organs. Another one or two incisions are made on the lower abdomen through which other instruments can be inserted. After the operation is completed, the tubes and instruments are withdrawn. The tiny incisions are sutured, and there is very little scarring.

If surgery can't be done by laparoscopy, the surgeon makes a horizontal (bikini) incision 4 to 6 inches (10 to 15 cm) long in the abdomen right above the public hairline. This is called a *laparotomy*.

Even when a laparotomy is performed, most women are out of bed and walking around within 3 days. Within a month or two, a woman can slowly return to normal activities, such as driving, exercising, and working.

Risks

All surgery, especially under general anesthesia, carries certain risks, such as the scarring, hemorrhaging, infection, and reactions to the anesthesia. Pelvic surgery can also cause internal scarring, which can lead to discomfort years afterward.

salpingitis Inflammation of the FALLOPIAN TUBE (which in Latin is "salpinx"). The tube may become inflamed as the result of the spread of an internal infection (such as a sexually transmitted disease), and may eventually spread to the peritoneal cavity, causing peritonitis. The tube also may become inflamed as the result of an infection spread from the outside, such as from the neighboring appendix. An infection spreading to the tube from the outside may have less of a harmful effect on the delicate interior structures of the fallopian tubes.

If salpingitis begins while a woman is wearing an INTRAUTERINE DEVICE, the IUD should be removed.

salpingitis isthmica nodosa   An abnormal inflammatory condition of the FALLOPIAN TUBE where it attaches to the UTERUS, which leads to a thickening of the tubal wall as a result of tiny growths from the inside of the tube. The fallopian tubes contain lumps that may lead to an ECTOPIC PREGNANCY before the tubes become fully blocked.

Diagnosis

A HYSTEROSALPINGOGRAM will reveal very small channels off the main tube, which may eventually become blocked.

Treatment

Surgery can unblock the tube; the procedure is called a tubal resection Reanastomosis, in which the abnormal path of the tube is removed. Up to 70% of women may expect to conceive after surgery, if they have no other infertility factors.

salpingolysis   Surgery performed to remove adhesions that restrict the movement and function of the FALLOPIAN TUBES. The surgery is usually performed by LAPAROSCOPY or LAPAROTOMY. Scissors, electrocautery and lasers are some of the surgical tools used in the procedure.

salpingo-oophorectomy   The surgical removal of a FALLOPIAN TUBE and an OVARY to treat ovarian or other gynecological cancers, infections, or ENDOMETRIOSIS. If only one tube and ovary are removed, the woman may still be able to conceive and carry a pregnancy to term.

If the procedure is performed through a LAPAROSCOPE, the surgeon can avoid a large abdominal incision and can shorten recovery.

With this technique, the surgeon makes a small cut through the abdominal wall just below the navel. General anesthesia is usually used; if there are no complications, the patient can leave the hospital the same day. This type of operation offers a much shorter recovery time.

If a laparoscope isn't used, the surgeon must make an incision 4 to 6 inches long (LAPAROTOMY) into the abdomen, either extending vertically up from the pubic bone toward the navel or horizontally (the "bikini incision") across the pubic hairline. The scar from a bikini incision is less noticeable, but sometimes a vertical incision is required because it provides greater visibility while operating. If performed through a laparotomy incision, salpingo-oophorectomy is more major surgery that requires three to 6 weeks for full recovery.

If both ovaries are removed in a premenopausal woman, the sudden loss of estrogen will trigger an abrupt premature menopause that may trigger "surgical menopause"—symptoms of hot flashes, vaginal dryness, painful intercourse, and loss of sex drive. In addition, women who lose both ovaries also lose the protection these hormones provide against heart disease and osteoporosis. Women who have had their ovaries removed are seven times more likely to develop coronary heart disease and much more likely to develop bone problems at an early age than are premenopausal women whose ovaries are intact. For these reasons, some form of estrogen replacement therapy (ERT) may be prescribed to relieve the symptoms of surgical menopause and to help prevent heart and bone disease.

In addition, to help offset the higher risks of heart and bone disease after loss of the ovaries, women should get plenty of exercise, maintain a low-fat diet, and ensure that intake of calcium is adequate.

A woman's reaction to the removal of her fallopian tubes and ovaries depends on a wide variety of factors, including her age, the condition that required the surgery, her reproductive history, and a previous history of depression.

Women who have had many gynecological surgeries or chronic pelvic pain seem to have a higher tendency to develop psychological problems after the surgery.

salpingostomy   Surgical repair made to the FALLOPIAN TUBES to open the fimbria on the outer ends. (If the tube itself is open and just the fimbria are stuck together, the operation to free them is called a FIMBRIOLYSIS.)

The ultimate success of the operation depends on how much the tubes' walls have become scarred and thickened, how severe the loss of the fine hairs on the cells lining the tubes, and where the tube itself is blocked. When tubes are severely damaged, up to a third of pregnancies that result after the operation occur inside the tube itself because the fertilized egg gets stuck.

Between 5% and 10% of women who have a salpingostomy each year will eventually be able to become pregnant and have a baby; the results depend on how badly damaged the tubes are and whether the woman has already had one attempt at salpingostomy.

salpingotomy   A laparoscopic surgical operation to open a blocked FALLOPIAN TUBE in which a temporary opening is made along the length of the fallopian tube. A salpingotomy is usually performed to treat an ECTOPIC PREGNANCY.

scrotal ultrasound   An imaging technique used to diagnose suspected abnormalities of the scrotum using harmless, high-frequency sound waves to form an image. The sound waves are reflected by scrotal tissue to form a picture of internal structures. The procedure is not invasive and involves no radiation.

Ultrasound of the scrotum is the most important imaging method to evaluate disorders of the TESTICLES and surrounding tissues. It is used when a patient has acute pain in the scrotum, an absent or undescended testicle, an inflammation problem, testicular torsion, fluid collection, abnormal blood vessels, or a lump in the testicles.

The patient lies on his back on an examining table as the technologist gently palpates the scrotum. A rolled towel is placed between the patient's legs to support the scrotum, and the penis is lifted up onto the abdomen and covered. After applying a gel on the scrotum to enhance sound transmission, the technologist places a transducer against the skin to create an image from reflected sound waves, which appear on a monitor screen. There is no discomfort from the ultrasound, but if the scrotum is very tender, even the slight pressure involved may be painful.

selective reduction   See MULTIFETAL REDUCTION.

semen   Fluid containing SPERM and a number of other substances, including water, simple sugars that nourish the sperm, alkaline chemicals that protect the sperm against the acidic environment of the urethra and vagina, and prostaglandins (fatty acid compounds that spur contractions in the muscles of the uterus and fallopian tubes and help the sperm's journey). Semen also contains vitamin C, zinc, cholesterol, and a few other compounds.

Although semen can carry bacteria or viruses of sexually transmitted diseases (including the AIDS virus), normal healthy semen doesn't contain any harmful substances.

Semen is normally translucent or whitish-gray. Blood found in semen (hematospermia) can color the semen pink to bright red to brownish red. The presence of blood in semen is abnormal. The presence of particles, nonliquified streaks of mucus, or debris also requires further evaluation.

semen analysis   A laboratory test used to assess SEMEN quality (SPERM quantity, concentration, form, and movement). In addition, the test measures semen fluid volume and whether or not white blood cells are present, which would indicate an infection. A normal ejaculate has more than 20 million sperm per milliliter; more than

50% of the sperm should be moving forward, and more than 30% should have normal shapes. The estimated cost is $25 to $35.

The man collects his semen by masturbating into a sterile collection cup; he should abstain from sex for 48 hours before analysis. Semen can't be collected during sex or from a latex condom because the latex may be toxic to sperm, and most of these condoms are also coated with the potent SPERMICIDE nonoxynol-9. If religious beliefs forbid masturbation, the doctor can recommend a silicon condom designed for specimen collection that doesn't harm sperm. This allows a man to produce a semen sample by intercourse.

Semen testing in a doctor's office or certified lab is done on fresh samples within 1 hour of collection. At least two semen samples collected on separate days by masturbation are recommended.

Each sample should be collected after not ejaculating for at least 48 hours, but not longer than 3 to 4 days. This helps the doctor get an idea of what the typical seminal fluid is like. Because sperm counts can vary, more than one sample may be necessary.

Process

The testing laboratory will provide a small container to use for the specimen. After the male partner ejaculates into the container, the sample must be taken immediately to the lab. Some labs ask the male partner to produce a specimen at the lab.

A general semen examination includes the time required for the semen to become liquid, its volume, consistency, and acidity. Microscopic evaluation of the ejaculate can determine the sperm count, motility (percentage of moving sperm), morphology (normality of shape), agglutination (clumping), and the presence of substances other than sperm, such as white blood cells or bacteria.

Standard lab results for sperm include:

Morphology: 50% to 60%
Motility: 50% or more with good forward progression

Sperm number: 20 million/ml or more
Volume: 1.0 to 5.0 ml or more

In addition, there should be no significant clumping or white or red blood cells, and no increased thickening of the seminal fluid.

semen viscosity   The liquid flow or consistency of the semen. Also known as liquefaction (liquid flow), semen viscosity can affect fertility. For example, the ejaculated semen of a normal man coagulates and then liquefies within 20 to 30 minutes. If this liquefaction is delayed for more than an hour, the sperm may become trapped in a jellylike mass.

Since the prostate gland produces the substance needed for liquefaction, "nonliquefying" semen may indicate a disorder of prostate gland function, such as an infection.

seminal vesicles   The paired glands in the male reproductive system at the base of the bladder that produce much of the SEMEN volume, including fructose (sugar) for nourishing the sperm and a chemical that causes the semen to coagulate on entering the vagina.

seminiferous tubules   In the TESTICLES, the network of tubes where SPERM are formed, mature, and move toward the EPIDIDYMIS.

septate uterus   A UTERUS divided into right and left halves by a wall of tissue called the septum. Women with a septate uterus have an increased chance of early pregnancy loss.

In this condition, the outside of the uterus is normal; the inside is divided into two halves. (In a BICORNUATE UTERUS, there is both a wall inside the uterus and a partial splitting of the outside, causing a "heart-shaped" uterus.) A woman with a UNICORNUATE UTERUS has only half of a uterus.

Of all these uterine abnormalities, the septate uterus has the highest rate of pregnancy loss.

Diagnosis

Uterine causes for repeated MISCARRIAGES are usually diagnosed with an X ray called a HYSTEROSALPINGOGRAM. In this test, dye is inserted into the uterus, and the X ray reveals the shape of the inside of the uterus. Sometimes a uterine abnormality may be diagnosed by either ultrasound or HYSTEROSCOPY, in which a small, lighted instrument is passed into the uterus.

Treatment

While a septate uterus may increase the chance for pregnancy loss, not all women with this problem will lose their pregnancies. Therefore, it is important to evaluate the size and location of the abnormality before proceeding with treatment.

In the past, major abdominal surgery was necessary, but that has been replaced by simpler hysteroscopic surgery that requires much shorter hospitalization and recovery time.

Serophene Brand name for CLOMIPHENE CITRATE.

Sertoli cell A testicular cell responsible for nurturing the immature SPERM. It secretes INHIBIN, a hormone that regulates production of FOLLICLE-STIMULATING HORMONE (FSH) from the pituitary gland. When stimulated by FSH, the Sertoli cell triggers sperm production.

sexually transmitted diseases and infertility Sexually transmitted diseases can lead to fertility problems as a result of inflammation in PELVIC INFLAMMATORY DISEASE in women and EPIDIDYMITIS in men. Therefore, if infertility is to be prevented, it's imperative to treat STDs early.

To decrease the risk of STDs, sexually active men and women should avoid multiple sex partners, use latex CONDOMS for contraception, and treat infections early. If one partner has an STD infection, both partners should be treated at the same time.

Female Infertility

Women get STDs more easily and experience more complications that include scarring, MISCARRIAGE, pelvic adhesions, blocked fallopian tubes, and ECTOPIC PREGNANCY. Severe cases of infection can lead to pelvic inflammatory disease, an inflammation of any one or all of the reproductive organs in a woman's pelvic cavity.

Male Infertility

Infections of the male genital tract may impair fertility. For example, diseases such as gonorrhea, tuberculosis, and some bacteria of the urinary tract may lead to blockages within the EPIDIDYMIS or VAS DEFERENS. In particular, large amounts of *E. coli* bacteria may interfere with sperm's ability to move and to kill immature sperm cells. Chronic bacterial infection of the semen may be an unsuspected factor in male infertility. Other diseases, such as mumps and syphilis, can inflame the testicles and lead to irreversible damage of the seminiferous tubules.

Infectious organisms such as *Chlamydia trachomatis,* ureaplasma urealyticum, herpes, mycoplasma, and cytomegalovirus also may cause inflammation of the urethra or the epididymis, or cause semen with few or abnormal sperm. However, researchers haven't confirmed a link between these organisms and infertility.

Treatment

The treatment of sexually transmitted diseases depends on the suspected infection. In the case of gonorrhea or chlamydia, oral antibiotics such as azithromycin or ofloxacin, or an injection of ceftriaxone followed by oral doxycycline, may be effective. Syphilis is usually treated with injections of penicillin.

sexual lubricants and infertility Some lubricants (such as K-Y Jelly) may have spermicidal properties and should not be used by couples who are interested in getting pregnant. However, even lubricants without SPERMICIDES may interfere with proper sperm movement. Using body oils and creams is not a good idea either, because they can also trap sperm.

Couples interested in conceiving a child should use only water-based lubricants. The best choice is to use only natural lubricants.

sexual positions and fertility Many believe that the missionary position (man on top) offers the best chance of a successful conception because this position allows for the deepest penetration and therefore places SPERM closer to the cervix. Some encourage a woman to raise her hips with a pillow so the cervix is exposed to the maximum amount of semen and advise the woman to stay in bed for up to 30 minutes after sexual intercourse. However, no sexual position has been shown to be more or less effective in causing pregnancy.

Sheehan's syndrome The common term for postpartum hypopituitarism, a condition caused by profuse bleeding at the time of delivery. The severe blood loss leads to circulatory collapse, which then results in poor blood supply and damage to the pituitary gland. The pituitary gland is particularly susceptible to postpartum complications because it is relatively enlarged during pregnancy. Hypopituitarism is an abnormal condition caused by a deficiency of one or more hormones secreted by the pituitary gland.

Sims-Huhner test Another name for the HAMSTER PENETRATION ASSAY.

smoking and infertility Tobacco use has been shown to affect the reproductive capacities of both men and women; in fact, tobacco is an especially potent reproductive toxin.

Among women, smoking boosts the risk of MISCARRIAGE and low–birth weight babies, and increases the time it takes to conceive as well. Scientists aren't sure what the connection may be, but research suggests that smoking may affect ESTROGEN production and may deplete egg supply. Smoking also affects cervical mucus,

since mucus production depends on estrogen. Moreover, nicotine has been found in cervical mucus—and nicotine is toxic to sperm. Smoking can also speed up the onset of MENOPAUSE, which can shorten the period of time when conception can occur.

It's also known that smoking can interfere with FALLOPIAN TUBE health, embryo cleavage, and BLASTOCYST formation and implantation. In fact, women who begin smoking before age 16 and who smoke more than a half pack a day have a higher risk of tubal infertility; this risk rises even more if they have had more than five sex partners or ever used an IUD. In addition, women smokers have twice the risk of tubal pregnancy and more premature deliveries and miscarriages.

Smoking also can affect assisted reproductive technologies. Women who smoke tend to be less successful with IN VITRO FERTILIZATION than nonsmokers; 38% of female nonsmokers conceived in their first cycle of attempting pregnancy compared to 28% of smokers. Smokers were also three to four times more likely than nonsmokers to have taken more than a year to conceive.

Moreover, some studies suggest that smoking can affect fertility several generations later: Women whose mothers smoked during their pregnancies are less likely to produce a live baby.

Smoking also affects a man's fertility. Men who smoke produce fewer and less healthy sperm (the average smoker has a sperm count that is 15% lower than those of nonsmokers). Sperm movement also slows down in men smokers, who also have a much greater percentage of abnormally shaped sperm.

A study of smokers who were followed for between 5 and 15 months after stopping smoking reported that their sperm counts rose between 50% and 800%. This suggests that reduction in sperm count is reversible once the man stops smoking.

Society of Reproductive Endocrinologists An organization of REPRODUCTIVE ENDOCRINOLOGISTS that works to extend knowledge of human reproduction and endocrinology. The society is primarily concerned with endocrine diseases, fertility, and hormonal disorders. It is also involved in ASSISTED REPRODUCTIVE TECHNOLOGY (ART), professional development, obstetrics, physician referrals, and reproductive health. Contact: Society of Reproductive Endocrinologists, c/o American Society for Reproductive Medicine, 1209 Montgomery Highway, Birmingham, AL 35216; phone: (205) 978-5000.

Society for Reproductive Endocrinology and Infertility

An organization dedicated to providing excellence in reproductive health through research, education, and patient care. The website provides for referrals to REPRODUCTIVE ENDOCRINOLOGISTS by state.

Membership requires certification by the American Board of Obstetrics and Gynecology in both obstetrics and gynecology and the subspecialty of reproductive endocrinology. Associate members have completed fellowship training in reproductive endocrinology, and are waiting to complete the Subspecialty Board Examination process. Contact SREI at their website: http://www.socrei.org/.

Society of Reproductive Surgeons

This specialty group of the AMERICAN SOCIETY FOR REPRODUCTIVE MEDICINE (ASRM) has more than 300 members throughout the United States. The Society of Reproductive Surgeons was founded in 1984 to serve as a forum for members of ASRM with special interest and competency in reproductive surgery. The society tries to promote excellence in gynecologic and urologic reproductive surgery by providing and encouraging professional education, by lay education, and by fostering research.

Doctors must complete a fellowship either in reproductive endocrinology or reproductive surgery and be in practice for at least 3 years to become eligible to join the society. A minimum caseload must be reproductive surgery for infertility, and two current members of the society who have performed surgery with them must approve their membership. Physicians who became members prior to 1989 were admitted based on their training and experience in reproductive surgery before formal fellowship training was established. See also REPRODUCTIVE SURGEON; REPRODUCTIVE SURGERY. Contact: The Society of Reproductive Surgeons, 1209 Montgomery Highway, Birmingham, AL 35216-2809; phone: (205) 978-5000, ext. 118; website: http://www.reprodsurgery.org/.

sonohysterography A type of diagnostic test (also called fluid ultrasound or hydrosonography) used to reveal the uterine cavity. The procedure is performed in the office without anesthesia. Advances in ultrasound have provided significant improvements in the ability to evaluate the UTERUS, ovaries, and FALLOPIAN TUBES.

A thin catheter is inserted into the uterus through the vagina, and a transvaginal ultrasound is then performed while saline is injected into the uterus. The fluid distends the uterus, revealing any fibroids, adhesions, or small polyps that could be missed with a HYSTEROSALPINGOGRAM (HSG).

The use of specialized protein solutions and color-flow Doppler ultrasound allows the doctor to visualize the liquid as it travels through the fallopian tubes and disperses in the abdomen. While this technique avoids X-ray exposure, the cost of the dye and color-flow Doppler ultrasound equipment limits use of this technique.

As the uterus is distended, there may be some cramping, which goes away after the procedure is finished. Lesions revealed by the test can't be treated at the same time, but the procedure is quick and costs much less than a HYSTEROSCOPY.

sperm The microscopic cell that carries the male's genetic information to the female's egg. Sperm is also known as the male reproductive cell or the male gamete. Sperm develop in seminiferous tubules found within the TESTICLES.

Human spermatozoa were first seen under the microscope by Leeuwenhoek as late as 1674, and scientific proof that the sperm fertilizes the egg to produce pregnancy was first available in 1779. Yet theories about semen were quite popular in centuries past.

The production of sperm (called SPERMATOGE-NESIS) is a complicated process of cell division that begins in the testicles, when very immature cells divide and eventually mature into tadpole-shaped spermatozoa (or sperm cells). Each sperm cell has half of its bearer's genetic material, and each contains mitochondria to power its tail during the journey to fertilize an egg. Sperm production usually occurs among groups of cells. Such groups (generations) of sperm pass through the same developmental stages together. The entire sperm production process takes about 2 1/2 months, so that sperm maturing now may have been affected by risk factors that were present 2 or 3 months ago.

Mature spermatozoa travel from the testicles into the EPIDIDYMIS, a C-shaped storage chamber next to the testes composed of a 20-foot coiled tube. Here they continue to increase in motility (movement) and mature. The sperm's journey through the epididymis takes about 3 weeks, at which point they pass into one of two muscular channels called the vas deferentia (a single channel is called a VAS DEFERENS). Each rigid vas deferens makes up part of the spermatic cord. Right before ejaculation, fluid from the prostate gland and seminal vesicles mix with the sperm from the epidymis to form semen, which is forced through the urethra during orgasm.

The process of sperm formation is controlled by hormones that are delicately balanced between the secretions of the testes, thyroid, adrenal glands, pituitary, and hypothalamus. Hormones that are specifically involved in spermatogenesis include

- testosterone: produced by the LEYDIG CELLS of the testes; needed for sperm manufacture
- follicle-stimulating hormone (FSH): produced by the pituitary that targets SERTOLI CELLS during spermatogenesis

- LUTEINIZING HORMONE (LH): produced by the pituitary, regulated by Gn-RH to stimulate testosterone production
- GONADOTROPIN-RELEASING HORMONE (Gn-RH): produced by the hypothalamus
- PROLACTIN produced by the pituitary; increased prolactin may decrease Gn-RH, lowering testosterone

sperm, immature (germ cell)   A sperm that has not matured and gained the ability to swim. During illness or infection, there may be many immature sperm.

sperm agglutination   Sperm clumping caused by antibody reactions or by infection.

spermatocele   Benign cysts in the scrotum, from the term *spermato* ("of SPERM") and *cele* ("cavity"). These very common growths often need no treatment, since they are not malignant. They are most often confused with hydroceles, another benign cystic disease of the scrotum.

Normally, every male has two TESTICLES within the scrotum that produce TESTOSTERONE and sperm. After sperm are produced in the testicles, they migrate into the EPIDIDYMIS, a small tubular gland behind the testicle about 1.5 inches long, where they mature for about 6 weeks. Eventually the sperm migrate through the epididymis to the vas deferens, the single tube that carries the sperm toward the prostate gland.

Cause

It is in the epididymis that the spermatoceles arise. For any of a number of reasons (trauma, infection, and birth defects), one of the tubes of the epididymis stops transporting sperm properly. As a result, one end of the tube begins to widen into a small cyst, which continues to enlarge. In many instances spermatoceles remain small, called "epididymal cysts." At other times, the spermatoceles continue to grow up to 5 to 6 inches or larger. Most of the time spermatoceles are painless. However, they can enlarge enough to make clothing uncomfortable, or at least tight-fitting with certain types of clothing.

Treatment

Spermatoceles don't go away without treatment, but most of the time they can simply be left alone and they will cause no pain, nor will they typically become invasive. If the spermatocele does require treatment, surgical removal is required. Surgery is usually done as outpatient, and requires less than an hour to perform. A general spinal or even local anesthetic can be used for the procedure. Most patients will need to stay off their feet for 3 to 5 days and reduce activity for a week.

Risks of the surgery include bleeding, pain, and infection, as is associated with any surgical procedure. The unique risks include recurrence of the spermatocele. Since the epididymis is left in place, there is the possibility of another duct blocking at a later time. The recurrence rate is about 5%. If the epididymis is removed with the spermatocele, the recurrence rate is lower, but then there is an slight increase in risk of damage to the blood supply to the testicle.

Because the epididymis is an integral part of the sperm transport system, any surgery done near the epididymis could cause occlusion of the duct, similar to having a vasectomy on that side. If fertility is not a concern, then epididymal trauma is not a risk. If the patient is still considering having children, spermatocelectomy should be put off until all childbearing is completed. Hormone problems after spermatocele removal is a very unlikely event and would only occur in the rare event that the blood supply to the testicle is damaged.

spermatocele, artificial An artificial, surgically created pouch used to collect sperm from men with irreversible tubal blockage.

spermatogenesis The medical term for SPERM production. Sperm is produced in a cyclic manner. The entire sperm-producing cycle takes about 100 days. Therefore, any treatment to improve sperm production can only be properly tested after waiting for about 100 days. If there is too much male hormone being produced, then the pituitary gland cuts back its production of LUTEINIZING HORMONE. This is called a feedback system; it helps the body regulate exactly how much stimulation is needed to keep normal testicular function going, both with regard to the production of male hormones and with regard to the production of spermatozoa.

sperm antibody test See ANTISPERM ANTIBODY TEST.

sperm bank A service that maintains frozen SPERM samples. Sperm donation is most often used to treat infertility related to low or absent sperm. Donors are matched by physical and other attributes. Most sperm banks require a physician referral. Semen samples cost between $100 and $250.

In the United States, donating sperm is a commercial enterprise, and donors are paid. There are more than 400 sperm banks in the United States, some of which are licensed and regulated by the states; however, licensing and standards are still fairly voluntary.

Current sperm bank standards require initial and interval testing for infectious diseases, including AIDS, syphilis, and hepatitis B and C. Donors also may be tested for chlamydia and gonorrhea. Because a donor's sperm could be infected with a disease such as AIDS or hepatitis, before the test turns positive most banks freeze and quarantine sperm for 6 months while the donor undergoes repeated testing for these diseases. The semen is released when the tests are negative for at least 180 days after the donation.

Confidentiality

Most sperm banks keep information about donors confidential. More recently, a few sperm banks now agree to release information about the donors to children born as a result of donor insemination, once they reach 18. The Sperm Bank of California in Berkeley was the first bank to offer this service, releasing the name, address, phone number, social security number, driver's license number, and hometown of donors. This "sunshine" policy is still fairly unusual in the United States, although it may become more common over time. In Sweden, open donor identity has been mandatory since 1989.

Sperm banks also vary on the amount of donor characteristics they will reveal to the infertile couple. Some banks offer just a brief physical description and a medical history, whereas others provide detailed questionnaires including donor hobbies, IQ, education, personality, occupation, and reasons for becoming a donor.

Superbaby Sperm

By 1980, at least one "superbaby" sperm bank was established in order to allow Nobel Prize winners to sell their sperm. Twelve years later, two more sperm banks in California began to specialize in selling the sperm of "gifted" men. One bank, the Repository for Germinal Choice, affiliated with the Foundation for the Advancement of Man, provides detailed descriptions of each donor for approved applicants.

Offspring Limits

Many sperm banks also limit the number of children who can be born as a result of insemination from one donor. (This is done to reduce the chance of closely related biological children inadvertently marrying.) While there is no legal requirement, most banks set a limit of five children per state and another five out of state. (It is possible, however, that the same donor may provide semen to another sperm bank, thus exceeding the recommended limit.) As a result of this potential problem, some countries (such as England and Sweden) maintain a central registry that limits the total number of children from one donor's semen.

Process

Most sperm banks can deliver sperm anywhere from a few days to a few weeks, depending on their own requirements; often, it's possible to send sperm directly to the home, but a few banks will only ship to a physician.

sperm count   The number of SPERM in the ejaculate, also called sperm concentration and given as the number of sperm per milliliter. A low sperm count is called OLIGOSPERMIA.

A general sperm count as part of a fertility evaluation should include the total density or count and the motile density. The motile density is perhaps the most important part of the semen analysis, as it reports the total number of sperm thought capable of progressing from the site of sperm deposition to the site of FERTILIZATION. This value is essential in both allowing a determination regarding whether or not a semen analysis is "normal," as well as in providing prognostic information should advanced reproductive medical assistance be required.

A sperm count of 20 million/ml or above is considered normal. However, about 20% of men with proven fertility have sperm counts below 20 million.

sperm filtering   A technique in which spunglass fibers are put into a syringe with SPERM, so that the sperm will be required to pass through the fibers. In theory, the dead sperm should stick to the filter and not make it through. This is a highly experimental procedure with unconfirmed success rates.

spermicide   An agent that kills SPERM, used as a type of BIRTH CONTROL METHOD. Available as foams, gels, films, creams, or suppositories, these preparations are most effective when used with a barrier form of birth control such as a CONDOM or DIAPHRAGM. They work by creating an environment in which sperm can't survive, damaging and killing sperm in the vagina. Therefore, the sperm are not able to travel from the vagina into the UTERUS and FALLOPIAN TUBES, where FERTILIZATION usually takes place.

Some people think of vaginal spermicides as a barrier method and use them alone, but it's best to use a spermicide with a condom or diaphragm. Vaginal spermicides when used alone are much less effective in preventing pregnancy than birth control pills or the IUD, or spermicides used with another form of birth control, such as CERVICAL CAPS, condoms, or diaphragms. Studies have shown that when spermicides are used alone, pregnancy usually occurs in 21 of each 100 women during the first year of spermicide use. The number of pregnancies is reduced when spermicides are used with another method, especially the condom. Discuss with a doctor what the options are for birth control and the risks and benefits of each method.

Products must be inserted into the vagina about 20 minutes before sex and remain effective for only about 1 hour. More foam, cream, or jelly must be inserted for each episode of intercourse.

Despite earlier beliefs to the contrary, government studies released in 1999 showed that nonoxynol-9 does not kill or stop the growth of the AIDS virus (HIV).

The safety of using spermicides in the rectum, anus, or rectal area is not known. However, no side effects or problems have been reported that are different from those reported for use in the vagina. Vaginal spermicides are available without a prescription.

sperm morphology One part of a SEMEN ANALYSIS that indicates the number or percentage of sperm in the sample that have been formed normally. The higher the percentage of misshapen sperm, the less likely FERTILIZATION can take place.

To assess sperm morphology, the sperm are stained and checked under a microscope using special criteria such as length of the sperm head's width and length, size of the midpiece, length of the tail, and any irregularities in the head contour. Adding colored stains to the sperm allows the observer to distinguish important normal characteristics as well as abnormal findings.

Sperm shape is determined by an average scoring of at least 100 cells, and it's considered normal if more than half of the sperm have an oval head, a length of 3 to 5 mm, and a width of 2 to 3 mm, with a customary midpiece and tail. A newer system called strict morphology is more stringent, with 15% the lower limit of normalcy, although some consider "normal" to be 5% or greater.

Several different types of sperm have been identified and characterized, grouped into one of four main categories: normal forms, abnormal head, abnormal tail, and immature germ cells.

Normal Forms

Normal sperm have oval head shapes, an intact midsection, and an uncoiled, single tail.

Abnormal Heads

Sperm with "abnormal heads" may include those with too large or small a head or no identifiable head at all. Tapering sperm heads, teardrop shapes, and duplicate or double heads also have been seen. A totally abnormal looking sperm is called an "amorphous" change.

Abnormal Tails

These abnormalities include coiling and bending of the tail, broken tails of less than half normal length, or double, triple, and quadruple tails. Droplets along the tail may indicate an immature sperm.

Immature Germ Cells

White blood cells in the semen should rarely be seen. It is very difficult to tell the difference between an immature germ cell and a white blood cell. Because the presence of white blood cells in the semen can be an important issue to recognize, anyone with a sperm count noting "many immature germ cells" needs to make sure that those cells are not in fact white blood cells.

sperm motility The ability of SPERM to swim (especially the sperm's forward propulsion). Sperm motility is one part of an overall assessment of sperm quality; poor sperm motility means the sperm will have a difficult time swimming toward the egg and penetrating it.

Structurally normal sperm swim faster and straighter than abnormal sperm—roughly 48 to 96 mm/second. The quality of sperm movement is based on a classification system of 0 to 4, wherein 0 represents no movement, and 4 represents excellent forward progression; for example, a semen sample with 60% motility would be characterized as "3+ to 4." A finding of decreased sperm motility is called ASTHENOZOOSPERMIA. A total absence of moving sperm is called NECROZOOSPERMIA.

During motility testing, the laboratory will note any sign of sperm "clumping" (agglutination) during microscopic evaluation. Clumping can keep the sperm from swimming properly through the cervical mucus and can prevent them from attaching to the egg. Increased agglutination may suggest an inflammatory condition (such as a bacterial infection) or an immune system abnormality.

Sperm may "clump" head-to-head, tail-to-tail, or head-to-tail, but tail-to-tail clumping is usually followed up with tests for ANTISPERM ANTIBODIES.

sperm-mucus interaction test   See POSTCOITAL TEST.

sperm penetration   The ability of the sperm to break through the egg so it can deposit the genetic material during fertilization.

sperm penetration assay   See HAMSTER PENETRATION ASSAY.

sperm production   See SPERMATOGENESIS.

sperm separation   See SPERM WASHING.

sperm washing   A technique used to separate SPERM cells from the seminal fluid, resulting in a small volume of highly concentrated sperm used for INTRAUTERINE INSEMINATION treatments. Sperm washing removes chemicals from the semen, such as prostaglandin, which causes uterine cramping. Washing is now a standard procedure in any IVF/GIFT-like procedure.

The sperm are separated from the semen by a process that involves mixing semen with a sterile fluid and being spun in a centrifuge. This removes the proteins and enzymes that protect the sperm's head, enabling it to enter the petri dish or fallopian tube fully capacitated.

The sperm are then mixed with a small amount of sterile fluid, which is used for the insemination. Washing sperm in this way may also increase the sperm's ability to fertilize the egg.

Spinnbarkeit   The stretchability of cervical mucus; the stringy quality that occurs at midcycle under the influence of estrogen. See also POSTCOITAL TEST.

split ejaculate   A method used to concentrate the SPERM for insemination, separating the semen into two portions. The first portion of the ejaculate, which is rich in sperm, and the second portion, which contains mostly seminal fluid.

sponge   The sponge is a donut-shaped polyurethane birth control device containing the spermicide NONOXYNOL-9 that is inserted into the vagina to cover the cervix, much like a DIAPHRAGM. A woven polyester loop is attached for easy removal.

The sponge is a low-cost, nonprescription product that protects for multiple acts of sex for 24 hours. It must be left in place for at least 6 hours after sex for contraceptive protection, but no more than 30 hours after insertion because of the slight risk of toxic shock syndrome.

Once so popular a form of birth control it became a famous joke on the TV comedy *Seinfeld*, the Today sponge was taken off the market in 1995 for financial—not health—reasons. The sole manufacturer (Whitehall Laboratories of

Madison, N.J.) had decided it would cost too much to correct manufacturing problems the FDA had discovered at the old factory where the sponge was made. (The FDA stressed that there never was any problem with Today's safety, just with the factory.)

Some 116,000 American women had been using Today in 1995 when its manufacturer stopped production, which had made it the most popular choice among methods that didn't require a doctor's visit. The only other woman-controlled nonprescription choices were spermicide and the female CONDOM; unlike those options, the sponge could be inserted up to 24 hours before sex and didn't require new applications for repeated intercourse. With its low risk of side effects, the sponge was attractive to women who didn't want to have to be fitted by a doctor, who had problems with prescribed hormonal contraceptives, or who enjoyed its ease of insertion.

Competing sponges were sold in France, Canada, and a few other countries, but once Today was off the U.S. market, no contraceptive sponge had been sold in this country. Allendale Pharmaceuticals of New Jersey is awaiting final FDA approval to market the sponge. Because the FDA never revoked the Today's approval, getting it back on the market was expected to be a quick process.

The sponge is available in Canada as Protectaid.

Stein-Leventhal disease Another name for POLYCYSTIC OVARY SYNDROME (PCOS). The condition is named after the two physicians who first described the condition.

sterility A condition that results in the absolute inability to reproduce. It is often confused with the term "infertility," which simply means the inability of a couple to achieve a pregnancy after trying for 1 year. While millions of people are infertile, most are not sterile—they simply have reduced fertility potential.

sterilization A permanent contraceptive option intended for people who don't want children in the future. It's considered permanent because reversal requires major surgery that may not be successful. In general, male sterilization (VASECTOMY) is less expensive and less risky than female sterilization (TUBAL LIGATION).

Tubal Ligation

To sterilize a woman, a doctor blocks the FALLOPIAN TUBES so that the SPERM and egg can't meet. Sterilization is usually done under general anesthesia with LAPAROSCOPY to block both fallopian tubes. The most common laparoscopic technique involves burning—and thereby destroying—a segment of the tube. In another technique, the physician uses mechanical clips or bands to block the tube. Both methods are effective, but the mechanical technique has a slightly higher failure rate. However, the mechanical technique is easier to reverse.

Sometimes a tubal ligation is not done through laparoscopy but by making a larger incision (LAPAROTOMY). It also may be done after a cesarian section. If so, the tubes are typically tied with suture and cut.

Complications of laparoscopic tubal ligation are rare, but they may include infection or damage to the bowel or blood vessels, or problems related to general anesthesia.

Vasectomy

Vasectomy involves cutting the tube that carries the sperm from the testicle to the penis called the VAS DEFERENS. Vasectomy is a quick operation (usually under 30 minutes) with the potential of only minor postsurgical complications such as bleeding or infection.

It may take several weeks to reduce sperm numbers to zero. Typically, a man should ejaculate 15 times after a vasectomy before he's infertile. It's best to use some sort of backup birth control method until a doctor can verify that the sperm count is zero.

stillbirth The death of a fetus between the 20th week of gestation and birth. A pregnancy that ends before the 20th week is called a MIS-CARRIAGE rather than a stillbirth.

Women who have had a stillborn child usually have a good chance of carrying a future pregnancy to term.

Causes

A number of factors increase the risk of stillbirth, including a mother who is over age 35, has poor nutrition, smokes, gets inadequate prenatal care, and abuses alcohol or drugs.

In addition, several disorders can cause stillbirth. They include

- pre-eclampsia and eclampsia: disorders of late pregnancy characterized by high blood pressure, fluid retention, and protein in the urine
- diabetes
- hemorrhage
- fetal abnormalities caused by infectious diseases such as syphilis, toxoplasmosis, German measles (rubella), and influenza
- severe birth defects: responsible for about 20% of stillbirths
- postmaturity: pregnancy beyond 41 weeks

stress and infertility Although infertility is a highly stressful experience, there is very little evidence that stress can *cause* infertility. However, it is certainly true that recurrent cycles of hoping to get pregnant followed by crushing disappointment, along with the high costs and low success rates of medical treatment, can lead to depression, anxiety, and frustration. Some scientists believe that such negative emotions can contribute to the failure to conceive, while others insist that such feelings are probably a response to, rather than the cause of, infertility.

In rare cases, high levels of stress in women can change hormone levels and cause irregular OVULATION. Some studies have shown that high stress levels may also cause fallopian tube spasm in women and decreased sperm production in men.

It is true that stress can boost activity of many body organs, leading to faster heart rate, higher blood pressure, and faster respiration, as well as sweaty palms and cool, clammy skin. Chronic stress can also cause depression and result in changes in the immune system and sleep patterns.

However, it is quite common to experience severe stress as a *result* of infertility. Research has shown that women undergoing treatment for infertility have a higher level of stress than those women struggling with life-threatening illnesses such as cancer and heart disease.

When diagnosed with infertility, many couples may no longer feel in control of their bodies or their plans and goals. Most couples are used to planning their lives and believe that if they work hard at something, they can achieve it. The experience of infertility can be a shock to that notion of self-control. In addition, infertility testing and treatments can be physically, emotionally, and financially stressful. A couple's intimacy may be destroyed by the infertility experience. Trying to coordinate doctor appointments with careers can also increase pressures on infertile couples.

subzonal sperm insemination (SUZI) SPERM injected into the subzonal space between the outer covering of the egg (ZONA PELLUCIDA) and the egg itself. Prior to 1992, experts thought that the sperm cell membrane had to merge with the egg cell membrane during microinjection, so SUZI was used. FERTILIZATION then took place normally, but there were relatively few births as a result of this procedure.

In 1992, Belgium scientists pioneered the sperm microinjection technique called INTRACY-TOPLASMIC SPERM INJECTION (ICSI), in which a single sperm is injected all the way into the egg; as a result, success rates were better than SUZI, which is now rarely used.

success rates   One of the most confusing issues related to reproductive technology is understanding how successful any particular FERTILITY CLINIC has been. This confusion stems from the fact that success rates vary depending on the reason for the infertility, the types of patients, and the way the pregnancy rate is reported.

For example, pregnancy rates can be reported by cycle, by patient, or by procedure, all of which give different results. Because of a number of factors that differ from one program to another, it's not a good idea to compare different fertility programs by using statistics alone. In fact, because of the wide variation in practice patterns and which couples have been included and excluded, the American Society for Reproductive Medicine (ASRM) has issued a specific warning against comparing programs using statistics prepared by the U.S. Center for Disease Control.

The most critical factor that affects a clinic's success rate is the decision about which couples to treat. Unfortunately, inclusion and exclusion criteria for any individual clinic are not reported to the CDC.

In 1995, more than 11,000 women who received ART treatments gave birth to 16,000 babies out of nearly 60,000 treatment cycles. Baby delivery rates from IN VITRO FERTILIZATION, the most common ART, were about 22.5% per procedure. In general, the success rates with IVF are lower for older women, couples with multiple fertility factors, women with uterine defects, smokers, and those who have a bulging-shaped fallopian tube. Age is the most important determinant; a recent report found that there were no pregnancies using ART after age 46. One study suggested that the best predictor of success is the responsiveness of the OVARY TO FERTILITY DRUGS, and that even older women might be good candidates for IVF if hyperstimulation produces a sufficient number of FOLLICLES. Other studies, however, indicate that quality, not quantity, is the problem in older women.

There are several examples of how selection criteria for treatment can affect the results. Some clinics offer treatment to almost everyone—even those couples who probably won't have much chance of success. Other centers discourage older patients, or encourage them to use donor eggs. Still other programs have an age cutoff and won't treat older women at all. In addition, clinics that offer advanced treatment to patients who might become pregnant with simpler treatments will appear to have higher success rates.

The number of embryos transferred also can affect a clinic's success rate. It's obvious that the more embryos transferred to a woman's uterus, the more likely it is that she will become pregnant. Unfortunately, this also increases the risk of higher-order births, which can pose significant risks to both mother and child. In order to limit this significant risk, the American Society for Reproductive Medicine (ASRM) recommends a limit of no more than three embryos to be transferred on average to women younger than 35 years of age.

However, despite the ASRM recommendation, the 1996 CDC report reveals that the average number of embryos transferred to women younger than 35 was 3.9, ranging from a low of 1.0 to a high of 5.9.

superovulation   Stimulation of multiple ovulation with FERTILITY DRUGS; also known as controlled OVARIAN HYPERSTIMULATION.

support groups for infertility   An infertility support group can help couples reduce their sense of isolation and understand that their experience and emotions are normal. The groups can help the infertile couple learn to express feelings, get help making decisions about how far to take infertility treatment, and discover new ways to cope that make the experience easier.

The largest support group for infertility problems is RESOLVE, an organization that helps couples find and select an infertility specialist, learn how to meet other people with similar concerns, and where to find other resources for more information. The group also offers a 24-hour helpline, a regional infertility specialist referral list, and insurance advocacy.

surrogate mother A woman who is artificially inseminated and carries to term a baby who will be raised by its genetic father and his partner.

swim-up technique A useful diagnostic procedure that also can be used to remove SPERM from SEMEN. It has some advantages to SPERM WASHING because the live sperm will swim up to the culture media leaving behind most of the debris, although some may float up into the medium.

The strongest sperm, which are those at the top of the medium, can be collected for IN VITRO FERTILIZATION or ARTIFICIAL INSEMINATION. A good swim test yields about .5 million very active sperm.

Synarel See NAFARELIN.

syphilis A sexually transmitted disease that can cause recurrent MISCARRIAGE in the second trimester. Latent syphilis does not cause symptoms, so a test for this disease is a standard assessment during pregnancy. An infected pregnant woman has about a 40% chance of having a stillbirth or giving birth to a baby who dies shortly after birth.

Syphilis is a complex disease caused by the bacterium *Treponema pallidum*. The syphilis bacterium is passed sexually from person to person through direct contact with a syphilis sore, usually on the external genitals, vagina, anus, or in the rectum. Sores also can occur on the lips and in the mouth. Pregnant women with the disease can pass it to the babies they are carrying. Syphilis can't be spread by toilet seats, door knobs, swimming pools, hot tubs, bath tubs, shared clothing, or eating utensils.

Symptoms

The time between picking up the bacterium and the start of the first symptom can range from 10 to 90 days. The primary stage of syphilis is marked by a single sore (chancre) that is usually firm, round, small, and painless; it appears at the spot where the bacterium entered the body. The chancre lasts between 1 and 5 weeks, and will heal on its own.

If untreated, the infection progresses to the secondary stage. This begins when a rough, "copper penny" rash appears on both the palms and the bottoms of the feet. The rash also may appear as a prickly heat rash, as small blotches or scales all over the body, as a bad case of acne, moist warts in the groin, slimy white patches in the mouth, sunken dark circles the size of a nickel or dime, or as pus-filled bumps like chicken pox. Some of these signs on the skin look like symptoms of other diseases. Sometimes the rashes are so faint they are not noticed. Rashes typically last 2 to 6 weeks and clear up on their own. In addition to rashes, second-stage symptoms can include fever, swollen lymph glands, sore throat, patchy hair loss, headaches, weight loss, muscle aches, and tiredness. The disease can be transmitted during either the first or second stage.

In the latent (hidden) stage, the bacterium remains in the body and begins to damage the brain, nerves, eyes, heart, blood vessels, liver, bones, and joints. About a third of the time, this damage appears many years later. In the late stage, the patient becomes paralyzed and experiences gradual blindness, madness, impotency, heart problems, and tumors. These may be serious enough to cause death.

Diagnosis

The bacterium can be detected by a blood test, which is accurate, safe, and inexpensive. A low level of antibodies will stay in the blood for months or years after the disease has been successfully treated, and antibodies can be found by subsequent blood tests. Because untreated syphilis in a pregnant woman can infect the fetus and possibly result in fetal death, every pregnant woman should have a blood test for syphilis.

In the United States, nearly 38,000 cases of syphilis were detected by health officials in 1998, including 7,000 cases of primary and secondary syphilis and 800 cases of congenital syphilis in newborns. More cases occur each year than come to the attention of health officials. The eight states with the highest 1998 syphilis rates were located in the southern region of the United States. These states had rates two to five times higher than the national rate. In 1998, 28 counties accounted for 50% of all primary and secondary syphilis cases.

Treatment

One dose of penicillin will cure a person who has had syphilis for less than a year; more doses are needed for someone who has had it for longer than a year. A baby born with the disease needs daily penicillin treatment for 10 days. Persons who receive syphilis treatment must not have sex with new partners until the syphilis sores are completely healed. See SEXUALLY TRANSMITTED DISEASES AND INFERTILITY.

syngamy The process that occurs when two sets of chromosomes from the egg and SPERM join together during FERTILIZATION. The chromosomes now number 46.

take-home baby rate Another name for the "live birth rate," the most important figure to check when comparing FERTILITY CLINICS. The take-home baby rate is a very good indication of a program's success, since the goal of fertility treatment is the birth of a live baby.

The rate should reflect the number of women who take babies home, not the number of babies brought home. If one woman has four babies, it's still one success, not four. See also SUCCESS RATES.

teratospermia Abnormal SPERM.

teratozoospermia Abnormal SPERM.

testicles Also known as testes, this pair of SPERM-producing glands are located in the scrotum (the sac holding the testes). The testes are responsible for the secretion of the male hormone TESTOSTERONE. For a man to be fertile, at least one testis must be able to manufacture sperm.

The testes are made up of supportive tissue, a network of ducts known as the SEMINIFEROUS TUBULES, and LEYDIG CELLS. Within each testis, the sperm are produced in the seminiferous tubules, the membranes of which contain primitive "germ" cells that eventually become sperm. The sperm then move through the EPIDIDYMIS, a coiled tube that begins at the top of each testis and descends along its length. The tail of the epididymis connects with a larger, muscular duct called the VAS DEFERENS, which continues upward for roughly 14 inches until it reaches the

area behind the bladder. There, at the base of the prostate (a gland that surrounds the neck of the bladder and urethra and adds a secretion to semen), the ends of the vas deferens join with a pair of pouches called seminal vesicles. The seminal vesicles and prostate produce seminal fluid to sustain the sperm.

The united vas deferens and seminal vesicles become the ejaculatory ducts. Both ejaculatory ducts enter the prostate gland, where they direct the ejaculate—sperm-containing semen—into the urethra, the tube that extends from the bladder to the end of the penis and passes urine or semen out of the body.

testicular biopsy A surgical procedure used to take a small sample of testicular tissue for microscopic examination to see if SPERM are present and able to be retrieved. This test may be needed if a man has no sperm in semen (AZOOSPERMIA) with apparently normal testes and VAS DEFERENS.

A testicular biopsy will reveal whether or not the lack of sperm is due to testicular failure (no functional sperm-producing tissue) or obstruction of the pathways from the testes to the urethra. Lack of sperm in a man with soft, small testes and a borderline FOLLICLE-STIMULATING HORMONE level is very likely to be caused by testicular failure. In this case, a biopsy is needed only when confirmation is absolutely essential.

This test is used to diagnose male fertility problems when no other means is available, because the biopsy procedure itself may be traumatic to the testes. After the test, the patient may need to wear an athletic supporter for several days and to refrain from sexual activity for 1 or 2 weeks.

The tissue is examined under a microscope and may reveal the following patterns:

- *normal.* If testicular tubules and sperm production seem normal despite a lack of sperm in the ejaculate, this means that sperm are being produced but aren't being ejaculated. In this case, doctors may suspect an obstruction or absence of the ducts from the testicle to the prostate. This problem could be treated by microsurgery.

- *sperm maturation arrest.* Problems can occur during any of a series of steps that sperm go through during maturation. Once the problem is diagnosed, treatments can help sperm mature fully, but the prognosis in this event is not good.

- *hypospermatogenesis.* Some men have all the elements for sperm production but don't produce many sperm. This problem can exist together with a problem with maturation of sperm.

- *germ cell aplasia.* If the man has no germ cells in his testicles, he won't produce sperm. There is no treatment for this disorder. Couples can either choose donor sperm insemination or adoption.

- *other conditions.* In addition to the above problems, a doctor may discover evidence of earlier infections, problems with LEYDIG CELLS (the testicular cell that produces testosterone), or testicular cancer. See also MALE FACTOR INFERTILITY.

testicular cancer and infertility There may be a link between INFERTILITY and testicular cancer, according to the results of one Danish study. Rates of testicular cancer (which affects about 1 in 500 men) have increased steadily since the 1930s, while the quality of sperm has reportedly declined over the past few decades.

The study of 30,000 Danish men with poor-quality sperm showed that there was a strong link between male subfertility and a higher risk of testicular cancer. The findings, reported in the British medical journal *The Lancet,* support earlier research that found similar results. All men of couples with fertility problems were 1.6 times more likely to develop testicular cancer than the Danish male population in general. Men who had abnormal sperm had a 2-fold to 3-fold risk of getting the disease. The scientists also found that men with poor-quality sperm were more likely than other men to develop cancer of the abdominal cavity and digestive organs.

Denmark, Switzerland, and Norway have the highest rates of testicular cancer in the world. It is the most common in men aged 25 to 29 years old.

An estimated 20% of cases have a genetic component. Doctors suspect that environmental factors and exposure to higher levels of the female hormone estrogen before birth are contributing factors to the increase in the disease. If detected early, testicular cancer has a 90% to 95% cure rate. See also RADIATION; TESTICULAR TUMORS; MEDICATIONS AND INFERTILITY.

testicular enzyme defect A congenital enzyme defect that prevents the testes from responding to hormonal stimulation.

testicular failure, primary A congenital, developmental, or genetic problem resulting in a testicular malformation that prevents SPERM production.

testicular failure, secondary Testicular damage that occurs after birth as a result of drug side effects, prolonged exposure to toxic substances, or swollen blood vessels surrounding the testicles that create a pool of stagnant blood (VARICOCELE).

testicular feminization An enzymatic defect that prevents a man from responding to the male hormone TESTOSTERONE. Such a man will look like a woman, but tests will reveal a normal

XY male chromosome pattern. Testosterone levels will be in the normal male range, and the ovaries are in fact testicular tissue.

testicular injury and infertility An injury to the testes may cause male INFERTILITY, especially if the trauma is followed by a decrease in the size of the injured TESTICLE or the appearance of ANTISPERM ANTIBODIES in the semen. Experts suspect that in this case, infertility is caused by an immune reaction due to penetration of sperm through the "blood-testis barrier," exposing them to the immune system.

Testicular injury may be caused by a physical blow, by twisting, or by damage that takes place on a cellular level, such as with a repeated infection.

testicular sperm extraction Testicular sperm extraction (TESE) allows men with a blocked or absent SPERM duct (vas deferens) to father a child through IN VITRO FERTILIZATION (IVF) as easily as if there were no obstruction to the sperm passage at all.

TESE makes IVF the treatment of choice for moderate or severe MALE FACTOR INFERTILITY. Even men who have had a VASECTOMY have a better chance of fathering a child with TESE and INTRACYTOPLASMIC SPERM INJECTION (ICSI) than with trying to reverse the vasectomy.

In the TESE procedure, the doctor inserts a thin needle directly into the testicle under local anesthesia and without making a skin incision. Pieces of testicular tissue as thin as a hair are removed during the procedure, which takes only about 15 to 30 minutes.

Sperm are extracted from the tissue and each egg is injected with a single sperm using the ICSI technique.

TESE is simple, low-cost, safe, and relatively pain free. Most men can have the procedure and return to normal activity right away. TESE is a good choice not only because of the very high success rates with ICSI but also because, unlike vasectomy reversal, the procedure allows the man to retain his vasectomy for future contraception.

testicular stress pattern A SEMEN ANALYSIS result showing low SPERM production, poor sperm movement, and poor sperm shape. The pattern may be related to testicular failure or illness.

testicular torsion The twisting of the spermatic cord that contains the blood vessels that supply the testicles. Testicular torsion most often starts during adolescence, and is acutely painful.

Cause

Torsion is caused by abnormally loose attachments of tissues that are formed during fetal development. This type of twisting can be complete, incomplete, or intermittent. Spontaneous "detorsion" (untwisting) can occur, which makes diagnosis difficult.

Diagnosis

SCROTAL ULTRASOUND can distinguish this condition from inflammatory problems such as an inflammation of the EPIDIDYMIS (EPIDIDYMITIS).

Treatment

Testicular torsion is a surgical emergency. A surgeon must operate as soon as possible to avoid permanent damage to the testes. See TESTICULAR INJURY AND INFERTILITY.

testicular tumors INFERTILITY problems are common in men who have been treated for testicular tumors. The rate of testicular tumor is especially high among men with undescended testes (CRYPTORCHIDISM), which is one reason why hormone therapy or surgical correction of an undescended testis in childhood is often recommended. Even though the increased risk of cancer remains after such treatment, the testes are more easily examined for potential malignancies when they are in the correct position in the scrotum.

Moreover, infertility problems are common among men who have been treated for cancer. RADIATION and chemotherapy with certain drugs such as cyclophosphamide, chlorambucil, and mustine is very toxic to the tissue that produces sperm cells. This is why freezing of sperm before beginning radiation or chemotherapy treatment is common. See also TESTICULAR CANCER AND INFERTILITY; MEDICATIONS AND INFERTILITY.

testosterone The primary male hormone responsible for secondary sex characteristics and for supporting the sex drive. Testosterone is also necessary for SPERM production.

A steroid hormone, testosterone is secreted from the LEYDIG CELLS of the testes in males and from the adrenal cortex and ovaries in females. In men, the pituitary hormone LH (LUTEINIZING HORMONE) stimulates testosterone production and secretion.

Testosterone levels can be assessed by a simple blood test, Normal values for men are 437 to 707 ng/dl; normal values for women are 24 to 47 ng/dl (ng/dl = nanograms per deciliter).

Abnormal testosterone test results could indicate KLINEFELTER'S SYNDROME, POLYCYSTIC OVARY SYNDROME, or TESTICULAR CANCER. A doctor also might order a testosterone test to rule out hypopituitarism, prolactinemia, or TESTICULAR FAILURE.

test-tube baby The common term that describes a baby conceived through ASSISTED REPRODUCTIVE TECHNOLOGY. See also BROWN, LOUISE.

TET See TUBAL EMBRYO TRANSFER.

therapeutic insemination by donor (TID) This is a type of ARTIFICIAL INSEMINATION in which sperm from a donor are placed in a woman's cervix or uterus.

Donors are usually carefully screened to comply with the AMERICAN SOCIETY OF REPRODUCTIVE MEDICINE standards and to match for characteristics similar to those of the parents or whatever other characteristics the patient desires.

thyroid gland problems and infertility See HYPER/HYPOTHYROIDISM.

thyroid function tests Blood tests used to evaluate how effectively the thyroid gland is working. These assessments include tests of the thyroid-stimulating hormone (TSH), thyroxine (T4), triiodothyronine (T3), thyroxine-binding globulin (TBG), triiodothyronine resin uptake (T3RU), and the long-acting thyroid stimulator (LATS).

These tests can help diagnose an underactive (hypothyroidism) or overactive (hyperthyroidism) thyroid and monitor response to thyroid therapy.

Most doctors consider the sensitive TSH test to be the most accurate measure of thyroid activity. By measuring this hormone, doctors can determine even small problems in thyroid activity before a patient complains of symptoms.

TSH triggers the thyroid gland to secrete the hormones thyroxine (T4) and triiodothyronine (T3). T3 is normally present in very small amounts but has a significant impact on metabolism, and it's the active component of thyroid hormone.

The thyroxine-binding globulin (TBG) test measures blood levels of this substance, which is manufactured in the liver. TBG binds to T3 and T4, prevents the kidneys from flushing the hormones from the blood, and releases them when and where they are needed to regulate body functions.

The long-acting thyroid stimulator (LATS) test shows whether blood contains long-acting thyroid stimulator. Not normally present in blood, LATS causes the thyroid to produce and secrete abnormally high amounts of thyroid hormones and is associated with Graves' disease.

Not all laboratories measure or record thyroid hormone levels the same way. Each laboratory will provide a range of values that is considered normal for each test. Here are some acceptable ranges:

- Normal TSH levels for adults are 0.5 to 5.0 mU/l.
- Normal T4 levels are 4 to 11 ug/dl at 10 years and older. Normal T4 levels don't necessarily indicate normal thyroid function. T4 levels can register within normal ranges in a patient who is pregnant, has recently had contrast X rays, or who has nephrosis or cirrhosis.
- Normal T3 levels are 110 to 230 ng/dl in adulthood.
- Normal TBG levels are 1.5 to 3.4 mg/dl or 15 to 34 mg/l in adults.

thyroid-stimulating hormone (TSH)   TSH is a pituitary hormone that triggers the thyroid gland to secrete the hormones thyroxine (T4) and tri-iodothyronine (T3). T3 is normally present in very small amounts but has a significant impact on metabolism, and it's the active component of thyroid hormone. Tests of TSH are ordered if the doctor suspects fertility problems caused by too much or too little thyroid hormone. See also HYPER/HYPOTHYROIDISM.

tocolytic   A drug that relaxes smooth muscles and therefore interferes with uterine contractions; it is often used to stop premature labor.

torsion   The medical term for "twisting." Torsion of the TESTICLES inside the scrotum causes extreme pain and swelling, twists off the blood supply, and causes severe damage.

Torsion of the ovary may occur in a woman suffering from hyperstimulation, a complication of OVULATION INDUCTION. See also TESTICULAR INJURY AND INFERTILITY.

transvaginal ultrasound   A type of scan using high-frequency sound waves using a wandlike instrument inserted into the vagina to visualize the organs in the pelvis as well as the blood flow to the ovaries.

The test, is performed on an empty bladder in the prone position. The ultrasound technician inserts the wand and checks the ultrasound screen to visualize the images. It will be necessary for the technician to manipulate the wand from side to side in order to obtain the necessary pictures.

There may be some mild discomfort as the technician manipulates the wand, but the procedure should not be painful. See also TRANSVAGINAL ULTRASOUND ASPIRATION.

transvaginal ultrasound aspiration   A technique used to remove eggs from the OVARY for IN VITRO FERTILIZATION.

The doctor places a vaginal ultrasound probe and, with ultrasound guidance, the doctor passes a needle through the upper vagina into the ovaries. With a suction device connected to the needle, the egg and fluid within each FOLLICLE is aspirated.

This procedure usually takes about 10 to 15 minutes and requires about an hour of recovery afterward. The woman can usually return to normal activity the following day, and the risks are minimal. Not all follicles will have recoverable eggs, although most larger follicles do have an egg present. Any successfully fertilized eggs that are not needed for transfer in this first IVF cycle may be frozen (cryopreserved) for use in a later cycle.

In almost all cases, egg retrieval is performed using the vaginal ultrasound-guided aspiration. The procedure uses intravenous sedation, not general anesthesia; therefore recovery from both the procedure itself and the anesthesia is relatively easy. The ultrasound image allows more accurate aspiration attempts because the physician can guide the needle into each follicle in order to withdraw the egg.

In the past, eggs were retrieved using LAPAROSCOPY, which requires general anesthesia.

The procedure is riskier than vaginal ultrasound retrieval but is rarely used today. See also VAGINAL ULTRASOUND.

trophoblast The outer layer of an early embryo that supplies nutrition and helps foster implantation by eroding away the tissues of the UTERUS with which it comes in contact. This allows the embryo to sink into the cavity formed in the uterine wall.

TSH See THYROID-STIMULATING HORMONE.

tubal embryo transfer (TET) One form of ASSISTED REPRODUCTIVE TECHNOLOGY method in which an embryo is placed into a woman's FALLOPIAN TUBES during a tubal transfer procedure (LAPAROSCOPY). This procedure is not widely used today.

In this procedure, a woman is first given medications to stimulate multiple egg development. When the woman's follicles are mature, the doctor performs an aspiration procedure to remove the eggs from her ovaries and fertilize them in the laboratory. The embryos are cultured in the laboratory for 2 days. At that time, a laparoscopy is done to place the embryos in the woman's fallopian tubes.

The TET procedure is similar to standard IVF where embryos are replaced 3 days after retrieval. However, with IVF the embryos are replaced into the uterus, not the tubes.

Some studies have shown higher implantation rates with TET as compared to IN VITRO FERTILIZATION (IVF) with uterine embryo transfer or GIFT. Recent well-controlled studies have shown little benefit to this procedure. In the past, proponents of TET argued that enabling the embryo to reach the uterus via its natural route (the fallopian tube) rather than by embryo transfer through the cervix increased the likelihood of implantation and a successful pregnancy. They also stressed that TET would allow the embryos to travel down the fallopian tube on their own,

and so reach the uterus at the appropriate stage (about 5 days after transfer) when the uterus is best prepared, while IVF delivers an embryo directly into the uterus 2 or 3 days earlier. Accordingly, it was argued that TET was better for older women for whom IVF is not as successful.

Recently, a number of well-conducted studies have confirmed that the pregnancy rate per embryo transferred with TET is the same as that reported for IVF. Therefore, almost all experts believe there is hardly any justifiable reason for performing TET instead of to IVF.

Cost

TET costs more than IVF because two surgical procedures are involved in an ultrasound egg retrieval and a laparoscopy to replace the embryos. Tubal-assisted reproduction procedures such as TET, GIFT, and ZIFT are not ever likely to be cost effective because of the additional cost of laparoscopy.

Success Rate

For high-quality IVF labs with reproductive endocrinologists skilled at uterine embryo transfer, there is no good evidence that pregnancy rates are better with TET compared with IVF, which costs less and is much less invasive. TET may be indicated when the embryos can't be passed through the cervix, thereby preventing a uterine transfer.

tubal insufflation A test to see if a woman's FALLOPIAN TUBES are open. In the procedure, the doctor will pass a colored dye through the cervix, UTERUS, and fallopian tubes during LAPAROSCOPY to check the tubes.

It is similar to an HYSTEROSALPINGOGRAM X-ray procedure, but it is performed while the woman is under general anesthesia for laparoscopy. After the dye has been inserted through the cervix into the uterus, if the tubes are blocked the gas or dye will accumulate in the uterus.

One potential limitation of this test is that even when a blockage is identified, it's not possible to figure out its precise location, which is why a hysterosalpingogram may add further information.

tubal ligation   Female STERILIZATION. In this procedure, the FALLOPIAN TUBES are blocked to prevent the egg from meeting SPERM. Commonly known as "having the tubes tied," this procedure is 99% effective in preventing pregnancy.

In many cases, women choose to have the procedure performed immediately after giving birth. If the delivery was by cesarean section, the procedure can be performed directly and quickly.

When tubal ligation is not done after delivery, it can be performed on an inpatient or outpatient basis, either under general or local anesthesia and tranquilizers, using LAPAROSCOPY. A special surgical tool called a LAPAROSCOPE allows a doctor to see the internal organs without the large incision that would once have been necessary. With another instrument, the doctor clips, ties, or seals each of the fallopian tubes.

Complications

Because tubal ligation is a more involved operation than VASECTOMY, there is more potential for complications. Complications include possible infection, internal trauma, or internal bleeding. These complications are rare, but a woman should discuss them with her doctor before she decides to undergo the procedure. The woman must know how to clearly tell if she is experiencing complications before she leaves the doctor's office, clinic, or hospital. Fever should be immediately reported to the doctor.

Pregnancies are rare in women who have been sterilized, but if they occur they may pose certain risks.

In the Future

A number of new types of approaches to tubal sterilization are currently being developed and may be introduced in the coming decade.

- Chemical scarring: Two chemical combinations are used for tubal sterilization in China. One is phenol (carbolic acid), combined with a thickening agent. The other is phenol, combined with quinacrine. The chemicals are used to damage the fallopian tubes so that scar tissue eventually blocks the tube.

- Chemical plugs: Canada and the Netherlands have approved permanent nonsurgical tubal sterilization through the introduction of chemicals into the fallopian tubes, such as methylcyanoacrylate (MCA, also known as Krazy Glue).

- Silicone plugs: A reversible, nonsurgical method of tubal sterilization using liquid silicone that is injected into the fallopian tubes. The silicone hardens and blocks the tube with a rubbery plug that can be removed later.

- Cryosurgery: Liquid nitrogen can freeze the connection between each fallopian tube and the uterus so that scar tissue blocks the tubes and prevents fertilization of the egg.

tubal ligation, reversal of   About 10% of women who have had TUBAL LIGATION (sterilization) later change their minds. Between 75% and 90% of the time, it is possible to reverse female sterilization. However, only about 60% to 75% of women who have had a tubal ligation reversed are able to get pregnant.

The success of the reversal depends on how the original sterilization procedure was done, how much of the tube remains after the sterilization, and how experienced the surgeon is at reversal. Tubes originally blocked with rings or clips often sustain less damage than if the sterilization was done by destroying the tubes by cauterizing (burning) them. The reversal of a tubal ligation is difficult; it is best performed by a surgeon who specializes in this type of microsurgical technique.

A reversal of a tubal ligation requires a major surgical operation called a LAPAROTOMY. Once the abdomen is opened, the surgeon removes the damaged part of the fallopian tube and sews the remaining sections together. This type of surgery typically requires a hospital stay and several weeks of recuperation.

tubal patency tests   The most common test to make sure the fallopian tubes are functioning is a special X ray using a contrast dye called a HYS-TEROSALPINGOGRAM. This test is scheduled immediately after a menstrual period but before OVULATION occurs. The dye is injected through the cervix, which then fills the UTERUS and flows into the FALLOPIAN TUBES.

Because the dye stretches the uterus, it can be uncomfortable, so painkillers can be given beforehand. If the tubes are blocked, pressure may build up and contribute to the pain. The procedure only takes a few minutes.

LAPAROSCOPY allows the doctor to look directly at the fallopian tubes while the patient is anesthesized, using a telescopic instrument inserted through a small incision near the navel. See also TUBAL PROBLEMS AND INFERTILITY.

tubal problems and infertility   The FALLOPIAN TUBES are active, muscular organs that retrieve the egg from the ovary and coax it toward the uterus and oncoming sperm. If scar tissue restricts the tube's mobility or if infection has stripped the tiny cilia from the tubal lining, the tube cannot perform its vital job. Problems with the fallopian tubes are the leading cause of female fertility problems. As a result of the rise in cases of PELVIC INFLAMMATORY DISEASE, sexually transmitted infections, and ENDOMETRIOSIS, tubal problems today account for half of female infertility.

Cause

A number of different problems can impair the fallopian tubes. When infection and disease attack the lining of the tubes, they may not function normally. Scarred by old wounds, the fallopian tubes can no longer retrieve the egg and move it along toward the uterus. Infection and

damage from ectopic pregnancy may damage the delicate hairs along the inner tubal walls. When this happens, sperm can't meet egg, and fertilization can't occur. If the tubes are obstructed only partially, sperm may be able to meet egg, but the developing embryo can become trapped inside the tube and cause a painful and even life-threatening ectopic pregnancy.

The PID epidemic alone is robbing the fertility of hundreds of thousands of women each year. Up to 60% of women who have antibodies to chlamydia are unaware that they ever had an infection. Fortunately microsurgery, laser surgery, and IN VITRO FERTILIZATION techniques can restore fertility to many of those women.

Diagnosis

There are a variety of tests that can help diagnose tubal problems, such as an X ray of the tubes (HYSTEROSALPINGOGRAM), ultrasound (SONOHYSTEROSGRAPHY), or a telescopic investigation of the abdomen (LAPAROSCOPY), and any of them can provide an excellent look at tubal problems for women who have had a history of repeated vaginal infections or who have had one or more episodes of PID or postpartum infection. It may also be useful for women with unexplained infertility, or those who have had a history of abdominal surgery, ruptured appendix, or ectopic pregnancies.

tubal reanastomosis   Surgical correction of previously "tied" tubes (female sterilization). Success rates depend on several things, including where the tubes have been rejoined, how much tissue was available to reconnect, the length of tube after the procedure, and quality of the tube lining in general. Microsurgical reconnection provides a greater success rate.

Before the surgery, experts recommend that a couple be tested to make sure there is enough sperm, that ovulation is normal, and that the lining of the uterus is normal.

A HYSTEROSALPINGOGRAM (HSG) may help make sure there are no problems in the uterine cavity; an HSG also can find out how much of the tube is open.

The surgery is typically scheduled for right after the end of a menstrual period, when blood flow through the tube is at its lowest.

The location of the site of the rejoined tubes is critical to getting pregnant afterward. For most tubal sterilization procedures, the obstruction will be near where the tube is connected to the uterus, which is also where most fertilization occurs.

After the surgery, the doctor will be able to confirm if both tubes were reconnected and if they were open at the conclusion of the reanastomosis. A follow-up HSG should be done after the next period a month later to determine if the tubes have healed and remained open.

tubocornual anastomosis   Surgery performed to remove a blocked portion of the FALLOPIAN TUBE and to reconnect the tube to the uterus (sterilization reversal). Tubouterine implantation may also be performed to remove fallopian-tube blockage near the uterus and reimplant the tube in the uterus. See also TUBAL ANASTOMOSIS.

tuboplasty   Surgical procedure to repair the FALLOPIAN TUBES.

Turner's syndrome   A genetic defect involving the absence of all or part of one of the sex chromosomes (X). It is associated with short stature and other medical problems.

Since two normal chromosomes are needed to produce normal ovaries, Turner's syndrome (also called monosomy-x) is associated with sexual immaturity and OVARIAN FAILURE. In this condition, the ovaries appear only as small streaks in the pelvis. About 1 in every 2,000 baby girls has Turner's syndrome, but the frequency is much higher in spontaneously aborted fetuses.

The condition first may be recognized in a newborn baby, a child, a teenager, or, rarely, in an adult. Those affected require special medical surveillance throughout life.

Symptoms
Turner's syndrome not only involves the ovaries but also affects many body systems. For example, serious heart and thyroid problems may occur.

Diagnosis
Turner's syndrome can be diagnosed by a blood test called karyotype. The test determines the makeup of the chromosomes, specifically assessing the sex chromosomes (X).

Treatment
While children with Turner's syndrome usually have enough growth hormone, they do increase their rate of growth with the addition of human growth hormone therapy. Oral replacement of estrogen hormones at the appropriate age will promote pubertal development. Although infertility can't be changed, pregnancy may be possible through egg donation.

Turner's Syndrome Society   Founded in 1987, the Turner's Syndrome Society of the United States is a young organization with more than 38 chapters and groups across the country. The society's mission is to increase public awareness and understanding of Turner syndrome and work together with health care professionals to better understand the condition through research and communication. Contact: Turner's Syndrome Society, 1313 Southeast 5th Street, Suite 328, Minneapolis, MN 55414 USA; phone: (800) 365-9944; website: www.turner-syndrome-us.org.

ultrasound Use of high-frequency sound waves that are reflected off solid tissues to give an image of internal body structures. This device is used to detect and count FOLLICLE growth (and disappearance) in many fertility treatments and to detect and monitor pregnancy.

ultrasound and infertility Ultrasound scans use high-frequency sound waves to bounce off the pelvic organs; the reflected sound waves are received by a probe called a transducer, and a computer is used to reconstruct the waves into black-and-white images on a monitor.

Today, the standard ultrasound technique for infertility uses vaginal ultrasound in which a slender probe is inserted into the vagina to scan the pelvic organs. This is much more comfortable for patients than the old abdominal approach, and gives much sharper and clearer pictures since the probe is much closer to the pelvic structures.

The ultrasound provides clear pictures of the uterus and the ovaries so that the doctor can diagnose early pregnancy, fibroids, OVARIAN CYSTS, and ECTOPIC PREGNANCY. This type of ultrasound scan is not very helpful in determining whether or not the fallopian tubes are normal.

The basic procedure for most infertility treatment is the follicular scan, which allows the doctor to determine when an egg matures and when a woman ovulates. Repetitive scans can follow the growing follicle and watch for when it has ruptured.

The doctor also can check the thickness of the uterine lining and therefore get a good idea of how much ESTROGEN a woman is producing. The quality of the egg is based on the thickness and brightness of the uterine lining on the ultrasound scan.

One of the most common problems that an ultrasound scan will reveal is an ovarian cyst (a fluid-filled sac in the ovary). It begins during OVULATION, when a follicle may grow but not rupture and release an egg. Instead of being reabsorbed, the fluid within the follicle remains and forms a cyst. Most of the time, ovarian cysts aren't related to a disease, and they disappear on their own. These function tests are different from other conditions involving cystic ovaries, such as POLYCYSTIC OVARY SYNDROME, endometriotic cysts, or ovarian tumors.

Since an ultrasound picture is really little more than a shadow, a doctor must be skilled at interpreting the image. Simple cysts have thin walls and look like a large black bubble on the screen. Cysts that contain blood (for example, CHOCOLATE CYSTS found in women with ENDOMETRIOSIS) will appear white inside; they are described as "complex masses."

The chance of developing a follicular cyst is higher among infertile women taking drugs like CLOMIPHENE CITRATE, or hMG for ovulation induction.

Ovarian cysts usually disappear within 2 months on their own, but if the cyst is bigger than 6 cm or lasts longer than 6 weeks, further testing may be needed.

Ultrasound scans can be done by a radiologist, a gynecologist, or an infertility specialist. The benefit of having scans done by an infertility specialist is that immediate decisions about treatment can be made based on the scan findings.

There have been advances in ultrasound technology in recent years. Using sonosalpingography, doctors can now assess a woman's fallopian tubes by introducing a fluid into the tubes through the uterus and watching the movement of the bubbles into the tubes and out into the abdomen. Since this test can be done in a fertility clinic and doesn't involve X-ray radiation, it may be a good choice for assessing that the tubes are normal. However, the standard method for tubal testing remains HSG and laparoscopy.

The newest ultrasound machines have Doppler attachments that allow a doctor to assess blood flow. Color Doppler allows blood flow to be mapped in color on the monitor. While still only a research tool, the color Doppler may provide important information for assessing the infertile patient in the coming years.

Using sophisticated microprocessors, the newest dimensional ultrasound machines allow the doctor to reconstruct the image for a three-dimensional view. While this provides excellent pictures, experts aren't sure if this technique will be useful for infertility.

Ultrasound also offers infertile patients newer treatment options previously unavailable. Modern surgical techniques have become less and less invasive. From LAPAROTOMY to laparoscopy, and now to ultrasound-guided procedures, the newest ultrasound methods lower costs, shorten hospital stays, lower risk of complications, and provide a better chance of maintaining fertility. Ultrasound-guided procedures can be used to treat a variety of problems, including

- egg retrieval for IN VITRO FERTILIZATION
- aspirating ovarian cysts
- treating ectopic pregnancy
- ultrasound-guided tubal embryo and gamete transfer for IVF and GIFT techniques
- Treatment of blocked tubes with ultrasound-guided tubal catheterization

underwear and infertility　High temperatures have been shown to lower SPERM production.

Tight clothing (jockey shorts) prevents the scrotal temperature from being lower than core body temperature and may impair sperm production. See also HEAT AND INFERTILITY.

undescended testicles　The common term for CRYPTORCHIDISM.

unicornuate uterus　An abnormality in which the UTERUS is one-sided and smaller than usual. Since the ovaries form separately from the uterus, they are generally normal in these patients.

Only about 7% of the abnormalities of the uterus are unicornuate. It is still possible for a woman with this condition to get pregnant, and the prognosis without treatment is excellent. Many patients with a unicornuate uterus are never diagnosed, and therefore the published rates of reproductive failure may be too high.

About 7% of women who have some type of birth defect involving the uterus have a unicornuate uterus. Total abnormalities of the uterus occur in about 1 in 200 to 600 fertile women.

ureaplasma urealyticum　A bacterial infection without symptoms that is sexually transmitted between partners. The bacteria can survive in the reproductive tract for many years until a patient is specifically tested for the infection.

Any woman who experiences infertility, recurrent pregnancy loss, pelvic pain, premenstrual symptoms, or vaginal symptoms should be tested for this infection, since it can lead to a wide range of infertility problems, including tubal disease, recurrent MISCARRIAGES, decreased sperm movement and count, and poor POSTCOITAL TESTS.

Treatment requires antibiotics prescribed by the physician to specifically treat this infection. Fourteen days or more after completing the medication, the patient receives a repeat test. If the culture returns positive again, it may be necessary to administer treatment with alternative antibiotics. Ninety percent of infections are effectively treated with the first course of antibiotics.

urinalysis and male infertility   A complete urinalysis may help to determine MALE FACTOR INFERTILITY.

Significant numbers of sperm in a urine sample suggest retrograde ejaculation. High numbers of white blood cells may indicate an infection in the PROSTATE GLAND or elsewhere in the urinary tract. See also EJACULATION, RETROGRADE.

urinary luteinizing hormone (LH) test
LUTEINIZING HORMONE (LH) is released by the pituitary gland to stimulate the ovaries to produce and release eggs each month during the menstrual cycle. The LH test measures the amount of LH in the urine and identifies the LH SURGE that occurs just before OVULATION.

Urinary LH is detected with a self-administered test kit (also called an ovulation predictor kit) that senses a higher level of LH in the urine. A sample of the woman's first morning urine is tested with the materials provided in the kit. By monitoring levels of LH and watching for the surge, a woman can time sexual intercourse to coincide with ovulation so as to increase the chance that the egg will be fertilized.

The level of LH in the urine will vary depending on at what point during the menstrual cycle the sample was taken. LH levels will be highest around the time of ovulation, about halfway between a woman's menstrual periods, and lower during the rest of the month. Likewise, postmenopausal women will have higher LH levels.

LH levels that don't rise at midcycle may indicate the absence of ovulation. Additional lab tests may be needed in this situation.

A urine LH detection kit is also available for use at home. These are sometimes called "ovulation tests" and are similar to home pregnancy tests. A sample of the woman's first morning urine is tested with the materials provided in the kit. By monitoring levels of LH and watching

for the "surge," a woman can time sexual intercourse to coincide with ovulation so as to increase the chance that the egg will be fertilized.

urofollitropin (Metrodin, Fertinex)   The generic name for a highly purified form of urinary FSH (FOLLICLE-STIMULATING HORMONE) used to stimulate follicle growth and development. Extracted from the urine of postmenopausal women, urofollitropin stimulates the follicles and can be used with HUMAN CHORIONIC GONADOTROPIN to produce the LH and FSH surges that trigger ovulation. It is generally used for women with polycystic ovaries when clomiphene citrate has failed.

The most potent form of urofollitropin is Fertinex, which was approved by the U.S. Food and Drug Administration in 1996. Compared to METRODIN, PERGONAL, or HUMAGON, Fertinex is 100 times more pure in FSH potency.

First introduced outside the United States in 1993, this highly purified formulation of FSH quickly became the most popular hormone treatment for infertility in many countries, including Germany, the United Kingdom, France, Italy, Spain, and Sweden. The manufacturing process for Fertinex, developed by the Ares-Serono Group, results in an FSH product of very high purity and consistency. FSH is the primary natural hormone that stimulates development and maturation of follicles.

urologist   A doctor who specializes in evaluating and treating disorders of the kidneys, urinary tract, bladder, and male reproductive organs. These doctors, who are certified by the American Board of Urology, can provide evaluation, diagnosis, and possible treatment of male infertility problems.

urology   A surgical specialty that deals with diseases of the male and female urinary tract and the male reproductive organs. The specialty also includes surgical care of the male and female adrenal glands. In the treatment of infertility, urology covers diagnosis and treatment of ERECTILE DYSFUNCTION (impotence), TESTICULAR CANCER, sexually transmitted diseases, and injury to urologic organs.

Although urology is classified as a surgical specialty, a knowledge of internal medicine, pediatrics, gynecology, and other specialties is required by the urologist because of the wide variety of clinical problems encountered. In recognition of the wide scope of urology, the American Urological Association has identified seven subspecialty areas, including pediatric urology, urologic oncology (cancer), renal transplantation, male infertility, urinary tract stones, female urology (urinary incontinence and pelvic outlet relaxation disorders), and neurourology (including erectile dysfunction).

uterine factors and infertility Problems with the UTERUS are the cause of infertility in about 5% to 10% of infertile couples. Uterine problems can influence fertility either by providing a poor environment for an egg, or by preventing the egg or embryo from implanting into the wall of the uterus.

A variety of conditions can adversely affect the uterus, including structural problems such as fibroids, adhesions, or polyps. These growths can distort or shrink the size of the uterus, interfering with the organ's blood supply. Although fibroids are very common in many women, when they become a certain size or grow in certain areas within the uterus, they may interfere with conceiving, implantation, or the ability to sustain the pregnancy the full 9 months.

Fibroids that grow inside the cavity of the uterus can wear away the lining so that an embryo can't implant. Growths inside the muscle wall won't interfere with conception, but if they get big enough they can interfere with the growth of the baby by affecting blood supply. Fibroids that actually protrude into the outer surface of the uterus can press on the fallopian tubes and interfere with their ability to retrieve an egg.

ENDOMETRIOSIS (a condition in which tissue from the uterus migrates outside the organ) also can affect fertility. Up to 35% of women having an infertility exam are actually found to have endometriosis, which can be inherited as a specific chromosomal abnormality.

Other problems with the lining of the uterus can affect fertility, such as infections or scarring from previous D&C procedures or abortions. Prenatal DES exposure may also affect the uterus and interfere with fertility.

Problems related to the uterus are generally evaluated first with a HYSTEROSALPINGOGRAM, followed by either HYSTEROSCOPY or LAPAROSCOPY, depending on the suspected cause of the problem.

uterus Part of the female reproductive system that holds and feeds a fetus until birth (also known as the womb).

The normal uterus develops from the conjunction of two Müllerian ducts of the same size, shape, and growth potential. But if the ducts aren't the same size, or if they grow at different rates, a unicornuate uterus develops. If the fusion is abnormal, a BICORNUATE UTERUS may develop. If the midline septum is not absorbed, a SEPTATE UTERUS results.

uterus, anteflexed A uterus that tilts forward. This is a normal position of the uterus.

uterus, anteverted A uterus that tilts toward the front of the abdomen; this is a normal position for the uterus.

vagina The female organ for the discharge of menstrual flow and for sexual intercourse, and the passageway through which the fetus is delivered. This muscular canal is lined with mucous membranes that extend from the outside of the body between the vulva and anus to the cervix of the uterus.

vaginal adenosis A specific abnormality of the vagina in women whose mothers took the medication DIETHYLSTIBESTEROL (DES) during pregnancy prior to 1971. In DES daughters who have vaginal adenosis, the growth of their vaginal lining is slowed. Although these changes are not precancerous, the cervical area where this occurs may develop cancer.

Experts recommend that DES daughters have frequent PAP SMEARS and colposcopy (a test using a magnifying scope to look at the vagina and cervix for signs of precancer cell growth.)

vaginal contraceptive film A vaginal SPERMICIDE contained in a paper-thin translucent sheet that contains a chemical that kills sperm (NONOXYNOL-9). The 2-inch by 2-inch contraceptive is simple to use and does not require a prescription.

After hands are washed with soap and water and dried the sheet is placed on or near the cervix inside the vagina, where it dissolves in seconds. Although it's effective for 1 hour, a woman must wait for at least 15 minutes after insertion before having sex. A new sheet is required before each episode of sexual intercourse. The contraceptive sheet may be used alone or with a

DIAPHRAGM or CONDOM, and protects against getting some sexually transmitted diseases.

While easy to use, the film is not as effective as some other contraceptives. Moreover, the film does not protect a woman from the AIDS virus or other infections. See also BARRIER METHODS; BIRTH CONTROL METHODS; SPERMICIDE.

vaginal contraceptive foam A SPERMICIDE (usually NONOXYNOL-9) in a foamy base that is inserted into the vagina before having sex. While it can be used alone, it's most effective when combined with another barrier method, such as a CONDOM or a DIAPHRAGM. Foam is a good method of backup birth control when taking birth control pills or when breast-feeding.

In addition, foam can be used as an emergency measure when a condom breaks. In this event, an applicator of foam can be inserted into the vagina as quickly as possible, followed by a call to the doctor about emergency birth control.

Contraceptive foam works by killing sperm directly and by preventing them from traveling up through the vagina and meeting an egg. When used alone, contraceptive foam is 80% to 90% effective, which means that 10 to 20 out of every 100 women who use only contraceptive foam will become pregnant. However, a woman who uses contraceptive foam with a condom every time can boost effectiveness to almost 100%. That means that fewer than 1 out of every 100 women who use foam and condoms will become pregnant.

Contraceptive foam can help protect against some sexually transmitted diseases, although nonoxynol-9 cannot protect against HIV, the virus that causes AIDS. Contraceptive foam is simple to use and inexpensive, and doesn't require a prescription. However, some couples object to the perfume or its taste; other find that the spermicide in the foam may cause itching, swelling, or burning.

vaginal ultrasound An ultrasound procedure used to determine follicular development and to guide the retrieval of eggs.

vaginitis An irritation in the vagina that often causes an abnormal discharge that can be caused by infections, lack of ESTROGEN, irritants, or allergies. Vaginitis is one of the most common reasons women seek health care; most women have it some time in life—often more than once. While usually it is not serious, it can be annoying and uncomfortable.

Frequent vaginitis may indicate the presence of pelvic adhesions and tubal blockage from other infections. It can be linked to infertility by interfering with SPERM penetration of the cervix. Symptoms may interfere with the ability or desire to have sex.

Symptoms

Vaginal irritation or an abnormal vaginal discharge, which may have an unpleasant odor (especially right after sex). There may be vaginal itching or burning, irritation, and a need to urinate more often than usual.

Cause

Vaginitis is most often caused by a bacterial, fungal, or parasitic infection. Between 20% to 25% of the vaginitis cases are caused by Candida, and about 75% of all women get a vaginal yeast infection at least once. In between 80% to 90% of the cases, it is caused by an overgrowth of the yeast *Candida albicans;* the remaining cases are caused by other species of candida. It isn't known what causes the yeast overgrowth, although antibiotics can inadvertently kill normal bacteria in the vagina and cause an overgrowth of candida.

Candida vaginitis is not considered a sexually transmitted disease because candida species are commonly found in the healthy vagina. Vaginal yeast infections tend to occur more frequently in women who

- are pregnant
- are diabetic and not controlling their disease
- take birth control pills, antibiotics, or corticosteroids
- have had previous candida infections
- have frequent sex
- have AIDS
- douche
- use perfumed feminine hygiene sprays
- wear tight clothing
- use vaginal sponges or an IUD

Some women have four or more attacks per year ("recurrent vaginal candidiasis").

Trichomoniasis accounts for 15% to 20% of the cases of vaginitis; about 2 to 3 million American women get trichomoniasis each year. Trichomoniasis is a sexually transmitted disease that occurs in both men and women and is caused by an infection with the single-celled parasite *Trichomonas vaginalis.* Infection with *T. vaginalis* is often associated with other sexually transmitted diseases and assists the spread of the AIDS virus.

Vaginitis also may be caused by allergic reaction, irritation, injury, low estrogen levels, and certain diseases.

Diagnosis

To diagnose vaginitis, the doctor examines the vagina and takes a sample of vaginal discharge for tests and microscopic analysis. Diagnosis may be difficult because there are many different causes of vaginitis. Women who think that they have vaginitis should consider seeing their doctor to get an accurate diagnosis. Many women assume that they have a yeast infection and take over-the-counter medicines without first consulting their doctors.

A diagnosis of candida vaginitis is made after finding a normal vaginal pH (4 to 4.5) and the presence of many yeast cells in the sample of vaginal discharge or growth of yeast on laboratory media. A trichomoniasis diagnosis is made when the parasites are found in the vaginal discharge either by microscopic examination or in laboratory cultures.

Treatment

Trichomoniasis is treated with either a large, single dose of metronidazole or with a smaller dose taken twice daily for 1 week. Male sexual partners of women with trichomoniasis also must be treated. Candida vaginitis is most often treated by medicated gels, creams, or suppositories applied directly to the vagina. The antifungal drugs used to treat Candida vaginitis include oral fluconazole (Diflucan), butoconazole (Femstat), clotrimazole (Gyne-lotrimin, Mycelex), miconazole (Monistat), and ticonazole (Vagistat). Most require only one or a few days of therapy to be effective. Women who have recurrent Candida infections may receive treatment for several weeks and then some form of a long-term preventative treatment.

Vaginitis is a disease with minor symptoms, and most women respond well to medications. Certain untreated vaginal infections can lead to more serious conditions such as PELVIC INFLAMMATORY DISEASE, ENDOMETRITIS, postsurgical infections, and spread of the AIDS virus.

Prevention

Vaginal infections may be prevented by following these suggestions. A woman should

- not take nonprescription yeast infection treatments unless she was diagnosed with candidiasis before and recognizes the symptoms
- not douche because it may disturb the balance of organisms in the vagina and spread them into the reproductive system
- thoroughly dry herself after bathing and remove a wet bathing suit promptly
- avoid wearing tight clothing
- wear cotton underwear
- clean DIAPHRAGMS, CERVICAL CAPS, AND SPERMICIDE applicators after use
- avoid sexually transmitted disease
- wipe from front to back after a bowel movement to avoid spreading bacteria to the vagina

vaginosis An infection that occurs when the normal balance of bacteria in the vagina changes, leading to an overgrowth of some bacteria normally found in the vagina. It is loosely associated with infertility, MISCARRIAGE, preterm birth, and low-birth weight babies.

Symptoms

Usually there is a heavy vaginal discharge. It is grayish and frothy and has an unpleasant odor.

Cause

The occurrence of bacterial vaginosis is difficult to determine, but studies have proposed that 10% to 41% of women have had it at least once; it's highest among African-American women and those who have had multiple sexual partners. Vaginosis is lowest among Asian women and women with no history of sexual contact with men. Bacterial vaginosis is not considered a sexually transmitted disease, although it can be acquired by sexual intercourse.

Bacterial vaginosis is not caused by a particular organism but is a change in the balance of normal vaginal bacteria for unknown reasons. Patients with vaginosis have very high numbers of bacteria such as *Gardnerella vaginalis*, *Mycoplasma hominis*, *Bacteroides* species, and *Mobiluncus* species.

Diagnosis

Vaginosis can be diagnosed by microscopic examination of the discharge. It may also be tested with chemicals.

Treatment

Treatment is optional when the infection is mild.

varicocele Dilated veins within the scrotum that create a pool of stagnant blood and is the most frequently diagnosed cause for poor SEMEN quality and MALE FACTOR INFERTILITY.

While only 10% to 15% of all men have varicoceles, the condition is found in about a third of those evaluated for male infertility. Therefore, although not all men with varicoceles are infertile, a significant number of infertile men have a varicocele. Experts aren't sure why varicoceles affect sperm, but they suspect that the dilated vein raises the temperature in the scrotum, leading to sperm abnormalities that cause male infertility.

Cause

A varicocele is caused when blood flows backward and pools, due to malfunctioning or missing valves in the spermatic veins. Because of the long, top-to-bottom route of the internal spermatic vein on the left side of each testis, more than 90% of varicoceles occur on the left.

Diagnosis

For a correct diagnosis, the patient should be examined standing up so that the doctor can compare the cord structures in both testicles. Then the patient may be asked to exhale forcefully with a closed nose and mouth, which will make an existing varicocele more prominent. The doctor will examine the scrotum while the patient is lying down as well. Sometimes varicoceles also can be seen with the naked eye, but small varicoceles may be detectable only with advanced technology, such as an ultrasound.

Treatment

Surgical correction is usually recommended for an infertile man only when semen quality problems can't be explained any other way, or in the case of shrinking size or pain in the testicles. The surgery (called VARICOCELECTOMY) involves tying off the affected spermatic veins. Some varicose veins that are identified during X ray can be treated by sealing off the vein with a blood clot.

Both methods may be performed on an outpatient basis, using regional or local anesthesia.

There are few side effects from surgical correction, and the operation often improves semen quality. However, the exact role of varicocele repair in the infertility evaluation is not uniformly agreed upon by experts.

varicocelectomy Removal of a swelling (VARICOCELE) in the scrotum caused by veins that have dilated and filled with blood. Blood tends to pool in these swollen veins, raising the temperature in the testes and interfering with SPERM production. Abnormal sperm counts, movement and shape are associated with varicoceles. About 15% of all men have varicoceles, but the incidence can be as high as a third of men who are infertile. About 30,000 men are treated every year in the United States with this safe, routine procedure.

Not every man with varicoceles needs corrective surgery, but when no other cause can be found for poor sperm quality and no significant female problems are identified, a varicocelectomy may be a good idea.

Fortunately, surgical procedures can be performed to tie off damaged veins and restore sperm production to normal. The surgery is designed to relieve discomfort in the scrotum, reduce congestion around the testicles, and improve quality and amount of sperm production.

Between 50% and 80% of men find that their semen quality improves after a varicocelectomy, and about 40% succeed in impregnating their partners.

Procedure

Varicocelectomy is considered a minor surgical procedure using either regional or local anesthesia. During the operation, an incision is made in the scrotum, and abnormal veins are cut and tied. The dilated veins that form the varicocele are cut free and removed, and the skin is closed with sutures that will be absorbed by the body. Complications such as bleeding or infection are uncommon.

The link between varicoceles and male infertility is controversial. There is scant medical literature that proves the value of varicocelectomy to treat infertility.

vas deferens, congenital absence of The absence at birth of the two vas deferens, which move SPERM along from the testes to the ejaculate. It is a cause of obstructive AZOOSPERMIA (lack of sperm). The vas deferens on each side is usually affected. This causes infertility, although it can be overcome by extracting sperm from the testicles as a prelude to IN VITRO FERTILIZATION.

This condition is usually caused by a gene for CYSTIC FIBROSIS. There is a test to uncover any abnormal genes; should the abnormal gene for cystic fibrosis be found, the woman also should be screened to predict the chance of cystic fibrosis in the offspring. (Cystic fibrosis will result only if both parents have the recessive gene for the condition.)

vasectomy The surgical separation of the vas deferens (the tube that carries sperm from the testicles to the urethra in the penis) as a means of permanent birth control. This surgery does not affect the man's ability to achieve orgasm or ejaculate. There will still be a fluid ejaculate, but there will be no sperm in this fluid. Although this surgery is relatively minor, because it is intended to be permanent, it should not be undertaken unless the man is completely certain that he will never want any more children.

When couples seek surgical sterilization, the vasectomy is often the procedure of choice because it is simpler than a woman's TUBAL LIGATION.

A vasectomy can be performed under local anesthesia in the doctor's office in about 30 minutes. After injecting an anesthetic in the scrotal area, the doctor locates the vas deferens (one in each testicle) and makes a small opening in the skin of the scrotal sac. Through this opening, the doctor withdraws a small segment of the vas deferens and surgically removes a short length of the tube. Either end is sealed with stitches. The severed ends are returned to the scrotum, and the outer incision is stitched closed. The procedure is then repeated on the other side.

After Surgery

The man spends a brief recovery period in the doctor's office. Strenuous activity such as heavy exercise should be avoided for the next few days. Some pain and swelling in the area of the incision is normal, but if the pain persists it should be checked out by a doctor. Doctors recommend wearing a scrotal supporter for 3 to 4 days after the procedure. An ice pack may be used to prevent or reduce swelling, and oral pain medications can usually easily manage the pain. Most men return to work within 2 to 3 days. Sex can be resumed about a week after the surgery.

The sperm count gradually decreases after vasectomy. Since the first 10 to 15 ejaculations after surgery may still contain sperm, the couple must use other types of birth control for a short period of time after the vasectomy. At 4 to 6 weeks, sperm should no longer be present in the semen, but a semen specimen must be examined and found to be totally free of sperm a month or more after vasectomy before the patient can rely on the vasectomy for birth control. Continued use of contraception is recommended until two to three sperm count tests are negative, indicating that the patient is sterile. See also BIRTH CONTROL METHODS.

vasography An X-ray study in which dye is injected into the vas deferens to reveal a block. It is usually used to check for an obstruction in men with no sperm (AZOOSPERMIA).

The procedure is done in an operating room under general anesthesia, where it can be combined with microsurgical correction if a block is found. A small vertical cut is made over the testis, which is then pulled forward. Using an operating microscope and microsurgical tools, the surgeon inspects the cavity of the vas for the presence of sperm-containing fluid. If no fluid is present, a flexible tube is passed through the vas to the EPIDIDYMIS, which is "milked" for fluid. If there is still no fluid, the seminal vesicle end of the vas is filled with a water or dye solution to confirm that this region is not blocked.

If a large amount of sperm-containing fluid is present when the vas deferens is opened, this indicates that there is probably a block in the seminal vesicle end of the vas. A catheter is passed up through the vas and is filled with water-soluble dye; the procedure is then repeated with the vas on the other side. If a blockage is found at the ejaculatory ducts, it is surgically corrected. If the vas deferens ends blindly, far away from the ejaculatory ducts, no further surgery is performed.

If a blockage is found in the groin region, the surgeon will surgically connect the unobstructed portions of the vas deferens.

If there are no sperm in the fluid from the vasography site, and there is no blockage at the seminal vesicle end of the vas, the vas may be cut and readied for vasoepididymostomy—a surgically made connection between the vas deferens and the epididymis.

vasovasostomy The reversal of a VASECTOMY. This operation repairs the severed vas deferens by reconnecting the ends to reestablish the flow of sperm. The reversal procedure is not a simple operation, since it involves connecting the two ends of both tubes, each with tiny openings.

If the vas deferens is blocked, the surgeon may try to connect the epididymis to an area in the vas that bypasses the blockage. Use of an experimental special glue instead of sutures may help reduce operation time and difficulty. Laser surgery may reduce operating time and cause fewer complications.

Reversal surgery is a major operation lasting 1 or 2 hours, a brief hospital stay, and 2 to 3 weeks recovery at home. It is far more expensive than a vasectomy; it's even more expensive if the procedure involves connecting the vas to the epididymis, which takes about 3 hours.

Even when the operation is successful and pregnancy is achieved, studies suggest that it may take up to a year after the surgery to conceive.

Reversal surgery is usually not reimbursed by insurance companies.

Success Rate

Pregnancy rate after a vasectomy reversal depends on several things, including the length of time that has passed since the vasectomy was first performed, the quality of fluid in the vas deferens, and whether there are any female problems with infertility. The longer the time that has elapsed since the vasectomy was done, the less successful a reversal will be.

Depending on the circumstances, a reversal can be successful as often as 75% of the time. However, if it has been between 3 and 8 years after a vasectomy, the prenancy rate drops to 53%, 9 to 14 years is 44%, and more than 15 years is 30%. The lower rates as time passes may be due to increasing chance for obstruction of the epididymis and the development of ANTISPERM ANTIBODIES.

The type of surgical technique also may affect the success of the reversal. Advanced microscopic techniques are increasing the chances of a reversal's success, but the rates still vary widely. In one small study, 89% of the procedures successfully reopened the tubes, and the pregnancy rate was 44%. These results were very similar, however, to those reported with macroscopic vasovasostomy, which uses magnification rather than microscopic tools. This less advanced technique has slightly lower success rates than microscopic procedures, but it is less expensive and has a shorter operating time than the newer techniques.

A successful reversal is more likely if the section removed during vasectomy was short, if the original procedure was performed on straight sections of the vas, and if the joined pieces were of equal size.

Reasons for Failure

A reversal of a vasectomy may not be successful even if the tubes have been successfully reattached. If the sperm count doesn't recover within a reasonable period after vasovasostomy, a secondary blockage of the epididymis is most often the cause. This can be corrected with a second procedure.

And while it's usually possible to reopen the epididymis, fertility may not be restored. After vasectomy, sperm continue to be produced, but instead of remaining in the reproductive passages, they leak into the body where the immune system perceives them as foreign invaders and develops antibodies to attack them. Even if a reversal is performed, such antibodies often persist.

Antibodies bind to specific parts of the sperm, such as the head or tail, and cause problems depending on where they attach. Sperm with these antibodies may stick together, fail to interact with cervical mucus, or fail to penetrate the egg.

High doses of corticosteroids may be useful in conjunction with intrauterine insemination for infertile men who show antibodies to their own sperm, although experts aren't sure how effective this is, and these drugs have potentially serious side effects with prolonged use. Some experts believe that in most cases the presence of these antibodies will not prevent conception unless a large percentage of sperm (70% or more for the most common antibody) is affected.

Assisted reproductive technologies are the best approach at this time for men with evidence of antisperm autoantibodies due to vasectomy or other causes.

Reoperations

If pregnancy fails after a reversal, in some cases a repeat operation may be effective. Success rates depend on several factors, including the doctor's skill, complications from the original operation, the effects of antisperm antibodies, and the time elapsed since vasectomy. Even though tubes are open and sperm is restored in as many as 85% of men, pregnancy rates still only average about 30%.

In one study, conception rates after reoperations were highest (80%) in couples who had

had children. The pregnancy rate was only 17% when men had remarried and were trying to have a child for the first time.

Damage to the epididymis occurs in about 75% of men who request a repeat operation after vasovasostomy failure. This requires an operation called vasoepididymostomy, which creates a bypass around the obstruction. Microscopic techniques are critical for the success of this procedure and require a specialist to perform them. Success rates are higher for repairing obstructions closer to the testicles because the epididymis is wider in this area. In general, pregnancy rates are around 20%. Damage in other ducts and small tubes are a major reason for vasoepididymostomy failure.

Fertility Treatments

ASSISTED REPRODUCTIVE TECHNOLOGIES (ART) or INTRAUTERINE INSEMINATION are available for men who want to conceive children after a failed vasectomy reversal. Some studies suggest that it may be cheaper to have ART instead of a vasectomy reversal. One 10-year analysis reported a pregnancy rate of 44% after reversal surgery, with a cost of more than $12,000, as compared to a 41% success rate and cost of $9,500 for those who banked sperm and had an average of three INTRAUTERINE INSEMINATION treatments.

For men whose vasovasostomy failed, however, a repeat procedure seems to be cheaper than beginning fertility treatments at that point.

INTRACYTOPLASMIC SPERM INJECTION (ICSI) is a very effective fertilization technique for men who have had vasectomies or failed reversal surgery. In this procedure, sperm are usually taken from the epididymis using a technique called EPIDIDYMAL SPERM ASPIRATION (MESA). The fertilized egg is then implanted in the woman.

VDTs and infertility   Some experts suspect that electromagnetic wave emissions from a computer screen (video display terminal or VDT) may be linked to infertility.

Studies of electromagnetic wave emissions, including those from computer displays, have been inconclusive. Nearly all monitors now comply with guidelines that reduce emissions, and laptop computers, which use liquid crystal display monitors, are completely safe.

In any case, experts usually advise women to avoid the side and back of computers where wave emission is strongest and sit as far from the front of the screen as possible.

venereal disease   Any infection that can be sexually transmitted, such as chlamydia, gonorrhea, ureaplasma, and syphilis. Many of these diseases will interfere with fertility, and some will cause severe illness. See also PELVIC INFLAMMATORY DISEASE; SEXUALLY TRANSMITTED DISEASES AND INFERTILITY.

Viagra   The first successful medication for ERECTILE DYSFUNCTION (impotence). In the United States, more than 5 million men have turned to Viagra to improve their sexual function, where it has been prescribed more than 16 million times.

This extremely popular drug, introduced in 1998, works by blocking the activity of a chemical that triggers a series of reactions in the body allowing men to have an erection. Neither an aphrodisiac nor a hormone, for most patients Viagra takes about 30 minutes to work and can last up to 4 hours. However, with Viagra a man must be sexually aroused to get an erection. If a man takes Viagra and isn't stimulated, nothing

will happen. An erection won't occur just by taking the pill.

Viagra leads to an improvement in erections for up to 82% of patients who take it, which means it works for more than 4 out of every 5 couples who try it. Viagra improves erections in most men regardless of how long they have had ED, what caused it, or how old they are.

Side Effects

The most common side effects are headache, facial flushing, and upset stomach. Viagra may also briefly cause bluish or blurred vision, or sensitivity to light. Patients should seek immediate medical help in the rare event of an erection lasting more than 4 hours.

However, Viagra isn't for everyone. Heart patients should make sure their doctors approve the use of Viagra. The drug should never be taken with any nitrate medicine, because blood pressure could suddenly drop to an unsafe or life-threatening level. Nitrates are found in many prescription medications that are used to treat angina (chest pain due to heart disease), including nitroglycerin sprays, ointments, skin patches or pastes, and tablets that are swallowed or dissolved in the mouth. Nitrates are also found in recreational drugs such as amyl nitrate or nitrite ("poppers").

vitelline membrane   Another term for the ZONA PELLUCIDA.

weight and infertility Weight (too much and too little) and excess exercise can affect fertility in significant ways.

Weight Loss

Low weight or a severe weight loss can lead to a drop in GONADOTROPIN-RELEASING HORMONE (Gn-RH) that the brain sends to the ovaries and testes to signal the release of GONADOTROPINS, which are critical for the development of eggs and SPERM.

The degree to which weight loss affects fertility will vary. In women who lose only a small amount of weight, the ovaries may still produce and release eggs, but the lining of the UTERUS may not be ready to receive a fertilized egg because of inadequate ovarian PROGESTERONE production (LUTEAL PHASE DEFECT). In more severe cases of weight loss, OVULATION does not occur, and menstrual cycles are irregular or absent. Low weight or weight loss in men can lead to a drop in sperm function or count.

If low weight or weight loss has been identified as the cause of infertility, the preferred treatment is to stop losing weight, or even to gain weight if needed. An alternative treatment is the use of medications such as gonadotropins to restore fertility. However, the use of these drugs can be complicated and expensive, and carries the risk of multiple pregnancies.

Obesity

While being very thin can lead to infertility, being overweight or obese also can affect hormonal signals sent to the ovaries or testes. Increased weight can boost insulin levels in women, which may cause the overies to over-produce male hormones and interfere with the release of eggs.

In cases of obesity, the best plan is to lose weight, but drugs such as CLOMIPHENE CITRATE or gonadotropins can be given as well. It is important to make sure that blood sugar levels are normal before trying to get pregnant and that there are no specific metabolic causes of obesity.

Excessive Exercise

Proper exercise and diet are important for maintaining good health, but too much exercise can lead to a drop in sperm production in men and the cessation of ovulation in women by decreasing the brain message to the ovaries and testes. While it's a good idea to get enough exercise, it's also possible to get too much exercise. This can lead to a drop in sperm production and the cessation of ovulation in women. However, in these instances, the amount of exercise must be quite high.

A normal exercise program will not affect fertility for most couples. While it's impossible to know just how much exercise is too much, it's generally believed that running more than 10 miles a week is considered too much when trying to conceive. The best way to treat fertility problems caused by too much exercise is to decrease or modify the amount of exercise.

wine and infertility See ALCOHOL AND INFERTILITY.

withdrawal A type of natural birth control in which a man will pull his penis out of the vagina before he ejaculates. This can work because pregnancy can't happen if SPERM is kept out of the vagina, but it's not considered very reliable. Of every 100 women whose partners use withdrawal, 19 will become pregnant during the first year of typical use. Of every 100 women whose partners use withdrawal, 4 will become pregnant during the first year of perfect use.

The reason withdrawal is not highly effective as a birth control method is because some fluid (pre-ejaculate) can leak out of the penis before ejaculation that contains enough sperm to cause pregnancy. Pregnancy is also possible if semen or pre-ejaculate is spilled on the vulva. In addition, withdrawal offers no protection against sexually transmitted infections.

The man who uses this method must withdraw his penis from the vagina before or when he feels he has reached the point when ejaculation can no longer be stopped or postponed. He ejaculates outside the vagina, being careful that semen does not spill onto his partner's vulva. However, some men can't tell when they are going to ejaculate, and some men ejaculate very quickly, before they realize it.

workplace hazards and infertility   Thousands of hazardous chemicals are produced and used in a wide variety of jobs, but only a few are known to harm the reproductive health of both men and women workers who are exposed to them. There are also physical and biological substances such as radiation and bacteria used in many workplaces that expose workers to other reproductive hazards. Most chemical substances and work situations have not been studied for their potential to damage human reproduction.

Exposure to certain substances on the job can prevent conception, change a person's sex drive, damage eggs or sperm, change the genetic material, or cause cancer or other diseases in the reproductive organs of men or women. As a result, some industries have implemented transfer policies that allow women workers to move out of areas with possible exposures when they are pregnant or thinking about becoming pregnant.

The harmful effects of a few substances in the workplace have been recognized for many years. More than 100 years ago, lead was discovered to cause MISCARRIAGES, stillbirths, and infertility in women pottery workers. It's important to remember that reproductive hazards don't affect every worker. Whether a man, a woman or her baby is harmed depends on how much of the hazard they are exposed to, when they are exposed, how long they are exposed, and how they are exposed. Workplace substances that affect workers can also harm their families. Without knowing it, workers can bring home harmful substances that can affect the health of other family members, both adults and children. For example, lead brought home from the workplace on a worker's skin, hair, clothes, shoes, tool box, or car can cause lead poisoning in family members, especially young children.

Women on the Job

A reproductive hazard could cause one or more health effects, depending on when the woman is exposed. For example, exposure to harmful substances during the first 3 months of pregnancy might cause a birth defect or a miscarriage. During the last 6 months of pregnancy, exposure to reproductive hazards could slow the growth of the fetus, affect the development of its brain, or cause premature labor. Reproductive hazards may not affect every worker or every pregnancy.

FEMALE REPRODUCTIVE HAZARDS	
Agent	**Observed Effects**
Ethylene glycol ethers (2-ethoxyethanol and 2-methoxyethanol)	Miscarriage
Carbon disulfide	Menstrual cycle changes
Lead	Infertility, miscarriage, low birthweight, developmental disorders
Ionizing radiation	Infertility, miscarriage, birth defects, low birthweight, childhood cancers, developmental disorders

Agent	Observed Effects
Prolonged standing, lifting	Miscarriage late in pregnancy, premature delivery

Harmful substances can enter the body by inhalation, contact with the skin, or ingestion (if workers do not properly wash their hands before eating, drinking, or smoking).

Men on the Job

Many people don't realize that a man's exposure to substances in the workplace can affect his ability to have healthy children. A number of workplace substances such as lead and radiation have been identified as reproductive hazards for men, but there is no complete list of reproductive hazards in the workplace. Scientists are just beginning to understand how these hazards affect the male reproductive system. Although more than 1,000 workplace chemicals have been shown to have reproductive effects on animals, most have not been studied in humans. In addition, most of the 4 million other chemical mixtures in commercial use remain untested.

Some reproductive hazards can stop or slow the production of sperm, so there will be fewer sperm present to fertilize an egg; if no sperm are produced, the man is sterile. If the hazard prevents sperm from being made, sterility may be permanent. Other hazards may alter the shape of sperm cells so that they have trouble swimming or lack the ability to fertilize the egg. Hazardous chemicals may collect in the epididymis, seminal vesicles, or prostate, where they may destroy sperm, change the way in which they swim, or attach to the sperm and be carried to the egg or the unborn child.

Reproductive hazards also can affect the chromosomes found in sperm. The sperm and egg each contributes 23 chromosomes at fertilization. The DNA stored in these chromosomes determines what we will look like and how our bodies will function. Radiation or chemicals may cause changes or breaks in the DNA. If the sperm's DNA is damaged, it may not be able to fertilize an egg; or if it does fertilize an egg, it may affect the development of the fetus. Some cancer treatment drugs are known to cause such

MALE REPRODUCTIVE HAZARDS (NATIONAL INSTITUTE OF OCCUPATIONAL SAFETY AND HEALTH)

Type of Exposure	Lowered Number of Sperm	Abnormal Sperm Shape	Altered Sperm Transfer	Altered Hormones/ Sexual Performance
Lead	X	X	X	X
Dibromochloropropane	X			
Carbaryl (Sevin)		X		
Toluenediamine and dinitrotoluene	X			
Ethylene dibromide	X	X	X	
Plastic production (styrene and acetone)		X		
Ethylene glycol monoethyl ether	X			
Welding		X	X	
Perchloroethylene			X	
Mercury vapor				X
Heat	X		X	
Military radar	X			
Kepone**		X		
Bromine vapor**				
Radiation** (Chernobyl)	X	X	X	X
Carbon disulfide				X
2,4-Dichlorophenoxy acetic acid (2, 4-D)		X	X	

* Studies to date show that some men experience the health effects listed here from workplace exposures. However, these effects may not occur in every worker. The amount of time a worker is exposed, the amount of hazard to which he is exposed, and other personal factors may all determine whether an individual is affected.

** Workers were exposed to high levels as a result of a workplace accident.

damage. However, little is known about the effects of workplace hazards on sperm chromosomes.

Finally, if a damaged sperm does fertilize an egg, the egg might not develop properly, causing a miscarriage or a possible health problem in the baby. If a reproductive hazard is carried in the semen, the fetus might be exposed within the uterus, possibly leading to problems with the pregnancy or with the health of the baby after it is born.

Z

ZIFT   See ZYGOTE INTRAFALLOPIAN TRANSFER.

Zoladex   The brand name for goserelin.

zona pellucida   The hard outer surface of the egg. The sperm must penetrate this outer surface before fertilization can occur.

zygote   The medical term for a fertilized egg (also, the embryo in the early stages of development).

zygote intrafallopian transfer (ZIFT)   One type of ASSISTED REPRODUCTIVE TECHNOLOGY (ART). In this procedure, as in IN VITRO FERTILIZATION (IVF) and GAMETE INTRAFALLOPIAN TRANSFER (GIFT), a woman's ovaries are first stimulated with GONADOTROPINS and monitored with blood tests and ultrasound, and when the eggs mature they are removed by a vaginal ultrasound oocyte retrieval. Sperm are collected, processed, and used to fertilize the egg in the lab. The resulting fertilized eggs, which have not yet divided, are called zygotes. In ZIFT, they are transferred into the woman's FALLOPIAN TUBES, rather than into the UTERUS.

ZIFT is very much like TUBAL EMBRYO TRANSFER (TET), except that the transfer to the fallopian tube occurs as soon as fertilization has been observed, and before the cells have divided and the embryo begins to develop.

ZIFT is rarely recommended as often as IVF, because IVF involves only one surgical procedure. The lack of data to support its superiority to IVF has limited its usefulness.

APPENDIXES

APPENDIX I
ORGANIZATIONS

ADOPTION

Adoptive Families of America
33 Highway 100 N.
Minneapolis, MN 55422
(800) 372-3300
http://www.adoptivefam.org

National nonprofit membership organization of 18,000 families and individuals and more than 250 adoptive parent support groups offers problem-solving help and information about the challenges of adoption to members of adoptive and prospective adoptive families; offers free "starter" kit, fact sheet, education, national magazine, aid to children, and advocacy.

Adoption Resource Exchange for Single Parents, Inc. (ARESP)
8605 Cameron Street, Suite 220
Silver Spring, MD 29010
(301) 585-5836
http://www.aresp.org

Nonprofit organization offering newsletter, information, referrals, and support to single parents interested in adoption.

American Academy of Adoption Attorneys
Box 33053
Washington, DC 20033-0053
(802) 832-2222
http://www.adoptionattorneys.org

National association of attorneys interested in the field of adoption law who promote adoption law reform and provide information on ethical adoption practices. Offers a newsletter, annual meetings, educational seminars, and directory.

Child Welfare League of America
440 First Street, NW, Suite 310
Washington, DC 20001
(202) 638-2952

Publishes the *National Adoption Resource Directory*, listing adoption agencies around the country.

Family Pride Coalition
P.O. Box 34337
San Diego, CA 92163
(619) 296-0199
http://www.familypride.org

Organization dedicated to helping gay, lesbian, bisexual, and transgendered couples adopt; provides information, support, and referrals.

Latin American Parents Association
P.O. Box 339
Brooklyn, NY 11234
(718) 236-8689
http://www.lapa.com

Provides information about adopting babies from Latin America.

National Adoption Center
1218 Chestnut Street
Philadelphia, PA 19107
(800) TOADOPT (not in PA); (215) 925-0200 (in PA)
http://www.adopt.org

Promotes adoption of children throughout the country (especially those with special needs).

National Adoption Information Clearinghouse
1400 Eye Street NW, Suite 600
Washington, DC 20005
(202) 842-1919
http://www.calib.com/naic/

Provides fact sheets, articles, and information about adoption, a computerized list of books, a directory of adoption agencies and other resources, and information on state and federal laws on adoption.

National Council for Adoption
1930 17th Street, NW
Washington, DC 20009
(202) 328-1200

Association of private adoption agencies that provides information, publications, and resource listings on adoption.

North American Council on Adoptable Children
970 Raymond Avenue #106
St. Paul, MN 55114
(612) 644-3036
http://www.nacac.org

National support group for adoptive parents that specializes in placing older, handicapped, and minority children.

OURS, Inc.
3333 Highway 100 North
Minneapolis, MN 55422
(612) 535-4829

National support group that provides information about licensed adoption agencies, with a focus on foreign adoptions.

ANDROLOGY

American Society of Andrology
P.O. Box 15171
Lenexa, KS 66285
(913) 541-9077
http://www.andrologysociety.com

Professional group that refers patients to andrologists across the country.

BIRTH CONTROL

AVSC International (formerly, the Association for Voluntary Surgical Contraception)
440 Ninth Avenue
New York, NY 10001
(212) 561-8000
http://www.avsc.org

Group that works worldwide to make reproductive health services safe and available, providing technical assistance, training, and information, with a focus on practical solutions. Provides information, support, referral, job information, publications, and working papers.

Planned Parenthood Federation of America
810 Seventh Avenue
New York, NY 10019
(212) 541-7800
http://www.plannedparenthood.org

Provides referral to local Planned Parenthood affiliates that may supply infertility diagnosis and counseling.

CUSHING'S DISEASE

National Cushing's Association
4645 Van Nuys Boulevard, 104
Sherman Oaks, CA 91403
(818) 788-9235; (818) 788-9239

National organization providing information and support to patients with Cushing's syndrome.

Cushing's Support and Research Foundation, Inc.
65 East India Row 22B
Boston, MA 02110
(617) 723-3824; (617) 723-3674
http://www.std.com/~csrf/

Relatively new organization offering a newsletter, a networking list, and information.

Pituitary Tumor Network Association
16350 Ventura Boulevard #231
Encino, CA 91436
(805) 499-9973
http://www.pituitary.com

Nonprofit group that supports and funds research on pituitary tumors and related pituitary disorders, providing information, publications, and support.

CYSTIC FIBROSIS

Cystic Fibrosis Foundation
6931 Arlington Road
Bethesda, MD 20814
(800) 344-4823
http://www.cff.org

A non-profit organization working to develop ways to control and cure CF. The group offers information, resources, and information on clinical trials.

DIETHYLSTILBESTROL (DES)

DES Action USA
1615 Broadway
Oakland, CA 94612

(510) 465-4011
http://www.desaction.org

Provides education and support to mothers, daughters, and sons exposed to the drug diethylstilbestrol (DES).

ENDOCRINOLOGY

The Endocrine Society
4350 East West Highway, Suite 500
Bethesda, MD 20814-4410
(301) 941-0200
http://www.endo-society.org

World's largest organization devoted to the research, study, and clinical practice of endocrinology, offering information, links to other sites, placement services, publications, and meetings relating to endocrinology.

National Adrenal Diseases Foundation
505 Northern Boulevard
Great Neck, NY 11021
(516) 487-4992
http://www.medhelp.org/nadf

A non-profit organization dedicated to providing support information and education to people with adrenal disease. The group also sponsors support groups and provides quarterly newsletters.

Thyroid Foundation of America
Ruth Sleeper Hall, Room RSL 350
40 Parkman Street
Boston, MA 02114
(800) 832-8321; (617) 726-8500
http://www.tsh.org

Non-profit group providing information, books, newsletters, and referrals to local thyroid specialists.

ENDOMETRIOSIS

Endometriosis Association
8585 North 76th Place
Milwaukee, WI 53223
(800) 992-3636 (in U.S.); (800) 426-2363 (in Canada)

Provides information on local support groups, crisis call assistance, and education and research programs regarding endometriosis.

Institute for the Study and Treatment of Endometriosis
2425 West 22nd Street
Oak Brook, IL 60523
(630) 954-0054

or
550 West Webster Avenue
Chicago, IL 60614
(773) 883-3880
http://www.endometriosisinstitute.com

A non-profit organization fostering research, education, and clinical advances in endometriosis.

GENETICS

National Society of Genetic Counselors
233 Canterbury Drive
Wallingford, PA 19086
(610) 872-7608
http://www.nsgc.com

Provides information on genetic counseling services and referrals.

IMPOTENCE (ERECTILE DYSFUNCTION)

Sexual Function Health Council
American Foundation for Urologic Disease
1128 North Charles Street
Baltimore, MD 21201
(410) 468-1800
http://www.afud.org
http:www.impotence.org

A health council of the American Foundation for Urologic disease that offers patient brochures on erectile dysfunction (impotence).

American Urological Association
1120 North Charles Street
Baltimore, MD 21201-5559
(410) 727-1100
http://www.auanet.org

A professional association for the advancement of urologic care. Website offers the latest information on urological conditions, including impotence.

American Association of Sex Educators, Counselors and Therapists (AASECT)
P.O. Box 238
Mount Vernon, IA 52314
http://www.aasect.org

Impotence Institute of America
8201 Corporate Drive, Suite 320
Landover, MD 20715
(800) 669-1603
http://www.impotenceworld.org

A division of the Impotence World Association, this group is a non-profit association dedicated to impotence education, and sponsors Impotence Anonymous.

INFERTILITY

American College of Obstetricians and Gynecologists Resource Center
409 12th Street, SW
P.O. Box 96920
Washington, DC 20090
(202) 638-5577

Provides information on a variety of medical conditions, including infertility at its resource center, including pamphlets, lists of ob-gyns in certain parts of the country, and answers to basic questions about infertility and women's health.

American Society for Reproductive Medicine
2140 11th Avenue South, Ste. 200
Birmingham, AL 35205
(205) 933-8494
http://www.asrm.com

A professional group devoted to advancing knowledge in reproductive medicine.

American Society of Andrology
74 New Montgomery, Suite 230
San Francisco, CA 94105
(415) 764-4823
http://www.andrologysociety.com

A unique partnership of scientists and clinicians interested in the study of male reproduction.

Fertility Plus
http://www.fertilityplus.org

Nonprofit website for patient information about infertility.

International Council on Infertility Information Dissemination
P.O. Box 91363
Tucson, AZ 85752
(520) 544-9548
www.inciid.org

A non-profit website dedicated to advocacy of the infertile customer.

RESOLVE, Inc.
1310 Broadway
Somerville, MA 02144

(617) 623-0744
http://www.resolve.org

Provides physician and IVF referrals, literature about aspects of infertility, newsletter, telephone counseling, and support groups.

INSURANCE

IVF-PALS Hotline
(800) IVF-PALS

Hotline that provides specific information about health insurance coverage for IVF.

MISCARRIAGE

Center for Loss in Multiple Birth, Inc.
c/o Jean Kollantai
P.O. Box 91377
Anchorage, AK 99509
(907) 222-5321
http://www.climb-support.org/

By and for parents throughout the United States, Canada, and beyond who have experienced the death of one or more, both, or all their children during a twin, triplet, or higher multiple pregnancy at birth. Provides newsletter, parent contact list, bibliography of information, and articles.

Compassionate Friends
The Compassionate Friends, Inc.
P.O. Box 3696
Oak Brook, IL 60522
(630) 990-0010; toll-free (877) 969-0010
http://www.compassionatefriends.org

Nonprofit group for parents who have lost a child of any age, including from miscarriage; offers resources, FAQs, magazine, newsletter, support, chapter locater, brochures, conferences, and links.

M.E.N.D. (Mommies Enduring Neonatal Death)
P.O. Box 1007
Coppell, TX 75019
(800) 695-MEND; toll-free (888) 695-MEND.
http://www.mend.org

Nonprofit organization offering Internet resources and free bimonthly newsletter; hosts three types of support groups: one for those who have recently lost a baby to miscarriage, stillbirth, and infant death; one for those who are considering becoming pregnant or are currently pregnant after a loss, and a "Daddies group" just for men.

SHARE – Pregnancy and Infant Loss Support, Inc.

Joseph Health Center
300 First Capitol Drive
St. Charles, MO 63301
(314) 947-6164

Provides information packets on miscarriage, still-birth, ectopic pregnancy, and neonatal death, references and articles, audiovisual material on grieving, bimonthly newsletter, a listing of parents in outreach groups, and support group referrals.

MULTIPLE BIRTH

The Center for Study of Multiple Birth (CSMB)

Suite 464
333 E Superior Street
Chicago, IL 60611
(312) 266-9093
http://www.multiplebirth.com/

Promotes and advances the health of women and children (particularly multiples) through education, research, and public service; offers resources, articles, research, news, and events.

Fullhouse MOMs

http://www.spindesign.com/fullhouse/

Nonprofit online support group designed to educate, assist, and support parents, expectant parents and legal guardians of multiple birth children; includes special activities, bulletin board, and links.

Mothers of Supertwins (MOST)

P.O. Box 951
Brentwood, NY 11717-0627
(631) 859-1110
http://www.mostonline.org

An international non-profit support group of families with triplets (or more), providing information, support, and empathy.

The National Organization of Mothers of Twins Clubs, Inc. (NOMOTC)

P.O. Box 23188
Albuquerque, NM 8792-1188
(505) 275-0955

Support group for parents of multiples, offering information, publications, research, referrals, special needs, and links.

The Triplet Connection

P.O. Box 99571
Stockton, CA 95209
(209) 474-0885
http://www.tripletconnection.org

A non-profit organization for multiple-birth families that provides vital information to those expecting triplets, quadruplets, quintuplets, or more, as well as encouragement, resources, and networking opportunities for families who are parents of larger multiples.

POLYCYSTIC OVARY SYNDROME

Polycystic Ovary Syndrome Association, Inc.

P.O. Box 80517
Portland, OR 97280
(877) 775-PCOS
http://www.pcosupport.org

A non-profit organization offering information, support, and conferences about PCOS.

REPRODUCTIVE HEALTH AND TECHNOLOGY

Association of Reproductive Health Professionals

2401 Pennsylvania Avenue NW
Suite 350
Washington, DC 20037-1718
(202) 466-3825
http://www.arhp.org

This non-profit medical organization offers education to physicians and patients about important reproductive health issues.

American Society for Reproductive Medicine

1209 Montgomery Highway
Birmingham, AL 35216
(205) 978-5000
e-mail: asrm@asrm.com

National organization of fertility specialists providing general information about infertility.

Society for Assisted Reproductive Technology (SART)

1209 Montgomery Highway
Birmingham, AL 35216
(205) 978-5000
http://www.sart.org
e-mail: asrm@asrm.com

An organization providing information on assisted reproductive technology. Website offers a fertility clinic locator for patients.

Society of Reproductive Endocrinologists (SRE)
1209 Montgomery Highway
Birmingham, AL 35216
(205) 978-5000

A membership society that works to extend knowledge of human reproduction and endocrinology.

Society of Reproductive Surgeons
1209 Montgomery Highway
Birmingham, AL 35216
(205) 978-5000
http://www.reprodsurgery.org

A forum for members of the American Society of Reproductive Medicine with Special interest in reproductive surgery. The group encourages research and education.

SEXUALLY TRANSMITTED DISEASES

American Social Health Association
P.O. Box 13827
100 Capitol Drive
Research Triangle Park, NC 27709-3827
(800) 230-6039; (919) 361-8400
http://www.ashastd.org

An organization that provides reliable information about sexually transmitted diseases.

SPERM BANKS

American Association of Tissue Banks
1350 Beverly Road, Suite 220-A
McLean, VA 22101
(703) 827-9582
http://www.aatb.org

Supplies a list of AATB-associated sperm banks in the United States and Canada.

SURROGACY

American Surrogacy Center
638 Church Street NE
Marietta, GA 30063
(770) 426-1107
http://www.surrogacy.com

An organization providing information on surrogacy and egg donation.

The Organization of Parents Through Surrogacy (OPTS)
P.O. Box 611
Gurnee, IL 60031
(847) 782-0224
http://www.opts.com

This organization provides information, networking and support for infertile couples, surrogate mothers, and professionals.

THYROID PROBLEMS

The American Thyroid Association, Inc.
Townhouse Office Park
55 Old Nyack Turnpike, Suite 611
Nanuet, NY 10954
http://www.thyroid.org

A nonprofit organization that promotes understanding of the thyroid and related diseases. The group fosters research, supports education, and guides public policy.

The Thyroid Foundation of America, Inc.
Ruth Sleeper Hall, RSL350
40 Parkman Street
Boston, MA 02114-2698
(800) 832-8321
http://www.tfaeweb.org/pub/tfa.

TURNER'S SYNDROME

The Turner's Syndrome Society
14450 T.C. Jester, Suite 260
Houston, Texas 77014, USA
(800) 365-9944
http://www.turner-syndrome-us.org

Nonprofit association offers support, information, bookstore.

UROLOGISTS

American Urological Association, Inc.
1120 North Charles Street
Baltimore, MD 21201
(410) 727-1100
http://www.auanet.org

Provides patient information pamphlets and referrals of those who can supply information about specific questions.

VAGINITIS

National Vaginitis Association
117 South Cook Street, Suite 315
Barrington, IL 60010
(800) 909-8745
http://www.vaginalinfections.org/index.html

WOMEN'S HEALTH

National Women's Health Resource Center
120 Albany Street
Suite 820
New Brunswick, NJ 08901
(877) 986-9473
www.healthywomen.org

The national clearinghouse for women's health information. The group has an extensive database of health resources, offers its National Women's Health Report, and maintains a website.

National Women's Health Network
514 10th Street NW, Suite 400
Washington, DC 20004
(202) 628-7814; (202) 347-1140
http://www.womenshealthnetwork.org

A nonprofit organization dedicated exclusively to women's health, offering information, resources, and a website.

APPENDIX II
HOT LINES

Emergency Contraception Hotline
(800) 584-9911

Fertilittext
(1-900) pregnant

A national telephone service providing recorded information and live consultation about fertility treatment and specialists.

IVF-PALS Hotline
(800) IVF-PALS

Provides specific information about health insurance coverage for IVF.

RESOLVE INC.
(617) 623-0744

APPENDIX III
READ MORE ABOUT IT

Aronson, Diane and Resolve. *Resolving Infertility: Understanding the Options and Choosing Solutions When You Want to Have a Baby.* New York: Harper Resource, 1999.

Berger, Gary, Marc Goldstein and Mark Fuerst. *The Couples Guide to Fertility: Techniques to Help You Have a Baby.* New York: Doubleday, 1995.

Bradstreet, Karen. *Overcoming Infertility Naturally.* Pleasant Grove, Utah: Woodland Publishing, 1994.

——. *Natural Treatments for Infertility.* Pleasant Grove, Utah: Woodland Publishing, 1997.

Kearney, Brian. *High Tech Conception.* New York: Bantam, 1998.

Marrs, Richard, Lisa Friedman Bloch and Kathy Kirtland Silverman. *Dr. Richard Marrs' Fertility Book.* New York: Dell, 1997.

Peoples, Debby, and Hariette Rovner Ferguson. *Experiencing Infertility: An Essential Resource.* New York: Norton, 2000.

HELPFUL NEWSLETTERS

Fertility Weekly
1087 Crooked Creek Road SE
Eatonton, GA 31024
(800) 705-7185

INCIID Insights
International Council on Infertility Information Dissemination
P.O. Box 91363
Tucson, AZ 85752
(520) 544-9548

Infertility Helper
36 Norwood Road
Toronto, Ontario M4E 2S2 (Canada)
(416) 690-9593

Newsletter of Resolve National
1310 Broadway
Somerville, MA 02144
(617) 623-0744

APPENDIX IV
HOW TO SELECT A FERTILITY SPECIALIST

1. Ask for a referral from your gynecologist, obstetrician, family doctor, or friends and relatives for recommendations.
2. Ask your local hospital or medical society for names. Contact local infertility support groups for information and emotional support.
3. Talk with several providers of infertility services before taking action so as to compare programs, gain more information about the field, and learn about different treatments.
4. Contact infertility programs first by telephone, study any literature, and then visit those that most interest you.
5. Try to select an infertility provider that you feel comfortable with and is convenient for you. Choose a program that is well established, has worked with many patients, and has a highly trained medical staff.

APPENDIX V
QUESTIONS TO ASK PROVIDERS

Once a couple selects an infertility provider, there are many questions to ask to make sure everyone is compatible. What follows are some of the most important questions to ask.

ABOUT THE SERVICE ITSELF

- What is your infertility service's success rate and how is it calculated?

- For established programs, what is your live birthrate per egg stimulation attempted?

- For new programs, what is your live birth rate plus ongoing pregnancies past 26 weeks per egg stimulation? Examine how each infertility service tabulates its success rate, and consider how meaningful these figures are.

- How long has your infertility service been in existence?

- How many patients have you treated?

- What is the training of your medical personnel?

- Is your infertility service associated with a medical board specializing in infertility? Do you have a doctor who is board-certified by the American Board of Obstetrics and Gynecology in the subspecialty of reproductive endocrinology? (This board certification provides recognition of tested expertise in IVF and GIFT procedures.)

ABOUT YOUR OWN PROCEDURE

- Tell the staff your individual circumstances. Then ask: Given our medical history, what are our chances of having a baby after undergoing a single egg-stimulation procedure?

- What is your success rate with couples who have had problems similar to ours?

- How successful have you been in helping couples with our specific problems?

- Can you send me written material about the particular procedure you are recommending?

- Can we talk with several former or current patients who have had problems similar to ours?

PAYING FOR TREATMENT

Fees can be high and insurance may not cover much (if any) of these procedures. Most infertility services won't require a payment all at once, but they will charge you as you advance through each step of the procedure. Review your health insurance to see how much (if any) of the procedures are covered. Ask the fertility center these questions:

- What are the fees for these procedures?

- How much will drugs cost?

- What is covered by insurance?

APPENDIX VI
INFERTILITY CLINICS

ALABAMA

ART Program of Alabama
Women's Medical Plaza
2006 Brookwood Medical Center Drive, Suite 508
Birmingham, AL 35209
(205) 870-9784

Center for Reproductive Medicine
3 Mobile Infirmary Center, Suite 312
Mobile, AL 36607
(334) 438-4200

University of Alabama at Birmingham IVF Program
618 South 20th, Suite 547
Birmingham, AL 35233
(205) 801-8225

University of South Alabama IVF and ART Program
307 University Boulevard, CCCB 326
Mobile, AL 36688
(334) 460-7173

ARIZONA

Arizona Center for Fertility Studies
8997 East Desert Cove Ave. 2nd Floor
Scottsdale, AZ 85260
(480) 860-4792
http://www.acfs2000.com

Arizona Reproductive Medicine and Gynecology Ltd
2850 North 24th Street, Suite 503
Phoenix, Arizona 85008
(602) 468-3840
http://www.conceive.com

Fertility Treatment Center
3200 North Dobson Road, Suite F-7
Chandler, AZ 85224
(480) 831-2445

IVF Phoenix
4626 East Shea Boulevard, Suite C-230
Phoenix, AZ 85028
(602) 996-2411

Mayo Clinic Scottsdale
Center for Reproductive Medicine
13737 North 92nd Street
Scottsdale, AZ 85260
(480) 614-6099

Samaritan Institute of Reproductive Medicine
Arizona Reproductive Medicine Specialists
1300 North 12th Street, Suite 520
Phoenix, AZ 85006
(602) 343-2767

Southwest Fertility Center
3125 North 32nd Street, Suite 200
Phoenix, AZ 85018
(602) 956-7481

University of Arizona Program of ART
Arizona Center for Reproductive Endocrinology
and Infertility
5190 Farness Drive, Suite 114
Tucson, AZ 85712
(520) 326-0001

West Valley Fertility Center
6525 West Sack Drive, Suite 208
Glendale, Arizona 85308
(623)561-8636
http://www.ihr.com

ARKANSAS

Intravaginal Culture Fertilization Program
500 South University, Suite 103
Little Rock, AR 72205
(501) 663-5858

University of Arkansas for Medical Sciences IVF
4301 West Markham, Slot 518
Little Rock, AR 72204
(501) 296-1705

CALIFORNIA (NORTHERN)

Alta Bates In Vitro Fertilization Program
2999 Regent Street #101A
Berkeley, CA 94705
(510) 649-0440
http://www.abivf.com

Astarte Fertility Center
450 Sutter Street, Suite 2215
San Francisco, CA 94108
(415) 773-3413
www.allaboutinfertility.com
or
2110 Forest Avenue, Suite B
San Jose, CA 95128
(408) 283-3721
www.allaboutinfertility.com

California North Bay Fertility Associates
1111 Sonoma Avenue, Suite 214
Santa Rosa, CA 95405
(707) 575-5831
www.cnbfma.com

Center for Male Reproductive Medicine
2080 Century Park East, Suite 907
Los Angeles, CA   90067
(310) 277-2873
www.malereproduction.com

Center for Surrogate Parenting
8383 Wilshire Boulevard, Suite 750
Beverly Hills, CA 90211
(323) 655-2007
www.eggdonor.com

Family Fertility Center
2855 Mitchell Drive, Suite 104
Walnut Creek, CA 94598
(925) 977-4850
www.surromother.com

Fertility Associates of the Bay Area
1700 California Street, Suite 570
San Francisco, CA 94109
(415) 673-9199
www.fertilityassociatessf.com
or

1260 S. Eliseo Street, Suite 201
Greenbrae, CA 94904
(415) 461-7812
www.fertilityassociatessf.com

Fertility Center of California
845 W. La Veta Avenue, Suite 104
Orange, CA 92701
(714) 744-2040
www.fertilityctr.com
or
6475 Alvarado Road, #109
San Diego, CA 92120
(619) 265-0102
www.fertilityctr.com

Fertility Physicians of Northern California
2516 Samaritan Drive, Suite A
San Jose, CA 95124
(408) 358-2500

Greater Valley Center for Reproductive Medicine
5400 Balboa Boulevard, Suite 220
Encino, CA 91316
(818) 461-1610

Huntington Reproductive Center
301 South Fair Oaks Avenue, Suite 402
Pasadena, CA 91105
(626) 440-9161

IGO Medical Group of San Diego
9339 Genesee Avenue, Suite 220
San Diego, CA 92121
(858) 455-7520

Infertility Clinic
Naval Medical Center, San Diego
34730 Bob Wilson Drive, Suite 100
San Diego, CA 92134
(619) 524-6218

Loma Linda University Center For Fertility and IVF
11370 Anderson Street, Suite 3950
Loma Linda, CA 92354
(909) 796-4851

Marin Fertility Medical Group
1100 South Eliseo Drive, Suite 107
Greenbrae, CA 94904
(800) 497-8889; (415) 464-8688
www.marinfertility.com

Northern California Fertility Medical Center
406 1/2 Sunrise Avenue, Suite 310
Roseville, CA 95661
(916) 773-2229
www.ncfmc.com

Northridge Center for Reproductive Medicine
18546 Roscoe Boulevard, Suite 240
Northridge, CA 91324
(818) 701-8181

NOVA In Vitro Fertilization Clinic
1681 El Camino Real
Palo Alto, CA 94306
(650) 322-0500
www.novaivf.com

Pacific Fertility Center
55 Francisco Street, Suite 500
San Francisco, CA 94133
(415) 834-3000
(888) 834-3095 Patient Resource Center
www.SFfertility.com

Reproductive Endocrine Associates
6719 Alvarado Road, Suite 108
San Diego, CA 92120
(619) 265-1800

Reproductive Partners-Long Beach
701 East 28th Street, Suite 202
Long Beach, CA 90806
(562) 427-2229

Reproductive Partners-Redondo Beach
510 North Prospect Avenue, Suite 202
Redondo Beach, CA 90277
(310) 318-3010

Reproductive Partners-San Diego
9850 Genessee Avenue, Suite 800
La Jolla, CA 92037
(858) 552-9177

Reproductive Science Center of the San Francisco Bay Area
3160 Crow Canyon Road, Suite 150
San Ramon, CA 94583
(925) 867-1800
www.rscbayarea.com
or
1999 Mowry Avenue, Suite I
Fremont, CA 94538
(510) 494-2000
www.rscbayarea.com

or
89 Davis Road, Suite 280
Orinda, CA 94563
(925) 254-0444
www.rscbayarea.com

Reproductive Specialty Medical Center
1441 Avocado Avenue, Suite 203
Newport Beach, CA 92660
(949) 640-7200

San Francisco Center for Reproductive Medicine
390 Laurel Street, Suite 205
San Francisco, CA 94118
(415) 771-1483
www.SFfertility.com

Scripps Clinic
10666 North Torrey Pines Road, MS314
La Jolla, CA 92037
(858) 554-8680

Smotrich Center for Reproductive Enhancement
6699 Alvarado Road, Suite 2306
San Diego, CA 92120
(619) 287-2222

Stanford Reproductive Endocrinology and Infertility Center
Stanford Hospital and Clinics
300 Pasteur Drive
Stanford, CA 94305
(650) 498-7911
www.stanfordivf.org

University of California, Davis Assisted Reproductive Technology Program
Department of Obstetrics/Gynecology
Ellison Ambulatory Care
4860 Y Street, Suite 2500
Sacramento, CA 95817
(916) 734-6930

UCLA Fertility Center
Department of Obstetrics/Gynecology
10833 Le Conte Avenue, 27-162 CHS
Los Angeles, CA 90095
(310) 825-9500

UCSF Fertility Group
350 Parnassus Avenue, Suite 300
San Francisco, CA 94117
(415) 476-2224.
www.ucsfivf.org

USC Reproductive Endocrinology and Infertility
1245 Wilshire Boulevard, Suite 403
Los Angeles, CA 90017
(213) 975-9990

Werlin-Zarutskie Fertility Centers
4900 Baranca Parkway, Suite 103
Irvine, CA 92604
(949) 726-0600

West Coast Fertility Centers
11160 Warner Avenue, Suite 411
Fountain Valley, CA 92807
(714) 513-1399

Woman to Woman Fertility Center
3201 Danville Boulevard, Suite 160
Alamo, CA 94507
(925) 820-9495

Zouves Fertility Center
901 Campus Drive, Suite 214
Daly City, CA 94015
(800) 800-1160
www.goivf.com

CALIFORNIA, SOUTHERN

Infertility and Gynecology Institute
18370 Burbank Boulevard, Suite 514
Tarzana, CA 91356
(818) 996-5550 or (805) 456-4868.
www.infertilityinstitute.com

Infertility, Gynecology and Obstetrics Medical Group of San Diego
9339 Genesee Avenue, Suite 220
San Diego, CA 92121
(858) 455-7520 (main switchboard operator)
(858) 455-1248 (access to the voice mail system, use #5 for directory)
www.ihr.com

Reproductive Medicine and Surgery Associates
Southern California Reproductive Center
450 N. Roxbury Drive
Beverly Hills, CA 90210
(310) 777-2393

Southern California Center For Reproductive Medicine
361 Hospital Road, Suite 333
Newport Beach, CA 92663
(949) 642-8727

West Coast Infertility Clinic, Inc.
250 N. Robertson Boulevard, Suite 403
Beverly Hills, CA 90211
(310) 285-0333
www.westcoastinfertility.com

COLORADO

Center for Reproductive Medicine
University of Colorado
4701 East 9th Avenue
University Pavilion 254 South
Denver, CO 80220
(303) 372-1483

Colorado Center for Reproductive Medicine
799 East Hampden Avenue, Suite 300
Englewood, CO 80110
(303) 788-8300

Colorado IVF at Rose
4600 East Hale Parkway, Suite 350
Denver, CO 80220

Colorado Springs Center for Reproductive Health
1625 Medical Center Point, Suite 290
Colorado Springs, CO 80907
(719) 636-0080

Conceptions Reproductive Associates
7720 South Broadway, Suite 580
Littleton, CO 80122
(303) 794-0045

Creating Families, Inc.
1395 Bellaire Street
Denver, CO 80220
(303) 355-2107
www.creatfam.com

Reproductive Genetics In Vitro
455 South Hudson Street
Level 3
Denver, CO 80246
(303) 399-1464

Rocky Mountain Center for Reproductive Medicine
1080 East Elizabeth
Fort Collins, CO 80524
(970) 493-6353

CONNECTICUT

Center for Advanced Reproductive Services, The
University of Connecticut Health Center
Dowling South Building
263 Farmington Avenue, Suite A330
Farmington, CT 06030
(860) 679-4580

Center for Fertility and Reproductive Endocrinology, The
New Britain General Hospital
100 Grand Street
New Britain, CT 06050
(860) 224-5695
www.nbgh.org/fertile.htm

New England Fertility Institute
1275 Summer Street, Suite 201
Stamford, CT 06905
(203) 325-3200

Yale University School of Medicine In-Vitro Fertilization Program
Department of Obstetrics/Gynecology
333 Cedar Street, Dana 2 Clinic Building
New Haven, CT 06510
(203) 785-4708

DELAWARE

The Center for Human Reproduction–Delaware, P.A.
Delaware Institute for Reproductive Medicine, P.A.
4745 Stanton-Ogletown Road, Suite 111
Newark, DE 19713
(302) 738-4600

Reproductive Associates of Delaware
4600 New Linden Hill Road, Suite 102
Wilmington, DE 19808
(302) 633-9533

FLORIDA

Advanced Reproductive Care Center, P.A.
10301 Hagen Ranch Rd, Suite 6
Boynton Beach, FL 33437
(561) 736-6006

Advanced Reproductive Technologies Program at University Community Hospital
3100 East Fletcher Avenue
Tampa, FL 33613
(813) 979-7956

Arnold Palmer Hospital Fertility Center
22 Underwood Street
Orlando, FL 32806
(407) 649-6995

Boca Fertility
875 Meadows Road, Suite 334
Boca Raton, FL 33486
(561) 368-5500
www.bocafertility.com

Center for Advanced Reproductive Endocrinology
6738 West Sunrise Boulevard, Suite 106
Plantation, FL 33313
(954) 584-2273
www.care-life.com

Center for Human Reproduction–Florida, The
2454 McMullen Booth Road, Suite 601
Clearwater, FL 33759
(727) 796-7705

Center for Infertility & Reproductive Medicine, P.A.
3435 Pinehurst Avenue
Orlando, FL 32804
(407) 740-0909

Fertility and IVF Center of Miami
8950 North Kendall Drive, Suite 103
Miami FL 33176-2197
(305) 596-4013
www.miami-ivf.com

Fertility Institute of Fort Lauderdale
4100 South Hospital Drive, Suite 209
Plantation, FL 33317
(954) 791-1442

Fertility Institute of Northwest Florida
1110 Gulf Breeze Parkway, Suite 202
Gulf Breeze, FL 32561
(850) 934-3900

Florida Institute for Reproductive Medicine
Baptist Medical Center
836 Prudential Drive, Suite 902
Jacksonville, FL 32207
(904) 399-5620; (800) 556 5620
www.firmjax.com

Florida Institute for Reproductive Science & Technology (F.I.R.S.T.)
9900 Stirling Road, Suite 300
Cooper City, FL 33024
(954) 436-2700

Genetics & IVF of Florida
Reproductive Medicine & Genetics
5500 Village Boulevard, Suite 103
West Palm Beach, FL 33407
(561) 697-4200

IVF Florida/Northwest Center for Infertility & Reproductive Endocrinology
2825 North State Route 7, Suite 302
Margate, FL 33063
(954) 247-6200

Palm Beach Fertility Center
9970 Central Park Boulevard, Suite 300
Boca Raton, FL 33428
(561) 477-7728

Reproductive Medicine and Fertility Center
615 East Princeton Street, Suite 225
Orlando, FL 32803
(407) 896-7575

Specialists in Reproductive Medicine & Surgery, P.A.
12611 World Plaza Lane, Building 53
Fort Myers, FL 33907
(941) 275-8118

South Florida Institute for Reproductive Medicine
6250 Sunset Drive, Suite 202
South Miami, FL 33143
(305) 662-7901

University of Florida/Park Avenue Women's Center
807 NW 57th Street
Gainesville, FL 32605
(352) 392-6200

University of Florida-Pensacola
5147 North Ninth Avenue
DePaul Medical Building 402
Pensacola, FL 32504
(850) 857-3733

Women's HealthCare Specialists IVF Miami
4302 Alton Road, Suite 900
Miami Beach, FL 33140
(305) 531-1480

GEORGIA

Atlanta Center for Reproductive Medicine
100 Stone Forest Drive, Suite 300
Woodstock, Georgia 30189

(770) 928-2276
www.acrm.com
or
960 Johnson Ferry Road, Suite 340
Atlanta, Georgia 30342
(404) 459-0403
www.acrm.com
or
743 Old Norcross Road
Lawrenceville, Georgia 30045
(770) 928-2276
www.acrm.com

Augusta Reproductive Biology Associates
812 Chafee Avenue
Augusta, GA 30904
(706) 724-0228

Emory Center for Reproductive Medicine and Fertility
20 Linden Avenue NE, Suite 4701
Atlanta, GA 30308
(404) 686-3229

Reproductive Biology Associates
5505 Peachtree Dunwoody Road, Suite 400
Atlanta, Georgia 30342
(404) 257-1900; (888) 722-4483
www.rba-online.com
or
790 Church Street Extension, Suite 330
Marietta, Georgia 30060
(770) 426-8822
www.rba-online.com
or
7444 Hannover Parkway South, Suite 225
Stockbridge, GA 30281
(678) 289-1034
www.rba-online.com
or
500 Medical Center Boulevard, Suite 350
Lawrenceville, GA 30045
(770) 277-3361
www.rba-online.com

HAWAII

Pacific IVF Institute
1319 Punahou Street, Suite 980
Honolulu, HI 96826
(808) 946-2226

Tripler Army Medical Center
1 Jarrett White Road

Tripler AMC, HI 96859
(808) 433-6845

ILLINOIS

Advanced Fertility Center of Chicago
30 Tower Court, Suite F
Gurnee, IL 60031
(847) 662-1818
www.advancedfertility.com

Advanced Institute of Fertility
Medical Institute of Fertility
1700 West Central Road 40
Arlington Heights, IL 60005
(847) 394-5437

Center for Human Reproduction
750 North Orleans Street
Chicago, IL 60610
(312) 397-8000
www.centerforhumanreprod.com

Fertility Centers of Illinois, S.C.
1585 N. Barrington Road
Professional Building II, Suite 305
Hoffman Estates, IL 60194
(847) 843-1510
www.fcionline.com
or
8651 West 159th Street, Suite 5
Orland Park, IL 60462
(708) 633-1999
www.fcionline.com
or
135 North Arlington Heights Road, Suite 195
Buffalo Grove, IL 60089
(847) 215-8899
www.fcionline.com
or
3703 West Lake Avenue, Suite 306
Glenview, IL 60025
(847) 998-8200
www.fcionline.com
or
750 Homewood Avenue, Suite 190
Highland Park, IL 60035
(847) 433-4400
www.fcionline.com
or
Lutheran General IVF Center-Park Ridge
Embroyology Laboratory
Lutheran General Hospital

1775 West Dempster Street, 1 South
Park Ridge, IL 60068
(847) 723-8785
www.fcionline.com
or
Illinois Masonic Medical Center Campus
2825 North Halsted Street, Suite 509
Chicago, IL 60657
(773) 472-4400
www.fcionline.com
or
1 S. 224 Summit Avenue, Suite 302
Oakbrook Terrace, IL 60181
(630) 889-7900
www.fcionline.com

IVF Illinois, Inc.
836 West Wellington
Chicago, IL 60657
(773) 296-7096

Midwest Fertility Center
4333 Main Street
Downers Grove, IL 60515
(630) 810-0212

Reproductive Health Specialists, Ltd.
9475 Bormet Drive (192nd)
Mokena, IL 60448
(815) 730-1100
www.reproductivespecialist.com
or
310 North Hammes, Suite #101
Joliet, IL 60435
(815) 730-1100
www.reproductivespecialist.com
or
675 W. North Avenue, Suite #212
Melrose Park, IL 60160
(708) 681-7390
www.reproductivespecialist.com

Rush Center for Advanced Reproductive Care
1725 West Harrison, 408 East
Chicago, IL 60612
(312) 997-2229

Rush-Copley Center for Reproductive Health
2020 Ogden Avenue, Suite 215
Aurora, IL 60504
(630) 978-6254

INDIANA

Advanced Fertility Group
201 North Pennsylvania Parkway, Suite 205
Indianapolis, IN 46280
(317) 817-1300

Associated Fertility & Gynecology
7910 West Jefferson, Suite 301
Fort Wayne, IN 46804
(219) 432-6250

Family Beginnings
7250 Clearvista Parkway, Suite 308
Indianapolis, IN 46256
(317) 841-2280

Indiana University Hospital
550 North University Boulevard
Indianapolis, IN 46202
(317) 274-4875

Midwest Reproductive Medicine
8081 Township Line Road, Suite 110
Indianapolis, IN 46260
(800) 333-1415

Reproductive Endocrinology Associates
2020 West 86th Street, Suite 310
Indianapolis, IN 46260
(317) 872-1515

Reproductive Surgery & Medicine, P.C.
8040 Clearvista Parkway, Suite 280
Indianapolis, IN 46256
(317) 841-2255

IOWA

Advanced Reproductive Care
The Iowa Women's Health Center
2 Boyd Tower
The University of Iowa Hospitals and Clinics
200 Hawkins Drive
Iowa City, IA 52242
(319) 356-8483
www.uihc.uiowa.edu/arc/

McFarland Clinic, P.C. Assisted Reproduction
1215 Duff Avenue
Ames, IA 50010
(515) 239-4414

Mid-Iowa Fertility, P.C.
3408 Woodland Avenue, Suite 302 West
Des Moines, IA 50266
(515) 222-3060

University of Iowa Hospitals and Clinics Center for Advanced Reproductive Care
200 Hawkins Drive
Department of Obstetrics/Gynecology BT 2004
Iowa City, IA 52242
(319) 356-8483

KANSAS

Center for Reproductive Medicine, The
2903 E. Central
Wichita, Kansas 67214
(316) 687-2112
www.kumc.edu/wichita/dept/wri/crm.html

Reproductive Medicine & Infertility
Shawnee Mission Medical Center
8800 West 75th Street, Suite 101
Shawnee Mission, KS 66204
(913) 432-7161

Reproductive Resource Center of Greater Kansas City, P.A.
12200 West 106th Street, Suite 120
Overland Park, KS 66215
(913) 894-2323
www.rrc-gkc.com

University of Kansas Medical Center
Women's Reproductive Center
3901 Rainbow Boulevard, 5th Floor
Kansas City, KS 66160
(913) 588-6272

KENTUCKY

Fertility & Endocrine Associates
1780 Nicholasville Road, Suite 402
Lexington, KY 40503
(606) 278-9151

Surrogate Parenting Associates, Inc.
for information on infertility and sterilization reversal:
225 Abraham Flexner Way, #501
Louisville, KY 40202
(502) 584-7787; (800) 766-0304
www.babies-by-levin.com
or
for surrogate parenting issues:
225 Abraham Flexner Way, #500
Louisville, KY 40202
(502) 584-7794
www.babies-by-levin.com

University of Kentucky Department of Ob/Gyn
800 Rose Street, Room C359
Lexington, KY 40536
(606) 260-1515

University Ob/Gyn Associates Fertility Center
Norton Healthcare Pavilion
315 East Broadway, First Floor
Louisville, KY 40202
(502) 629-3830

LOUISIANA

Center for Fertility & Advanced Reproductive Care, The
4720 South I-10 Service Road, Suite 309
Metairie, LA 70001
(504) 887-7001

Center for Fertility & Reproductive Health
2401 Greenwood Road
Shreveport, LA 71103
(318) 632-8270

Fertility and Laser Center
4720 South I-10 Service Road, Suite 100
Metairie, LA 70001
(504) 454-2165

Fertility Clinic
Tulane University Hospital and Clinic
1415 Tulane Avenue
New Orleans, LA 70112
(504) 588-2341

The Fertility Institute
6020 Bullard Avenue
New Orleans, LA 70128
(504) 246-8971
www.fertilityinstitute.com

MARYLAND

Center for Reproductive Medicine
9711 Medical Center Drive, Suite 214
Rockville, MD 20850
(301) 424-1904

Center for Surrogate Parenting
9 State Circle, Suite 302
Annapolis, MD 21401
(410) 990-9860
www.eggdonor.com

Fertility Center of Maryland
110 West Road, Suite 102
Towson, MD 21204
(410) 296-6400; (800) 405-4IVF
www.fertilitycentermd.com

Fertility and Reproductive Health Center, The
Robinwood Medical Center
11110 Medical Campus Road, Suite 211
Hagerstown, MD 21743
(301) 714-4100
www.frhcfertility.com

Greater Baltimore Medical Center (GBMC) Fertility Center
6569 North Charles Street, Suite 406
Physicians Pavilion West
Baltimore, MD 21204
(410) 828-2484
www.gbmc.org/p.cfm/womenshealth/fertilitycenter

Helix Center for ART
Union Memorial Hospital-Obstetrics/Gynecology
201 East University Parkway
Baltimore, MD 21218
(410) 554-2271

Johns Hopkins Fertility Center
10753 Falls Road, Suite 335
Lutherville, MD 21093
(410) 847-3650

Mid-Atlantic Fertility Centers
10215 Fernwood Road, Suite 301A
Bethesda, MD 20817
(301) 897-8850

Shady Grove Fertility
15001 Shady Grove Road, Suite 400
Rockville, MD 20850
(301) 340-1188
www.shadygrovefertility.com
or
116 Defense Highway, Suite 203
Annapolis, MD 21401
(410) 224-5500
www.shadygrovefertility.com

University of Maryland Medical School Center for Advanced Reproductive Technology
University of Maryland Medical System
405 West Redwood Street, 3rd Floor
Baltimore, MD 21201
(410) 328-2304

MASSACHUSETTS

Baystate IVF
Chestnut Surgical Center
759 Chestnut Street
Springfield, MA 01199
(412) 794-1950

Boston IVF
The Brookline Center
One Brookline Place, Suite 602
Brookline, MA 02445
(617) 735-9000
www.bostonivf.com
or
The Waltham Center
40 Second Avenue, Suite 300
Waltham, MA 02451
(781) 434-6500
www.bostonivf.com
or
The South Shore Center
2300 Crown Colony Drive
Quincy, MA 02169
(617) 793-1100
www.bostonivf.com

Center for Assisted Reproduction
Brigham & Women's Hospital
75 Francis Street, Tower 5C
Boston, MA 02115
(617) 732-4222

**Faulkner Center for Reproductive
Medicine**
1153 Center Street
Boston, MA 02130
(781) 326-9732

Fertility Center of New England, Inc.
Norfolk Place, 333 Elm Street, 3rd Floor
Dedham, MA 02026
(781) 326-9732
www.fertilitycenter.com
or
20 Pond Meadow Drive, Suite 101
Reading, MA 01867
(781) 942-7000
www.fertilitycenter.com
or
Wellesley Hills, MA Office
Wellesley Hills, MA
(781) 237-0080
www.fertilitycenter.com

or
33 Lyman Street, Suite 102B
Westboro, MA
(508) 366-5898
www.fertilitycenter.com

Hallmark Health Fertility Services
The Malden Hospital
100 Hospital Road
Malden, MA 02148
(781) 397-6540

**Massachusetts General Hospital Vincent
IVF Unit**
55 Fruit Street, VBK 210
Boston, MA 02114
(617) 724-3500

**New England Fertility and Endocrinology
Associates**
One Brookline Place, Suite 421
Brookline, MA 02445
(617) 277-1778

**The Reproductive Science Center
of Boston**
Deaconess Waltham Hospital
20 Hope Avenue
Waltham, MA 02454
(781) 647-6263

MICHIGAN

Ann Arbor Reproductive Medicine
4990 Clark Road, Suite 100
Ypsilanti, MI 48197
(737) 434-4871

**Beaumont Center for Fertility and
Reproductive Medicine**
3535 West Thirteen Mile Road, Suite 344
Royal Oak, MI 48073
(810) 551-0515

**Center for Reproductive Medicine
Hurley Medical Center**
2 Hurley Plaza, Suite 101
Flint, MI 48503
(810) 257-9714

**Center for Reproductive Medicine
Oakwood Hospital**
18181 Oakwood Boulevard, Suite 109
Dearborn, MI 48124
(313) 593-5880

Center for Reproductive Medicine Rochester Hills
3950 South Rochester Road, Suite 2300
Rochester Hills, MI 48307
(248) 844-8845

Fakih Institute of Reproductive Science & Technology (FIRST)
3950 South Rochester Road, Suite 2300
Rochester Hills, MI 48307
(248) 844-8840

Grand Rapids Fertility/Spectrum Health East
1900 Wealthy Street, Suite 315
Grand Rapids, MI 40506
(616) 774-2030

Henry Ford Reproductive Medicine
1500 West Big Beaver, Suite 105
Troy, MI 48084
(248) 637-4050

Infertility and Gynecology Center of Lansing, P.C.
1200 East Michigan Avenue, Suite 305
Lansing, MI 48910
(517) 484-4900

Michigan Reproductive & IVF Center
221 Michigan, NE, Suite 406
Grand Rapids, MI 49503
(616) 391-2558

Michigan State University Center for Assisted Reproductive Technology
1200 East Michigan Avenue, Suite 700
Lansing, MI 48912
(517) 364-5888

West Michigan Reproductive Institute, P.C.
885 Forest Hills Avenue, SE
Grand Rapids, MI 49546
(616) 942-5180

University of Michigan Medical Center
Taubman Center
1500 East Medical Center Drive, Suite 1442
Ann Arbor, MI 48109
(734) 763-4323

MINNESOTA

Center for Reproductive Medicine
2800 Chicago Avenue South, 3rd Floor
Minneapolis, MN 55407
(612) 863-5390

Mayo Clinic Assisted Reproductive Technologies
Charlton 3A
200 First Street, SW
Rochester, MN 55905
(507) 284-4520

Midwest Center for Reproductive Health, P.A.
Oakdale Medical Building
3366 Oakdale Avenue North, Suite 550
Minneapolis, MN 55422
(612) 520-2600

Reproductive Medicine and Infertility Associates, P.A.
360 Sherman Street, Suite 350
St. Paul, MN 55102
(651) 222-6050; (800) 440-7359
www.rmia.com

MISSOURI

Advanced Assisted Reproductive Technology Program
Center for Reproductive Medicine and Infertility
4444 Forest Park Avenue, Suite 3100
St. Louis, MO 63108
(314) 286-2400

Advanced Reproductive Specialists
Saint Luke's Hospital
226 South Woods Mill Road, Suite 64 West
Chesterfield, MO 63017
(314) 542-9422

Fertility Institute
226 South Woods Mill Road, 39 West
Chesterfield, MO 63017
(314) 205-8809

Mid-Missouri Center for Reproductive Health
1502 East Broadway, Suite 106
Columbia, MO 65201
(573) 443-4511

University of Missouri Hospital & Clinics–IVF Embryology Lab
Department of Obstetrics/Gynecology
1 Hospital Drive, N610 HSC
Columbia, MO 65212
(573) 882-7937

Infertility & IVF Center
3009 North Ballas Road, Suite 359C
St. Louis, MO 63131
(314) 225-5483

Infertility Center of St. Louis, The
St. Luke's Hospital
224 S. Woods Mill Road, Suite 730
St. Louis, MO   63017
(314) 576-1400

MISSISSIPPI

University of Mississippi Medical Center
Department of Obstetrics/Gynecology, Division of
Reproductive Endocrinology
2500 North State Street
Jackson, MS 39216
(601) 984-5330

Women's Specialty Center
501 Marshall Street, Suite 600
Jackson, MS 39202
(601) 948-6540; (800) 696-7059
www.ivfmississippi.com

NEBRASKA

Center for Reproductive Medicine
Department of Obstetrics/Gynecology
PO Box 983255
Omaha, NE 68198
(800) 981-5858

Reproductive Endocrinology/Infertility
8111 Dodge Street, Suite 237
Omaha, NE 68114
(402) 354-5210

NEVADA

Fertility Center of Las Vegas
8851 West Sahara, Suite 100
Las Vegas, NV 89117
(702) 254-1777

The Fertility Institutes
4275 Burnham Avenue, Suite 330
Las Vegas, NV 89119
(702) 458-6500
www.fertility-docs.com

**University Institute of Fertility
Nevada Fertility Center for Advanced
Reproductive Endocrinology and Surgery**
653 Town Center Drive, Suite 206
Las Vegas, NV 89144
(702) 341-6616

NEW HAMPHSIRE

Dartmouth–Hitchcock Medical Center
One Medical Center Drive
Lebanon, NH 03756
(603) 650-8162

Fertility Center of New England, Inc.
Cypress Medical Office Park, #9
Elliot Hospital
Manchester, NH
(603) 641-9899
www.fertilitycenter.com

NEW JERSEY

**Center for Advanced Reproductive
Medicine & Fertility**
Durham Center
One Ethel Road, Suite 107B
Edison, NJ 08817
(732) 339-9300

**Center for Human Reproduction of
New Jersey**
Fertility Institute of New Jersey & New York
400 Old Hook Road
Westwood, NJ 07675
(201) 666-4200

**Center for Reproductive Medicine at
Hackensack University Medical Center**
214 Terrace Avenue, 2nd Floor
Hasbrouck Heights, NJ 07604
(201) 393-7444

**Cooper Center for In-Vitro Fertilization, P.C.
Cooper Institute for Reproductive
Hormonal Disorders, P.C.**
8002E Greentree Commons
Marlton, NJ 08053
(856) 751-5575
www.jhcheck.com

Diamond Institute for Infertility
89 Milburn Avenue
Millburn, NJ 07041
(973) 761-5600
Fax: (973) 761-5100

East Coast Infertility and IVF, P.C.
200 White Road, Suite 214
Little Silver, NJ 07739
(732) 758-6511

Institute for Reproductive Medicine and Science, The
of Saint Barnabas Medical Center
Old Short Hills Road East Wing, Suite 403
Livingston, NJ 07039
(973) 533-8286

IVF New Jersey
1527 Route 27, Suite 2100
Somerset, NJ 08873
(732) 220-9060

IVF of North Jersey, P.A.
15-01 Broadway
Fair Lawn, NJ 07410
(973) 470-0303

North Hudson IVF
Center for Fertility and Gynecology
385 Sylvan Avenue
Englewood Cliffs, NJ 07632
(201) 871-1999

Princeton Center for Infertility & Reproductive Medicine
3131 Princeton Pike, Building 4, Suite 204
Lawrenceville, NJ 08648
(609) 895-1114

Reproductive Gynecologists, P.C.
Kennedy Health System
2201 Chapel Avenue West, Suite 206
Cherry Hill, NJ 08002
(609) 662-6662

Reproductive Medicine Associates of New Jersey
Morristown Office
111 Madison Avenue, Suite 100
Morristown, NJ 07962
(973) 971-4600
www.rmanj.com
or
West Orange Office
769 Northfield Avenue
Suite 228
West Orange, NJ 07052
(973) 325-2229
www.rmanj.com
or
Englewood Office
25 Rockwood Place
Englewood, NJ 07631
(201) 569-7773
www.rmanj.com

Robert Wood Johnson Medical School IVF Program
303 George Street, Suite 250
New Brunswick, NJ 08901
(732) 235-7300

Shore Institute for Reproductive Medicine
1608 Route 88 West, Suite 117
Brick, NJ 08724
(732) 840-1447

South Jersey Fertility Center, P.A.
512 Lippincott Drive
Marlton, NJ 08053
(856) 596-2233

NEW MEXICO

Center for Reproductive Medicine of New Mexico
201 Cedar Street, SE,
Presbyterian Professional Building LL20
Albuquerque, NM 87106
(505) 247-3333

Southwest Fertility Services
4705 Montgomery, NE, Suite 101
Albuquerque, NM 87109
(800) 577-7133; (505) 837-1510
www.southwestfertility.com

NEW YORK

Advanced Fertility Services, P.C.
1625 Third Avenue
New York, NY 10128
(212) 369-8700

Brandeis Center for Reproductive Health
606 Columbus Avenue, 2nd Floor
New York, NY 10024
(212) 362-4848

Brooklyn Fertility Center
55 Central Park West, Suite 1C
New York, NY 10023
(212) 721-4545

Brooklyn IVF
1355 84th Street
Brooklyn, NY 11228
(718) 283-8600

Capital Region Genetics & IVF at Bellevue Hospital
2210 Troy Road
Niskayuna, NY 12309
(518) 346-9544

Center for Reproductive Medicine and Infertility
505 East 70th Street, Suite 340
New York, NY 10021
(212.746.1762
www.ivf.org

Central New York Fertility Center
4850 Broad Street, Suite 1K
Syracuse, NY 13215
(315) 492-5376

Children's Hospital IVF Program
Infertility & IVF Associates of Western New York
4510 Main Street
Snyder, NY 14226
(716) 839-3057

Columbia Presbyterian Medical Center
Center for Women's Reproductive Care
at Columbia University
161 Fort Washington Avenue, 4th floor, Room 450
New York, NY 10032
(212) 305-4665

Division of Reproductive Endocrinology SUNY at Stony Brook
Health Science Center T9-080
Stony Brook, NY 11794
(516) 444-2737

The Fertility Institute at the Brooklyn Hospital
161 Ashland Place
Brooklyn, NY 11201
(718) 237-4593

Garden City Center for Advanced Reproductive Technologies
Yu-Kang Ying M.D., P.C.
394 Old Country Road
Garden City, NY 11530
(516) 248-8307

Institute For Reproductive Health and Infertility
1561 Long Pond Road, Suite 410
Rochester, NY 14626
(716) 723-7468

Leading Institute for Fertility Enhancement (L.I.F.E.)
130 Everett Road
Albany, NY 12204
(518) 482-1008

Long Island IVF Associates
625 Belle Terre Road, Suite 200
Port Jefferson, NY 11777
(516) 331-7575

Macleod Laboratory
65 E. 79th Street
New York, NY 10021
(212) 717-4444
www.fertilitysolution.com

Montefiore's Fertility & Hormone Center
20 Beacon Hill Drive
Dobbs Ferry, NY 10522
(914) 693-8820

New York Fertility Institute
1016 Fifth Avenue
New York, NY 10028
(212) 734-5555

New York Medical Services for Reproductive Medicine
784 Park Avenue
New York, NY 10021
(212) 744-4222

NYU Medical Center: In Vitro Fertilization, Reproductive Surgery & Infertility
First Avenue and 38th Street
New York, NY
(212) 263-8990
www.nyuivf.com

North Shore University Hospital Center for Human Reproduction
IVF Program: Ambulatory Building
300 Community Drive
Manhasset, NY 11030
(516) 562-2229

Offices for Fertility and Reproductive Medicine
88 University Place, 9th Floor
New York, NY 10003
(212) 243-5550

Reproductive Medicine Associates of New York, LLP
635 Madison Avenue, 9th floor
New York, NY 10022

(212) 756-5777
http://cobweb.aecom.yu.edu

Reproductive Medicine/IVF
1321 Millersport Road, Suite 102
Williamsville, NY 14221
(716) 634-4351

Reproductive Science Associates
200 Old Country Road, Suite 330
Mineola, NY 11501
(516) 739-2100
www.rsofny.com
                    or
Reproductive Science Associates
2500 Nesconset Highway, Building 19
Stony Brook, NY 11790
(631) 246-9100
www.rsofny.com

Strong Infertility and IVF Center
University of Rochester
601 Elmwood Avenue, Box 685
Rochester, NY 14642
(716) 275-1930

Westchester Fertility & Reproductive Endocrinology
136 South Broadway, Suite 100
White Plains, NY 10605
(914) 949-6677

Women's Health Center of Albany Medical Center
Division of Reproductive Endocrinology and Infertility
58-60 Hackett Boulevard
Albany, NY 12209
(518) 462-0084

NORTH CAROLINA

Duke University Medical Center Division of Reproductive Endocrinology and Infertility
Box 3143, Clinic 1-K
Durham, NC 27710
(919) 684-5327

Institute for Assisted Reproduction
1918 Randolf Road, 5th Floor
Charlotte, NC 28207
(704) 343-3400

North Carolina Center for Reproductive Medicine
The Talbert Fertility Institute

400 Ashville Avenue, Suite 200
Cary, NC 27511
(919) 233-1680

Program for Assisted Reproduction
Carolinas Medical Center 1000 Blythe Boulevard
Charlotte, NC 28203
(704) 355-3153

University of North Carolina ART Clinic
Department of Obstetrics/Gynecology, Division of Infertility
CB 7570 Manning Drive
Chapel Hill, NC 27514
(919) 966-1150

Wake Forest University Program for Assisted Reproduction
Department of Obstetrics/Gynecology
Medical Center Boulevard
Winston-Salem, NC 27157
(336) 716-2368

NORTH DAKOTA

MeritCare Medical Group Fertility Center
737 Broadway
Fargo, ND 58123
(701) 234-2700

OHIO

Akron City Hospital IVF Center
Summa Health System
525 East Market Street
PO Box 2090
Akron, OH 44309
(330) 375-3585

Bethesda Center for Reproductive Health and Fertility
10506 Montgomery Road, Suite 303
Cincinnati, OH 45242
(513) 745-1675; (800) 634-1222

Center for Reproductive Health
The University Hospital
Eden and Bethesda Avenues, ML0456
Cincinnati, OH 45219
(513) 584-0955

Cleveland Clinic Foundation
Department of Obstetrics/Gynecology
9500 Euclid Avenue, Desk-A81
Cleveland, OH 44195
(216) 444-8374

Fertility Center of Northwest Ohio
2142 North Cove Boulevard
Toledo, OH 43606
(419) 479-8830

Fertility Unlimited, Inc.
468 East Market Street
Akron, OH 44304
(330) 376-8353

Genetics & IVF Institute of Ohio
369 West 1st Street, Suite 120
Dayton, OH 45402
(937) 228-4483

**Greater Cincinnati Institute for
Reproductive Health at the Christ Hospital**
MOB 2, 2123 Auburn Avenue, Suite A-44
Cincinnati, OH 45219
(513) 585-4400

Miami Valley Hospital Fertility Center
One Wyoming Street
Dayton, OH 45409
(937) 208-2120

Ohio Reproductive Medicine
4830 Knightsbridge Boulevard, Suite E
Columbus, OH 43214
(614) 451-2280

The Reproductive Center
900 Sahara Trail
PO Box 3707
Youngstown, OH 44413
(330) 965-8390

University Fertility Institute
Camelot Women's Health Center
4775 Knightsbridge Boulevard, Suite 103
Columbus, OH 43214
(614) 442-5761

**University Hospitals of Cleveland
MacDonald Women's Hospital IVF Program**
11100 Euclid Avenue
Cleveland, OH 44106
(216) 844-1741

OREGON

Northwest Fertility Center
1750 Southwest Harbor Way, Suite 200
Portland, OR 97201
(503) 227-7799

**Oregon Health Sciences University
Fertility Program**
OHSU Fertility Consultants
1750 Southwest Harbor Way, Suite l00
Portland, OR 97201
(503) 418-3700
www.fertilityoregon.com

University Fertility Consultants
Oregon Health Sciences University
1750 Southwest Harbor Way, Suite 100
Portland, OR 97201
(503) 418-3700

OKLAHOMA

Henry G. Bennett, Jr., Fertility Institute
3433 Northwest 56th Street, Suite 200B
Oklahoma City, OK 73112
(405) 949-6060

**Presbyterian Hospital Laboratory for
Assisted Reproductive Technologies**
1000 North Lincoln Boulevard, Suite 300
Oklahoma City, OK 73104
(405) 271-9200

Tulsa Center for Fertility & Women's Health
1145 South Utica, Suite 1209
Tulsa, OK 74104
(918) 584-2870

PENNSYLVANIA

Abington Reproductive Medicine
1245 Highland Avenue, Suite 404
Abington, PA 19001
(215) 887-2010
www.abington-repromed.com

Allegheny General Hospital IVF Program
One Allegheny Center, Suite 280
Pittsburgh, PA 05212
(412) 359-1900

**Center for Reproductive Medicine at The
Bryn Mawr Hospital**
D Wing, Ground Floor
130 South Bryn Mawr Avenue
Bryn Mawr, PA 19010
(610) 526-8950

**Family Fertility Center
95 Highland Avenue, Suite 100**
Bethlehem, PA 18017
(610) 868-8600

The Fertility Center at Saint Clair Hospital
IVF Marrero
1050 Bower Hill Road, Suite 304
Pittsburgh, PA 15243
(412) 572-6565

Geisinger Medical Center's Infertility Center
Geisinger Health System Woman's Pavilion
Danville, PA 17822
(570) 271-5620

Infertility Solutions, P.C.
2200 Hamilton Street, Suite 105
Allentown, PA 18104
(610) 776-1217

Lehigh Valley Hospital Section of Reproductive Endocrinology and Infertility
401 North 17th Street, Suite 312
Allentown, PA 18104
(610) 402-9522

Northern Fertility and Reproductive Associates
Holy Redeemer Office
Holy Redeemer Office Building
1650 Huntingdon Park, Suite 154
Meadowbrook, PA 19046
(215) 938-1515

Penn State Geisinger Health System
The Hershey Medical Center
500 University Drive
PO Box 850, C3608
Hershey, PA 17033
(717) 531-6731

Pennsylvania Reproductive Associates
Women's Institute for Fertility, Endocrinology, and Menopause
819 Locust Street
Philadelphia, PA 19107
(215) 922-3173

Reprotech, Inc.
440 South 15th Street
Allentown, PA 18062
(610) 437-7000

Reproductive Endocrinology and Fertility Center
1 Medical Center Boulevard
Upland, PA 19013
(610) 447-2727

Reproductive & Medical Endocrine Associates, P.C.
7447 Old York Road
Melrose Park, PA 19027
(215) 635-4400
www.jhcheck.com

Reproductive Science Center of Greater Philadelphia
Reproductive Science Institute–Philadelphia
950 West Valley Road, Suite 2401
Wayne, PA 19087
(610) 964-9663

Reproductive Science Institute
950 West Valley Road, Suite 2401
Wayne, PA 19087
(610) 964-9663
www.rsiinfertility.com

Thomas Jefferson IVF Program
Ben Franklin House
834 Chestnut, Suite 300
Philadelphia, PA 19107
(215) 955-4018

Toll Center for Reproductive Sciences
1200 Old York Road, Suite 404
Abington, PA 19001
(215) 481-2349

University of Pennsylvania Medical Center
34th and Spruce Streets
Philadelphia, PA 19104
(215) 662-6560

University Women's Health Care Associates
University of Pittsburgh Physicians
300 Halket Street, Room 0673
Pittsburgh, PA 15213
(412) 641-4726

Women's Institute for Fertility, Endocrinology and Menopause
815 Locust Street
Philadelphia, PA 19107-5507
(215) 922-2206
www.womensinstitute.org
or
5217 Militia Hill Road
Plymouth Meeting, PA 19462-1247
(610) 834-1230
www.womensinstitute.org

PUERTO RICO

Centro de Fertilidad del Caribe
Torre San Francisco
369 Avenida De Diego, Suite 606
Río Piedras, PR 00923
(787) 763-2773

RHODE ISLAND

Women & Infants Hospital IVF Program
101 Dudley Street
1 Blackstone Place, First Floor
Providence, RI 02905
(401) 453-7500

SOUTH CAROLINA

Center for Women's Medicine
Reproductive Endocrinology and Infertility
890 West Faris Road, Suite 470
Box 32
Greenville, SC 29605
(864) 455-8488

Southeastern Fertility Center
1375 Hospital Drive
Mt Pleasant, SC 29464
(843) 881-3900
www.southeasternfertility.com

SOUTH DAKOTA

University Physicians Fertility Specialists
1310 West 22nd Street
Sioux Falls, SD 57105
(605) 782-2284

TENNESSEE

Appalachian Fertility and Endocrinology Center
2204 Pavilion Drive, Suite 307
Kingsport, TN 37660
(423) 392-6330

Center for Applied Reproductive Science
Johnson City Medical Center Office Building
408 State of Franklin Road
Johnson City, TN 37604
(423) 461-8880

The Center for Reproductive Health
326 21st Avenue North
Nashville, Tennessee 37203
(615) 321-8899

Center for Reproductive Medicine and Fertility
935 Spring Creek Road, Suite 205
Chattanooga, TN 37412
(423) 899-0500

Nashville Fertility Center
2400 Patterson Street, Suite 319
Nashville, TN 37203
(615) 321-4740

University Fertility Associates
909 Ridgeway Loop Road
Memphis, TN 38120
(901) 767-6868

TEXAS

Baylor Assisted Reproductive Technology
6550 Fannin, Suite 821
Houston, TX 77030
(713) 798-8232

Baylor Center for Reproductive Health
3707 Gaston Avenue, Suite 310
Dallas, TX 75246
(214) 821-2274

Center for Assisted Reproduction
1701 Park Place Avenue
Bedford, TX 76022
(817) 540-1157

Center for Reproduction at Gramercy
2727 Gramercy, Suite 200
Houston, TX 77025
(713) 661-3111

The Center for Reproductive Medicine
3506 21st Street, Suite 605
Lubbock, TX 79410
(806) 788-1212

Center for Women's Healthcare and Research
7400 Fannin, Suite 1130
Houston, TX 77054
(713) 797-9200

The Center of Reproductive Medicine
450 Medical Center Boulevard, Suite 202
Webster, TX 77598
(281) 332-0073

Cooper Institute for Advanced Reproductive Medicine
Green Park One Building

7515 South Main Street, Suite 580
Houston, TX 77030
(713) 794-0070; (877) 2-COOPER; (877) 226-6737
    or
Methodist Health Center
16651 Southwest Freeway, Suite 200
Sugar Land, TX 77479

Fertility Center of San Antonio
4499 Medical Drive, Suite 200
San Antonio, TX 78229
(800) 708-1869; (210) 692-0577
www.fertilitysa.com

Fertility Concepts
4499 Medical Drive, Suite 380
San Antonio, TX 78229
(210) 616-3303

Houston Infertility Clinic
1631 North Loop West, Suite 410
Houston, TX 77008
(713) 862-6181
www.infertilityivf.com

Institute for Women's Health
Advanced Fertility Laboratory
7940 Floyd Curl Drive, Suite 900
San Antonio, TX 78229
(210) 616-0680

National Fertility Center of Texas, P.A.
7777 Forest Lane, C-638
Dallas, TX 75230
(972) 566-6686

North Houston Center for Reproductive Medicine
530 Wells Fargo Drive, Suite 116
Houston, TX 77090
(281) 444-4784; (800) 444-0812
www.nhcrm.com

Presbyterian Hospital ARTS Program
8200 Walnut Hill Lane, 6th Floor
Dallas, TX 75231
(214) 345-2624

Reproductive Science Center of Dallas
Trinity IVF Program
Trinity Medical Center 308
4325 North Josey Lane, Suite 308
Carrollton, TX 75010
(972) 394-3699

South Texas Fertility Center
University of Texas Health Science Center at
San Antonio
8122 Datapoint Drive, Suite 1300
San Antonio, TX 78229
(210) 576-7575

Texas Fertility Center
3705 Medical Parkway, Suite 420
Austin, TX 78705
(512) 451-0149

Texas Institute for Reproductive Medicine and Endocrinology, P.A.
7400 Fannin, Suite 850
Houston, TX 77054
(713) 791-1874
www.hormoneproblems.com

Texas Technology University Health Sciences Center
IVF Program
Department of Obstetrics/Gynecology
3601 4th Street
Lubbock, TX 79430
(806) 743-1200

University of Texas Southwestern Fertility Associates
James W. Aston Ambulatory Care Center
Department of Obstetrics/Gynecology
5323 Harry Hines Boulevard
Dallas, TX 75235
(214) 648-8846

University of Texas Women's Health Center
6410 Fannin, HPB 350
Houston, TX 77030
(713) 704-5131

Wilford Hall Medical Center
Department of Obstetrics/Gynecology
2200 Bergquist Drive, Suite 1
Lackland AFB, TX 78236
(210) 292-7547

UTAH

Center for Advanced Reproductive Medicine
730 East 300 South
Springville, UT 84663
(801) 491-0556

Reproductive Care Center
1220 East 3900 South, Suite 4-G
Salt Lake City, UT 84124
(801) 268-7752

Utah Center for Reproductive Medicine
University of Utah Medical Center
50 North Medical Drive
Salt Lake City, UT 84132
(801) 581-4838

VERMONT

University of Vermont-IVF Program
Vermont Center for Reproductive Medicine
University of Vermont-IVF Program
Women's Health Care Service-FAHC
1 South Prospect Street
Burlington, VT 05401
(802) 847-0986

VIRGINIA

Beach Center for Infertility, Endocrinology and IVF, The
Virginia Beach, VA 23451
(757) 428-0002
www.beachcenter.com

Dominion Fertility and Endocrinology
46 South Glebe Road, Suite 301
Arlington, VA 22204
(703) 920-3890

Fertility and Reproductive Health Center, The
Annandale Square
4316 L Evergreen Lane
Annandale, VA 22003
(703) 658-3100
www.frhcfertility.com
or
Hospital Center Medical Plaza
1830 Town Center Drive, Suite 306
Reston, Virginia 22090
(703) 481-1500
www.frhcfertility.com

Fertility Institute of Virginia
10710 Midlothian Turnpike, Suite 331
Richmond, VA 23235
(804) 379-9000

Jones Institute for Reproductive Medicine
601 Colley Avenue
Norfolk, VA 23507
(800) 515-6637; (757) 446-7100
www.jonesinstitute.org

Lifesource Fertility Center
7603 Forest Avenue, Suite 204
Richmond, VA 23229
(804) 673-2273

Medical College of Virginia
1101 East Marshall Street
PO Box 980034, Sanger 11-022
Richmond, VA 23298
(804) 828-9638

The New Hope Center for Reproductive Medicine
1200 First Colonial Road, Suite 100M
Virginia Beach, VA 23454
(757) 496-5370

Shady Grove Fertility
3299 Woodburn Road, Suite 480
Annandale, VA 22003
(703) 876-0734
www.shadygrovefertility.com

University of Virginia ART Program
Northridge OB/GYN
2955 Ivy Road, Suite 304
Charlottesville, VA 22903
(804) 243-4590

WASHINGTON

Bellingham IVF
2980 Squalicum Parkway, Suite 103
Bellingham, WA 98225
(360) 715-8124

Center for Reproductive Endocrinology and Fertility
West 508 6th, Suite 500
Box 7
Spokane, WA 99204
(509) 462-7070

GYFT Clinic, P.L.L.C.
3582 Pacific Avenue, 3rd Floor
Tacoma, WA 98408
(206) 475-5433

Olympia Women's Health Capital Medical Center
403 Black Hills Lane, SW
Olympia, WA 98502
(360) 786-1515

Overlake Reproductive Health
1135 116th Avenue, NE, Suite 640
Bellevue, WA 98004
(425) 646-4700
www.fertileweb.com

Pacific Gynecology Specialists
1101 Madison Street, Suite 1500
Seattle, WA 98104
(206) 215-3200

**University of Washington Medical Center
The Fertility & Endocrine Center**
4225 Roosevelt Way, NE, Suite 101
Seattle, WA 98105
(206) 598-4225

**Virginia Mason Center for Fertility and
Reproductive Endocrinology**
1100 Ninth Avenue
PO Box 900-X11-FC
Seattle, WA 98111
(206) 223-6190

**Washington Center for Reproductive
Medicine**
1370 116th Avenue, NE, Suite 100
Bellevue, WA 98004
(425) 462-6100
www.seattleivf.com

WASHINGTON, D.C.

**Columbia Hospital for Women ART
Program**
2440 M Street, NW, Suite 401
Washington, DC 20037
(202) 293-6567

**The George Washington University Medical
Center IVF Program**
2150 Pennsylvania Avenue, NW, 6A241
Washington, DC 20037
(202) 994-4614

Reproductive Science Center
Walter Reed Army Medical Center
6900 Georgia Avenue, NW, Ward 43 Building 2,
Room 4304
Washington, DC 20307
(202) 782-5090

Shady Grove Fertility-Georgetown
3800 Reservoir Road, NW
3rd Floor-Gorman
Washington, DC 20007

(202) 784-1511
www.shadygrovefertility.com

WEST VIRGINIA

Center for Reproductive Medicine
West Virginia University Health Sciences Center
830 Pennsylvania Avenue, Suite 304
Charleston, WV 25302
(304) 344-1515

WISCONSIN

Advanced Institute of Fertility
Saint Luke's Medical Center
2801 W. Kinnickinnic River Parkway, Suite 535
Milwaukee, WI 53215
(414) 645-5437

Clinic of Obstetrics & Gynecology, Ltd.
8800 West Lincoln Avenue
West Allis, WI 53227
(414) 545-8808

Family Fertility Program
Appleton Medical Center
1818 North Meade Street
Appleton, WI 54911
(920) 738-6242

Gundersen/Lutheran Medical Center
1836 South Avenue
La Crosse, WI 54601
(608) 782-7300

**Medical College of Wisconsin, Department
of Ob/Gyn**
Froedtert E. Lutheran Memorial Hospital
9200 West Wisconsin Avenue
Milwaukee, WI 53226
(414) 257-5546

**Reproductive Specialty Center at IVF
Columbia, Columbia Hospital**
2315 North Lake Drive, Seton Tower, Suite 501
Milwaukee, WI 53211
(414) 289-9668

University of Wisconsin-Madison
Women's Endocrine Services
600 Highland Avenue, H4/630 CSC
Madison, WI 53792
(608) 263-1217

Women's Health Care, S.C.
721 American Avenue, Suite 304
Waukesha, WI 53188
(414) 549-2229

GLOSSARY

adhesions Attachment of adjacent organs by scar tissue. When adhesions occur in the fallopian tubes or inside the uterus, they can interfere with transport of the egg and implantation of the embryo in the uterus.

adnexa The region of the pelvis that includes the ovary, fallopian tube, and surrounding broad ligaments.

adrenal gland The endocrine gland lying over each kidney that is important in the production of androgens (male hormones). It is also responsible for producing the stress hormone cortisol.

agglutination Clumping together (as of sperm) often caused by infection, antibodies, or inflammation.

androgens Male sex hormones.

antibody Chemical produced by the body's immune system in response to a foreign substance (also called an antigen).

antigen A substance that triggers the formation of an antibody.

autoimmunity An immune reaction against a person's own tissues.

cannula A hollow tube that can be used for artificial insemination, among other procedures.

cauterize A process that destroys tissue with heat, cold, or caustic substances.

cervix The lower portion of the uterus that opens into the vagina.

chromosome The DNA threads in the cell that carry hereditary information. Humans have 46 chromosomes, 23 from the egg and 23 from the sperm.

cilia Tiny hairlike projections lining the inside surface of the fallopian tubes. The waving action of these "hairs" sweeps the egg toward the uterus.

cryocautery Destruction of tissue (cautery) by freezing.

cumulus oophorus The protective layer of cells surrounding the egg.

endometrial cavity The space inside the uterus lined by the ENDOMETRIUM.

endometrium The lining of the uterus that grows and sheds in response to estrogen and progesterone stimulation; the bed of tissue designed to nourish the implanted embryo.

epididymis A coiled, tubular organ attached to and lying on the testicle which stores the sperm before ejaculation.

fallopian tubes Hollow ducts through which a mature egg, released from the follicle, travels to the uterus. Fertilization usually occurs in the fallopian tubes.

follicles Fluid-filled sacs in the ovary which contain the immature eggs.

follicle-stimulating hormone (FSH) A hormone produced by the pituitary that acts to stimulate the development and maturation of follicles and eggs.

gamete A reproductive cell: sperm in men, the egg in women.

gene The unit of heredity made up of DNA.

gestation The medical term for pregnancy.

gonad The gland that makes reproductive cells and sex hormones: the testicles, which make sperm and testosterone, and the ovaries, which make eggs and estrogen.

gonadotropins   Pituitary hormones that control reproductive function, including follicle-stimulating hormone (FSH) and leutenizing hormone.

hirsute   The overabundance of body hair, such as a mustache or pubic hair growing upward toward the navel, found in women with excess androgens.

hypoestrogenic   Having lower-than-normal levels of estrogen.

hypospermatogenesis   Low sperm production.

karyotyping   A test performed to analyze chromosomes for the presence of genetic defects.

luteinizing hormone (LH)   A hormone produced by the pituitary that induces ovulation from the most mature follicle in the ovary.

meiosis   The cell division, peculiar to reproductive cells, which allows genetic material to divide in half. Each new cell will contain 23 chromosomes. The immature sperm and eggs each contain 23 chromosomes, so when they fertilize, the baby will have a normal complement of 46.

mitosis   The division of a cell into two identical cells in which all 46 human chromosomes are duplicated; the first division of the germ cell.

oligomenorrhea   Infrequent menstrual periods.

oligospermia   Having few sperm.

ovum   The egg, also known as the reproductive cell from the ovary, the female gamete, or the sex cell that contains the woman's genetic information.

panhypopituitarism   Complete pituitary gland failure.

pituitary gland   The master gland; the gland that is stimulated by the hypothalamus and controls all hormonal functions. Located at the base of the brain just below the hypothalamus, this gland controls many major hormonal factories throughout the body, including the gonads, the adrenal glands, and the thyroid gland.

placenta   The embryonic tissue that invades the uterine wall and provides a mechanism for exchanging the baby's waste products for the mother's nutrients and oxygen. The baby is connected to the placenta by the umbilical cord.

progesterone   The hormone produced by the corpus luteum during the second half of a woman's cycle. It thickens the lining of the uterus to prepare it to accept implantation of a fertilized egg.

recombinant product   A product made by genetically altered lab cells; this process ensures a pure, steady supply of the product.

salpingectomy   Surgical removal of the fallopian tube.

scrotum   The bag of skin and thin muscle surrounding the man's testicles.

secondary sex characteristics   The physical qualities that distinguish man and woman, such as beard, large breasts, and deep voice. Formed under the stimulation of the sex hormones (testosterone or estrogen), these characteristics also identify those people who have gone through puberty (sexual maturity).

seminal vesicles   Glands in the male reproductive system which produce much of the semen volume, including sugar for nourishing the sperm and a chemical that causes the semen to coagulate on entering the vagina.

seminiferous tubules   The testicular tubules in which the sperm mature and move toward the epididymis.

spermatogenesis   Sperm production in the testicles.

thyroid gland   The endocrine gland in the front of the neck that produces thyroid hormones to regulate the body's metabolism.

urethra   The tube that allows urine to pass between the bladder and the outside of the body. In the man this tube also carries semen from the area of the prostate to the outside.

uterus   The hollow, muscular organ that nourishes the fetus during pregnancy.

vas deferens   One of the tubes through which the sperm move from the testicles toward the seminal vesicles and prostate gland. These tubes are severed during a vasectomy performed for birth control.

X chromosome   The information in a cell that transmits the information necessary to produce a female. All eggs contain one X chromosome, and half of all sperm carry an X chromosome. When two X chromosomes combine, the baby will be a girl.

Y chromosome The genetic material that transmits the information necessary to produce a boy.

The Y chromosome can be found in half of a man's sperm cells. When an X and a Y chromosome combine, the baby will be a boy.

zygote The medical term for a fertilized egg (also, the embryo in the early stages of development).

BIBLIOGRAPHY

Aguillaume, Claude J., and Louise B. Tyrer. "Current status and future projections on use of RU-486." *Contemporary OB/GYN* 40/6 (1995): 23–40.

American Society of Anesthesiologists news release. "Regional anesthesia for egg retrieval increases in vitro fertilization pregnancies." Oct. 3, 2000.

Aronson, Diane. *Resolving Infertility: Understanding the Options and Choosing Solutions When You Want to Have a Baby.* Arlington, Mass.: Harper Resource, 1999.

Baber, R., H. Abdalla and J. Studd. "The premature menopause." *Progress in Obstetrics and Gynecology* (1993): 209–26.

Balasch, J. "Investigation of the infertile couple in the era of assisted reproductive technology: a time for reappraisal." *Human Reproduction* 15/11 (Nov. 2000): 2251–57.

Behr, B., J. D. Fisch, C. Racowsky, K. Miller, T. B. Pool, and A. A. Milki. "Blastocyst-ET and monozygotic twinning." *Journal of Assisted Reproductive Genetics* 17/6 (July 2000): 349–51.

Bergher, Gary S., Marc Goldstein, and Mark Fuerst. *The Couples Guide to Fertility.* New York: Doubleday, 1995.

Bevilacqua, K., D. Barad, J. Youchah, and B. Witt. "Is affect associated with infertility treatment outcome?" *Fertility and Sterility* 73 (2000): 648–69.

Boer-Meisel, M. E., E. R. te Velde, J. D. F. Habbema, J. W. P. F. Kaurdaun. "Predicting the pregnancy outcome in patients treated for hydrosalpinges: a prospective study." *Fertility and Sterility* 45 (1986): 23–29.

Boivin, J., J. E. Takefman, Tulandi, T., and Brender, W. "Reactions to infertility based on extent of treatment failure." *Fertility and Sterility* 63 (1995): 801.

Boulot, P., J. Vignal, C. Vergnes, H. Dechaud, J-M. Faure, and B. Hedon. "Multifetal reduction of triplets to twins: a prospective comparison of pregnancy outcome." *Human Reproduction.* 15 (2000): 1619–23.

Bradshaw, K. D., and B. R. Carr. "Modern diagnostic evaluation of the infertile couple." In Carr, B. R., and Blackwell, R. E., eds. *Textbook of Reproductive Medicine,* 1st ed. Norwalk, Conn.: Appleton & Lange, 1993.

Bree, Robert L., and D. T. Hoang. "Scrotal ultrasound." *Radiologic Clinics of North America* 34 (Nov. 1996): 1183–1205.

Brown, S. E., and others. "Evaluation of outpatient hysteroscopy, saline infusion hysterosonography, and hysterosalpingography in infertile women: a prospective, randomized study." *Fertility and Sterility* 74/5 (Nov. 1, 2000): 1029–34.

Carson, Sandra, Peter R. Casson, and Deborah Shuman. *Complete Guide to Fertility.* New York: Comtemporary Books, 1999.

Caton, Helen, Harold Buttram, and Damien Downing. *The Fertility Plan: A Holistic Program for Conceiving a Healthy Baby.* New York: Fireside, 2000.

Cooper, Susan, and Ellen Sarasohn Glazer. *Choosing Assisted Reproduction: Social, Emotional & Ethical Considerations.* Indianapolis: Perspectives Press, 1999.

Cundiff, G., B. R. Carr, and P. B. Marshburn. "Infertile couples with a normal hysterosalpingogram: reproductive outcome and its relationship to clinical and laparoscopic findings." *Journal of Reproductive Medicine* 40 (1995): 19.

Cunningham, F. Gary, et al. *Williams Obstetrics.* Stamford: Appleton & Lange, 1997.

Daley, Suzanne. "France provides morning-after pill to schoolgirls." *The New York Times* (Feb. 8, 2000): A1.

Darai, E., L. Dessolle, F. Lecuru and Soriano, D. "Transvaginal hydrolaparoscopy compared with laparoscopy for the evaluation of infertile women:

a prospective comparative blind study." *Human Reproduction* 15/11 (Nov. 2000): 2379–82.

DeBruyne, F., P. Puttemans, W. Boeckx, and I. Brosens. "The clinical value of salpingoscopy in tubal infertility." *Fertility and Sterility* 51 (1989): 339–40.

Dechaud, H., T. Anahory, N. Aligier, F. Arnal, H. Humeay, and B. Hedon. "Salpingectomy for repeated embryo non-implantation after in vitro fertilization in patients with severe tubal factor infertility." *Journal of Assisted Reproductive Genetics* 4 (2000): 200–65.

DeGroot, Leslie J., ed., et al. "Cushing's Syndrome." *Endocrinology. Vol. 2.* Philadelphia: Saunders, 1995.

Dodson, W. C., and A. F. Haney. "Controlled ovarian hyperstimulation and intrauterine insemination for treatment of infertility." *Fertility and Sterility* 55 (1991): 457.

Domar, Alice. *Healing Mind, Healthy Woman.* New York: Holt, 1996.

Dos Reis, R. M., and others. "Familial risk among patients with endometriosis." *Journal of Assisted Reproduction* 16 (1999): 500–03.

Ellertson, Charlotte. "History and efficacy of emergency contraception: beyond Coca-Cola." *Family Planning Perspectives* 28/2 (1996): 44–48.

Falcone, T., J. M. Goldberg, H. Margossian, and L. Stevens. "Robotic-assisted laparoscopic microsurgical tubal anastomosis: a human pilot study." *Fertility and Sterility* 73 (2000): 1040–42.

FDA. "FDA approves progestin-only emergency contraception." *The Contraception Report* 10/5 (1999): 8–10, 16.

———. "Prescription drug products; certain combined oral contraceptives for use as postcoital emergency contraception." *Federal Register* 62/37 (1997): 8609–12.

Felembam, Alaf, et al. "Laparoscopic treatment of polycystic ovaries with insulated needle cautery: a reappraisal." *Fertility and Sterility* 73/2 (2000): 266–69.

Fenster, Laura, et al. "Psychologic stress in the workplace and spontaneous abortion." *American Journal of Epidemiology* 142/11 (1995).

Fluker, M. R., J. E. Copeland, and A. Yuzpe. "An ounce of prevention: outpatient management of the ovarian hyperstimulation syndrome (OHSS)." *Fertility and Sterility* 73 (2000): 821–24.

Franks, S. "Medical progress: polycystic ovary syndrome." *New England Journal of Medicine* 333/13 (1995): 853–61.

Geva, E., I. Yovel, L. Lerner-Geva, and J. B. Lessing, "Intrauterine insemination before transfer of frozen-thawed embryos may improve the pregnancy rate for couples with unexplained infertility: preliminary results of a randomized prospective study." *Fertility and Sterility* 73 (2000): 755–60.

Gilman, Lois. *The Adoption Resource Book.* New York: Harper, 1998.

Glasier, Anna, and David Baird. "The side effects of self-administering emergency contraception." *The New England Journal of Medicine* 339/1 (1998): 1–4.

Gleicher, N., D. M. Oleske, I. Tur-Kaspa, A. Vidali, and V. Karande. "Reducing the risk of high-order multiple pregnancy after ovarian stimulation with gonadotropins." *New England Journal of Medicine* 343 (2000): 2–7.

Goldfarb, J. M., C. Austin, B. Peskin, H. Lisbona, N. Desai, J. R. Loret de Mola. "Fifteen years experience with an in-vitro fertilization surrogate gestational pregnancy programme." *Human Reproduction* 15 (2000): 1075–1076.

Gordeski G. L. "Premature menopause." *Menopause Management* (1997): 10–17.

Griffith, C. S., and D. A. Grimes. "The validity of the postcoital test." *American Journal of Obstetrics and Gynecology* 162 (1990): 615.

Grimes, D. A. "Intrauterine device and upper-genital-tract infection." *The Lancet* 356/9234. (Sep. 16, 2000): 1013–19.

Grossman, Richard A., and Bryan D. Grossman. "How frequently is emergency contraception prescribed?" *Family Planning Perspectives* 26/6 (1994): 270–71.

Guillebaud, John. "Time for emergency contraception with levonorgestrel alone." *The Lancet* 352/9126 (1998): 416.

Healy, Bernadine. *A New Prescription For Women's Health.* New York: Viking, 1995.

Hembree, W. C., P. Zeidenberg, and G. G. Nahas. "Marijuana's effect on human gonadal function." In Nahas, G. G., ed. *Marijuana: Chemistry, Biochemistry and Cellular Effects.* New York: Springer-Verlag, 1976, pp. 521–32.

Hennelly, B., R. F. Harrison, J. Kelly, S. Jacob, and T. Barrett. "Spontaneous conception after a successful attempt at in vitro fertilization/ intracytoplasmic sperm injection." *Fertility and Sterility* 73 (2000): 774–78.

Henshaw, Stanley K. "Abortion incidence and services in the United States." *Family Planning Perspectives* 30/6 (1998): 263–70, 287.

————, et al. "Recent trends in abortion rates worldwide." *International Family Planning Perspectives* 25. 1 (1999): 44–48.

Hornstein, M. D., O. K. Davis, J. B. Massey, R. J. Paulson, and J. A. Collins. "Antiphospholipid antibodies and in vitro fertilization success: a meta-analysis." *Fertility and Sterility* 73/2 (2000): 330–33.

Hsieh, Y-Y., H-D. Tsai, C-C. Chang, H-Y. Lo, and C-L. Chen. "Low-dose aspirin for infertile women with thin endometrium receiving intrauterine insemination: a prospective, randomized study." *Journal of Assisted Reproduction Genetics* 3 (2000): 174–77.

Isselbacher, Kurt J., ed., et al. "Cushing's syndrome etiology." In *Harrison's Principles of Internal Medicine*, 13th ed. 2/13, New York: McGraw-Hill, 1994.

Jansen, Robert. *Overcoming Infertility: A Compassionate Resource for Getting Pregnant.* New York: Freeman, 1997.

Kamada, M., et al. "Semen analysis and antisperm antibody." *Archives of Andrology* (Mar. to Apr. 1998): 117–28.

Kearney, Brian. *High-Tech Conception: A Comprehensive Handbook for Consumers.* New York: Bantam, 1998.

Kee, B. S., B. J. Jung, and S. H. Lee. "A study on psychological strain in IVF patients." *Journal of Assisted Reproduction Genetics* 17/8 (Sep. 2000): 445–48.

Kerin, J. F., Williams, and others. "Falloposcopic classification and treatment of fallopian tube lumen disease." *Fertility and Sterility* 57 (1992): 731–41.

Kerin, J., E. Surrey, L. Daykhovsky, and W. S. Grundfest. "Development and application of a falloposcope for transvaginal endoscopy of the fallopian tube." *Journal of Laparoendoscopy* 1 (1990): 47–56.

Kolata, Gina. "Morning-after contraceptive to be marketed." *The New York Times* (July 21, 1998): A12.

Khorram, O., S. S. Shapiro, and J. M. Jones. "Transfer of nonassisted hatched and hatching human blastocysts after in vitro fertilization." *Fertility and Sterility* 74 (2000): 163–65.

Kaiser Family Foundaton (1998, accessed Aug. 20, 1999). National Survey of Women's Health Care Providers on Abortion [Online]. http://www.kff.org/content/archive/1431/ru486_rel.html.

Lanzendorf, S. E., F. Nehchiri, J. F. Mayer, S. Oehninger, and S. J. Muasher. "A prospective, randomized, double blind study for the evaluation of assisted hatching in patients with advanced maternal age." *Human Reproduction* 13/2 (1998): 409–413.

Lark, S. *The Estrogen Decision; Self-Help Book.* Berkeley, CA: Celestial Arts, 1995.

Lauersen, N., and S. Whitney. *It's Your Body: A Woman's Guide to Gynecology.* New York. Putnam, 1993.

Lederer, K. J. "Transcervical tubal cannulation and salpingoscopy in the treatment of tubal infertility." *Current Opinions in Obstetrics/Gynecology* 5 (1993): 240–44.

Levron, J., A. Aviram-Goldring, I. Madgar, G. Raviv, G. Barkai, and J. Dor. "Sperm chromosome analysis and outcome of IVF in patients with non-mosaic Klinefelter's syndrome." *Fertility and Sterility* 74/5 (Nov. 1, 2000): 925–29.

Lewis-Jones, D. I., M. R. Gazvani, and R. Mountford. "Cystic fibrosis in infertility: screening before assisted reproduction: Opinion." *Human Reproduction* 15/11 (Nov. 2000): 2415–17.

Liebmann-Smith, Joan, Jacqueline Nardi Egan, and John Stangel. *The Unofficial Guide to Overcoming Infertility.* New York: Macmillan, 1999.

————. *In Pursuit of Pregnancy.* New York: Newmarket, 1987.

Lieman, H., and N. Santoro. "Premature ovarian failure: a modern approach to diagnosis and treatment." *The Endocrinologist* 7 (1997): 314–21.

Maguinness, S. D., and O. Djahanbaksh. "Salpingoscopic findings in women undergoing sterilization." *Human Reproduction* 7 (1992): 269–73.

Marconi, G., L. Auge, E. Sojo, E. Young, and R. Quintana. "Salpingoscopy: systematic use in diagnostic laparoscopy." *Fertility and Sterility* 57 (1992): 742–46.

Marrs, Richard, Lisa Friedman Bloch, Kathy Kirtland Silverman. *Dr. Richard Marrs' Fertility Book: America's Leading Infertility Expert Tells You Everything You Need to Know About Getting Pregnant.* New York: Dell, 1997.

Marshburn, P. B., and W. H. Kutteh. "The role of antisperm antibodies in infertility." *Fertility and Sterility* 61 (1994): 799.

McNeil, Donald G., Jr. "No more 'morning-after pills' at school, French court says." *The New York Times* (July 1, 2000): A6.

Mather, R. S., A. V. Akande, S. D. Keay, L. P. Hunt, and J. M. Jenkins. "Distinction between early and late ovarian hyperstimulation syndrome." *Fertility and Sterility* 73/5 (2000): 901–75.

Miller, Manya Deleon, and Ronald Clisham. *The Complete Fertility Organizer: A Guidebook and Record-Keeper for Women.* New York: Wiley, 1999.

Murphy, A. A., M. H. Zhou, S. Malkapuram, N. Santanam, S. Parthasarathy, and N. Sidell. "RU486-induced growth inhibition of human endometrial cells." *Fertility and Sterility* 74/5 (Nov. 1, 2000): 1014–19.

Pagana, Kathleen Deska, and Timothy James Pagana. *Mosby's Diagnostic and Laboratory Test Reference,* 3rd ed. St. Louis: Mosby–Year Book, 1997.

Paulson, R. J., and M. V. Sauer. "Counseling the infertile couple: when enough is enough." *Obstetrics and Gynecology* 78 (1991): 462.

Peoples, Debby, and Harriette Rovner Ferguson. *What to Expect When You're Experiencing Infertility.* New York: Norton, 1998.

Pizer, Frank, and Christine O'Brien Palinski. *Coping With a Miscarriage.* New York: Dial, 1980.

Population Council (1998, accessed Aug. 20, 1999). Medical Abortion with Mifepristone and Misoprostol [Online]. http://www.popcouncil.org/rhpdev/mifepristone_faq98.html.

Pouly, J. L., C. Chapron, H. Manhes, et al. "Multifactorial analysis of fertility following conservative laparoscopic treatment of ectopic pregnancy through a 223 series." *Fertility and Sterility* 56 (1991): 435–60.

Rajfer, Jacob. "Congenital anomalies of the testes and scrotum." In Patrick C. Walsh, ed., *Campbell's Urology.* Philadelphia: Saunders, 1998.

Resolve. *Environmental Toxins and Fertility.* Somerville, Mass.: Resolve, 1995.

Rodgers, H. C., D. R. Baldwin, and A. J. Knox. "Questionnaire survey of male infertility in cystic fibrosis." *Respiratory Medicine* 94/10 (Oct. 2000): 1002–03.

Rojansky, N., and others. "Seasonal variability in fertilization and embryo quality rates in women undergoing IVF." *Fertility and Sterility* 74 (2000): 476–81.

Rosenthal, M. Sara, and Masood A. Khatamee. *The Fertility Sourcebook.* Los Angeles: Lowell House, 1998.

Rozauski, Thomas, et al. "Surgery of the scrotum and testis in children." In Patrick C. Walsh, ed, *Campbell's Urology.* Philadelphia: Saunders, 1998.

Saleh, A., S. L. Tan, M. M. Biljan, and T. Tulandi. "A randomized study of the effect of 10 minutes of bed rest after intrauterine insemination." *Fertility and Sterility* 74 (2000): 509–11.

Schreurs, A., E. Legius, C. Meuleman, J. P. Fryns, and T. M. D'Hooghe. "Increased frequency of chromosomal abnormalities in female partners of couples undergoing in vitro fertilization or intracytoplasmic sperm injection." *Fertility and Sterility* 74 (2000): 94–96.

Scott, R. T., Jr., and G. E. Hoffmann. "Prognostic assessment of ovarian reserve." *Fertility and Sterility* 63 (1995): 1.

Scudamore I. W., B. C. Dunphy, and I. D. Cooke. "Falloposocpic comparison of unilateral and bilateral proximal tubal occlusive disease." *Human Reproduction* 9 (1994): 1516–18.

Sher, G., V. M. Davis, and J. Stoess. *In Vitro Fertilization: The A.R.T. of Making Babies.* New York: Facts On File, 1995.

Silber, S.J., L. Johnson, G. Verheyen, and A. Van Steirteghem. "Round spermatid injection." *Fertility and Sterility* 73 (2000): 897–900.

Silverman, Edward R. "First U.S. post-sex pill about to be sold: Belle Mead Firm, at FDA behest, set to test market and risk furor." *The Star-Ledger* (July 19, 1998): 1.

Sobel, Jack D. "Vaginitis." *The New England Journal of Medicine* 337 (Dec. 1997): 1896–1903.

Spandorfer, S. D., P. H. Chung, I. Kligman, H. C. Lie, O. K. Davis and Z. Rosenwaks. "Analysis of the effect of age on implantation rates." *Journal of Assisted Reproduction Genetics* 17 (2000): 303–06.

Speroff, L., R. H. Glass, N. G. Kase. *Clinical Gynecologic Endocrinology and Infertility,* 5th ed. Baltimore: Williams & Wilkins, 1994.

Spitz, Irving, et al. "Early pregnancy termination with mifepristone and misoprostol in the United States." *New England Journal of Medicine* 338/18 (1998): 1241–47.

Steele, E. K., N. McClure, and S. E. M. Lewis. "Comparison of the effects of two methods of cryopreservation on testicular sperm DNA." *Fertility and Sterility* 74 (2000): 450–53.

Stephen, J. A., I. E. Timor-Tritsch, J. P. Lerner, A. Monteagudo, and C. A. Alonso. "Ovarian stimulation and endometrial receptivity." *American Journal of Obstetrics and Gynecology* 182 (2000): 962–65.

———. "Amniocentesis after multifetal pregnancy reduction: is it safe?" *American Journal of Obstetrics and Gynecology* 182 (2000): 962–65.

Sukcharoen, N., T. Sithipravej, S. Promviengchai, V. Chinpilas, and W. Boonkasemsanti. "No differences in outcome of surgical sperm retrieval with intracytoplasmic sperm injection at different intervals after vasectomy." *Fertility and Sterility* 74 (2000): 174–75.

Talbot, Margaret. "The little white bombshell." *New York Times Magazine* (July 11, 1999): 39–43.

Task Force on Postovulatory Methods of Fertility Regulation. "Randomised controlled trial of levonorgestrel versus the Yuzpe regimen of combined oral contraceptives for emergency contraception." *The Lancet* 352/9126 (1998): 428–33.

Trantham, Patricia. "The infertile couple." *American Family Physician* (Sep. 1996): 1001–09.

Turkington, Carol A., and Susie Probst. *The Unofficial Guide to Women's Health.* New York: Macmillan, 1999.

Turiel, Judith Steinberg. *Beyond Second Opinions: Making Choices About Fertility Treatment.* Los Angeles: University of California Press, 1998.

Van Voorhis, B. J., A. Dokras, and C. H. Syrop. "Bilateral undescended ovaries: association with infertility and treatment with IVF." *Fertility and Sterility* 74/5 (Nov. 1, 2000): 1041–43.

Venezia, R., C. Zangara, C. Knight, and E. Cittadini. "Initial experience of a new linear everting falloposcopy system in comparison with hysterosalpingography." *Fertility and Sterility* 60 (1993): 771–75.

Walsh, Patrick C., et al. *Campbell's Urology.* Philadelphia: Saunders, 1998.

Warnock, J. K., J. C. Bundren, and D. W. Morris. "Depressive mood symptoms associated with ovarian suppression." *Fertility and Sterility* 74/5 (Nov. 1, 2000): 984–86.

Weschler, T. *Taking Charge of Your Fertility.* New York. HarperCollins, 1995.

Wilson, Jean D., ed., et al. "Hyperfunction: glucocorticoids: hypercortisolism (Cushing's syndrome)." In *Williams Textbook of Endocrinology,* No. 8. Philadelphia: Saunders, 1992, pp. 536–62.

Winikoff, Beverly, et al. "Acceptability and feasibility of early pregnancy termination by mifepristone-misoprostol: results of a large multicenter trial in the United States." *Archives of Family Medicine* 7 (July/Aug. 1998), 360–66.

Woodruff, J. D., and C. J. Pauerstein. *The Fallopian Tube: Structure, Function, Pathology and Management.* Baltimore: Williams & Wilkins, 1969.

World Health Organization. Task Force on Postovulatory Methods of Fertility Regulation. "Comparison of three single doses of mifepristone as emergency contraception: a randomised trial." *Lancet,* 353 (Feb. 27, 1999): 697–702.

Zech, H., P. Vanderzwalmen, Y. Prapas, B. Lejeune, E. Duba, and E. Schoysman. "Congenital malformations after intracytoplasmic injection of spermatids." *Human Reproduction* 15 (2000): 969–71.

Zouves, Christo, and Julie Sullivan. *Expecting Miracles: On the Path of Hope from Infertility to Parenthood.* New York: Holt, 1999.

INDEX